Research Methods
in Psychiatry

Third

Edited b

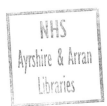

Gaskell

This publication is dedicated to the memory of Richard Harrington, whose
contribution to scientific methodology in child psychiatry was substantial
and highly productive but which sadly ended so prematurely.

Contents

Part III: Tools

Part IV: Special areas of research

Figures

Tables

Boxes

Contributors

German Berrios, Professor of the Epistemology of Psychiatry, University of Cambridge, Addenbrooke's Hospital, Cambridge CB2 2QQ

Patricia Casey, Professor of Psychiatry, Mater Misericordiae Hospital, Eccles Street, Dublin, Ireland

Mike Crawford, Reader in Mental Health Services Research, Department of Psychological Medicine, Division of Neuroscience and Mental Health, Imperial College, London W6 8RP

Yvonne Edmonstone, Consultant Psychotherapist, Royal Edinburgh Hospital, Morningside Terrace, Edinburgh EH10 5NF

Chris Freeman, Consultant Psychiatrist and Psychotherapist, Royal Edinburgh Hospital, Morningside Terrace, Edinburgh EH10 5NF

Susie Gibbs, Specialist Registrar in the Psychiatry of Learning Disability, Child and Adolescent Mental Health Service at Royal Hospital for Sick Children, Edinburgh EH9 1LL

Simon Gilbody, Senior Lecturer in Mental Health Services Research, Department of Health Sciences, University of York, York YO10 5DD

Richard Harrington, Late Professor of Child Psychiatry, Royal Manchester Children's Hospital, Pendlebury, Manchester M27 4HA

Matthew Hotopf, Professor of General Hospital Psychiatry, King's College London, Department of Psychological Medicine, Institute of Psychiatry, Weston Education Centre, Cutcombe Road, London SE5 9RJ

Tony Johnson, Senior Statistician, Medical Research Council Biostatistics Unit, Institute of Public Health, University Forvie Site, Robinson Way, Cambridge CB2 2SR

Neil Mayfield, Consultant in General Adult Psychiatry, Herdmanflat Hospital, Haddington, East Lothian EH41 3BU

Caroline Methuen, Teaching Fellow, Department of Psychological Medicine, Division of Neuroscience and Mental Health, Imperial College, London W6 8RP

Stephen Morley, Professor of Clinical Psychology, Academic Unit of Psychiatry, University of Leeds, 15 Hyde Terrace, Leeds LS2 9JT

Walter Muir, Reader in the Psychiatry of Learning Disability, Division of Psychiatry, Kennedy Tower, University of Edinburgh, Morningside Park, Edinburgh EH10 5HF **Ula Nur**, Statistician, Department of Psychological Medicine, Division of Neuroscience and Mental Health, Imperial College, London W6 8RP

David F. Peck, Clinical Psychologist, School of Health in Social Science, University of Edinburgh, Teviot Place, Edinburgh EH8 9AG

Atif Rahman, Wellcome Research Career Development Fellow and Honorary Consultant in Child Psychiatry, University Department of Child Psychiatry, Royal Manchester Children's Hospital, Pendlebury, Manchester M27 4HA

Deborah Rutter, Research Fellow, Department of Psychological Medicine, Division of Neuroscience and Mental Health, Imperial College, London W6 8RP

Philip Snaith, Late Senior Lecturer in Psychiatry, Academic Unit of Psychiatry, Department of Clinical Medicine, St James University Hospital, Leeds LS9 7TF

Rebecca Tipper, Consultant in Addiction Psychiatry, Borders Community Addictions Team, Galavale Lodge, Tweed Road, Galashiels TD1 1PF

Peter Tyrer, Professor of Community Psychiatry, Department of Psychological Medicine, Division of Neuroscience and Mental Health, Imperial College, London W6 8RP

Preface to the first edition

Chris Freeman and Peter Tyrer

For the past 3 years we have been running regular 2- and 3-day research methodology courses for psychiatric trainees. These courses have demonstrated the need for a basic text on research methodology that is sensitive to the aims and resources available to trainees and that is suitable for someone starting out on their first research project. We have found considerable enthusiasm for psychiatric research among junior psychiatrists and an impressive array of original and clinically relevant research ideas. Why then is there not more research carried out by psychiatric trainees? Firstly, an enthusiastic trainee needs an enthusiastic and knowledgeable supervisor and such an individual seems to be hard for many trainees to find. Secondly, it is difficult for those working in university centres with easy access to research facilities to appreciate the difficulties that some trainees have. For example, on a recent course we had one trainee who had a 4-hour round trip to visit a psychiatric library. Thirdly, trainees have many competing demands, such as the Membership examination, night duty, etc., and many projects appear to get started but never completed, or completed and the results never analysed and written up.

We hope that this book will be helpful at all stages of a research project, although it can never be a substitute for good supervision. Many of the chapters are written by psychiatrists who have acted as tutors on our research methodology courses and most of the authors have been involved in supervising trainees in their own training schemes. We feel confident, therefore, that they have written in a way that is accessible and understandable to trainees.

We have included extensive sections in the book on rating scales and again this reflects our experience both in individual supervision and from running courses. Some of the most frequently asked questions concern what is an appropriate scale to use, how to find the reference for it, and how long it will take to administer. We have not included sections on statistics. We feel that there are numerous small statistics books available that cover all the main statistical tests that are likely to be needed. We have emphasised in the book that consulting a medical statistician is important and that it is useful to do that before starting research, not once the results have been collected.

We hope then that this book will help trainees to get started, help them avoid many of the pitfalls that frequently occur in planning and carrying out research, help maintain their enthusiasm and carry them through to their first published paper.

We wish those beginning research luck in what at times can appear futile, depressing, tedious, and repetitive. However, it can also be an exciting endeavour, and we hope very much that the balance remains on the positive attributes.

Preface to the second edition

Chris Freeman and Peter Tyrer

Since the first edition of this book was published we have had many useful comments and suggestions for changes and improvements. We have done our best to accommodate these in this revised edition. There are new chapters by Dr German Berrios on the neglected art of writing a review article, considered by many to be much more difficult than writing an original paper, and historical aspects, the section on data collection and computer programs has been expanded, together with an additional glossary, and most of the chapters have been updated. In particular, meta-analysis is described in more detail and the sections on rating scales have been expanded in an attempt to keep pace with, or at least not lag too far behind, developments in a growing industry. We have also separated the book into two sections to aid quick reference and fit in with trainees' needs.

We are glad to note that promotion of research projects and critical awareness of their findings have been given increased priority in psychiatric training programmes. We trust that this book will continue to play a part in facilitating these, and that the standard probability level for successful research projects ($P = 0.05$, representing one successful project for every 20 begun) can be further increased.

Preface to the third edition

Chris Freeman and Peter Tyrer

We are pleased that this book still seems to have a place in the education of psychiatric trainees. In the past 10 years there has been a rapid shift towards evidence-based medicine and research methodology has moved in parallel with this. In this new edition we therefore have a new chapter on systematic reviews and an expansion on the statistical methodology related to evidence-based medicine. We are also aware that previous editions have perhaps focused too much on general psychiatric subjects and we therefore have new chapters on research methodology in child and adolescent psychiatry, in learning disability and in old age psychiatry. We also have a completely new chapter on qualitative methodology in psychiatry, a discipline that is becoming increasingly important as interventions become more complex and research questions more difficult to define simply. The chapter on epidemiology has also been completely revised to help trainees, who often start their research careers with a simple cross-sectional study in this area.

This edition is influenced greatly by the internet and by the need to improve research capabilities in poorer countries. With so much information now readily available online we do not feel it necessary to give so much detail on subjects such as rating scales, though we have tried to give some notion of the relative importance of scales that cover the same subject (mainly by giving their citation rates). We have also continued with a revision of our chapter on the use of computers in research and others on writing and publishing papers, as for many working in less favoured countries this is likely to remain a valuable text for those in very young research settings. The advantages of local peer review, research presentations in front of an informed critical audience and frank, open discussion before a paper is submitted are so often lacking and the text of this book, although a poor substitute, still has some value in enhancing published success (Tyrer, 2005). Our intention is still to guide the trainee from the genesis of a research idea to a published paper. There are still too many research projects that could in principle be published but which have not been, and we hope that this text may help to reduce these without going so far as to confirm the witticism 'a determined author can get any rubbish published'. There is really no excuse why worthwhile research should not be written up in a form that can achieve the aim of widespread dissemination.

We thank Sheila McKenzie for secretarial assistance and Dave Jago at the Royal College of Psychiatrists for continued encouragement.

Reference

Tyrer, P. (2005) Combating editorial racism in psychiatric publications. British Journal of Psychiatry, **186**, 1–3.

Part I

General considerations

CHAPTER 1

Getting started in research

Chris Freeman and Peter Tyrer

Research recognises no boundaries of class, culture or status. It is critical and iconoclastic, as indeed should be the psychiatric trainee. It is now recognised in most medical curricula that students should have some awareness of research methods during their training, not because they should become research workers, but for the simple reason that an understanding of research and its principles is an aid to better clinical practice. This also applies to other disciplines within mental health, in which we are glad to note research is coming much more to the fore. The history of medicine is littered with examples of mistakes made as a consequence of slavish adherence to dogmatic assertion, and psychiatry, as a late-developing medical discipline, has recapitulated many of the same mistakes in its short history.

Psychiatric trainees, whatever their research aspirations, need to learn how to observe and be sensitive to the unexpected. Most of the major advances in medicine have been made by following up chance observations in a logical and consistent way. Jenner's observation of cowpox, Fleming's of penicillin and Bowlby's of childhood separation did not require intellectual genius; they depended on observation untrammelled by preconceptions. All mental health professionals should be capable of this.

This chapter aims to give general guidelines to the trainee who would like to know how a research idea can be converted into an investigation that will yield a useful result. However, no amount of knowledge of research methods will necessarily create a good project. A good project arises from a good research question, and getting the right research question is perhaps the most important part of the whole project. It is therefore far better for the trainee to develop research notions or ideas which can then be shaped into research questions and testable hypotheses than to rely on someone else's suggestions or a casual review of the literature. Worse still, in this age of easy data access and storage, the fond belief that packing of large amounts of accumulated data into a large computer will deliver a Nobel prize bears no relation to the truth. If a research project is worth doing it is quite likely that it has already been done by somebody, so it is important from the onset to find out if indeed the proposed project is truly novel.

The aim of your research

This is the most important part of any research endeavour and is obviously independent of research methodology. A bad research idea will produce bad results no matter how good the methods used. In selecting an issue that seems to be appropriate for research, the following questions need to be asked before beginning. If they are not answered before you start, a great deal of hard work could be wasted.

Why do you want to do the research?

If the answer is only 'to get a publication for my curriculum vitae', the work is likely to fail as it will lack commitment. Research has to be of value to others if it is worth doing at all. The need to publish is understandable in a competitive age but should not be the only motivation. Table 1.1 gives some other motives for research, along with their probability of being realised.

If the work is worth doing, why hasn't it been done before?

Research workers sometimes complain that there are 'no good ideas left'. It is still common for research to be completed on subjects that lead to interesting results but which, on closer examination of the literature, turn out to have been published before. A good literature search is therefore essential before starting any project (see below). A replication study should be a planned exercise, not an accidental one.

Table 1.1 Reasons for doing research

Reason	Predicted probability of success P
Nobel Prize	≤0.000001
Knighthood	≤0.00001
Fame, prestige, glory	≤0.0001
Changing our views of the world	≤0.0001
Getting published	0.1
Helping to pass exams by learning research methods	0.2
Modifying practice (at least yours)	0.3
Getting a better job	0.7
Keeping a critical attitude	0.75
Enjoyment (sometimes)	0.8
Educating parts of the brain seldom exercised	0.9

What results do you expect from the research work?

This question needs to be answered for two important reasons. The first is that the results might be completely predictable before beginning the investigation and would not therefore contain the element of doubt which is essential to any research inquiry. For example, there is probably little point in carrying out an investigation to determine whether tall people weigh more than short people, even if there has been no previous published study in the scientific literature. However, there are many well-known beliefs that have not been formally tested (e.g. the effect of bloodletting by leeches) and whose investigation might provide some valuable insight. The second reason is the important one of bias. It is an unfortunate fact that research workers tend to find the results they expected before they started their work, and it is worthwhile making a note of your expectations before you start your research. This may need to be disclosed in published work when the results are presented.

What are the likely implications of your research, including both positive and negative findings?

Good research has significant implications whether the findings turn out to be positive or negative. However, a great deal of research seems to be carried out because it is technically feasible and can be performed within a short time span, even though it has little or no long-term implications. Many replication studies fall into this category, but these can be justified if the methodology is superior to that used in previous studies. In deciding on the implications, please take account of both negative and positive findings.

Do I need advice before I go any further?

Before starting any research project it is advisable to discuss it with others. Of course there are some single-minded people who will go ahead anyway and who regard all other advice as less relevant than that they can obtain themselves, but these people are in the minority. It is therefore a good idea to discuss your general ideas for the project with a colleague whom you both trust and respect before going any further. This will often save a great deal of trouble in the long term.

Reviewing the literature

The best starting point is a good review article, particularly a systematic review as this follows standard procedure (see Chapter 4). With the introduction of the internet there is really no reason now for researchers not to examine the literature fully before beginning a project. In addition to the standard searches of medical databases such as Medline, complex searches can be carried out using the ISI Web of Knowledge, which is available to most academic institutions and which allows complicated searches to be carried out very quickly. Another very useful source is the PsychLit database, which is now available in most countries and covers a wide range of psychological journals, many of which are not covered by Medline. This is also available in most university libraries.

Development of a hypothesis

When developing a hypothesis it is usually wise to follow the agnostic viewpoint of Carl Popper that science exists to disprove hypotheses rather than to prove them. Thus no hypothesis can be said to be right; the best hypothesis is the closest approximation to the truth that we have at present, but there is always the possibility that it will be replaced by another at a later date. For this reason, hypotheses that are tested in scientific research are usually null hypotheses (i.e. they predict a negative result). If a null hypothesis is disproved, then it is reasonable to entertain the opposite (positive) hypothesis until it is tested again.

Hypotheses must be precisely formulated questions rather than vague statements and much care is needed in preparing them. Examples are given below.

- Vague hypothesis: 'Does psychotherapy help patients with anorexia nervosa?'
- Precisely formulated hypothesis: 'Does psychotherapy in the form of cognitive therapy, when given for 10 weeks, lead to a significantly greater weight gain in patients with anorexia nervosa compared with those not receiving cognitive therapy?'
- Null hypothesis: 'There is no difference in the weight gain of patients with anorexia nervosa when treated with cognitive therapy compared with a control procedure'.

The design features of a clinical study

The chapters that follow will deal with research designs in greater detail, but it may be helpful to ask yourself the following at intervals as you plan your project.

- Is the objective of the study clearly and sufficiently described?
- Are clear diagnostic criteria used?
- Can you give a clear statement about the source of participants?
- Are you using concurrent controls rather than historical controls?
- Are the treatments well defined?
- Are you using random allocation, and, if so, what type?
- Will the trial be masked and, if so, how will this be ensured?
- Are there appropriate outcome measures?
- Using these measures, do you have defined criteria of outcome (particularly a primary outcome)?

- Have you carried out a power calculation (Chapter 8) to help determine the most appropriate sample size?

Organising supervision

A good supervisor is essential for a trainee who is performing research. At times it can be lonely and dispiriting carrying out research projects, especially when recruitment of participants grinds to a halt. Contact with the supervisor does not necessarily need to be frequent, although you are particularly likely to need help and constructive criticism when planning your study and at the writing up stage. Most good supervisors are extremely busy and it is important to use your supervision time fruitfully. The following section, 'Keeping a research diary', may help you with this. It is important that you and your supervisor negotiate exactly what is to be done at each stage and it is usually helpful for you to be given deadlines. Your supervisor does not necessarily need to be an expert in the field of your research. It is more important that they have a general appreciation of the research design and a critical enquiring attitude. Those in distant countries with no potential supervisor should try to get one from another country. With e-mail and improved communication there is no need for geographical boundaries to prevent such supervision.

Keeping a research diary

When you start a project it is useful to keep a notebook with a proposed time plan. At the beginning you need to include as much detail as possible about the course of the project, allowing time for the literature search, designing a protocol, submission to an ethics committee, recruitment of participants, collection of data and writing up the findings. You also need to note in the diary as many of your own predictable life events as possible (e.g. Christmas, annual holidays). If you allow for these in the planning of your research, you can fit blocks of research around them. For example, plan what is going to happen to patients when you are on holiday, and remember that it is unlikely you will be able to recruit new participants or get people to attend for follow-up around Christmas and New Year. Also allow for the fact that when you are in training you may have to move from post to post. Some of the issues that arise are outlined in Fig. 1.1.

As the research project progresses you should use the notebook to record all important decisions that you make: it can be very frustrating to reach the end of a project and have no idea why you decided to alter particular facets of the research or why a particular person was excluded. Retrospective adjustment of data is one of the most common, and most dangerous, exercises in research. Also write down any relevant and interesting anecdotes that occur as you go through the project. If you have a relatively complete research notebook, analysis of data and writing up will be much easier.

Date	Main stages of study	Study tasks	Life events
Oct. 06	Literature review	Medline/Psylit/ ISI Web of Knowledge searches	
Dec. 06	Initial protocol		Christmas holidays
Jan. 07	Pilot studies	Try questionnaire on individual patients	
Feb. 07	Submit to ethics committees		Revision
Mar. 07		Contact GPs and consultants	Exams
Apr. 07	Main study	Final draft of questionnaire ready	
Jun. 07		Give to GP patients Definite cases	
Jul. 07		Borderline cases Physically ill	Summer holiday
Aug. 07		Psychiatrically ill samples	New post in rotation
Oct. 07		Test–retest reliability study	Revision
Nov. 07			Exams
Dec. 07	Complete main study	Code and check all data	
Jan. 08	Analysis		
Feb. 08			New post in rotation
Mar. 08			Moving house
Apr. 08	Writing up	Deciding on authorship	
May 08	Submission of paper		
Jun. 08	Study ends		Present results at scientific meeting

Fig. 1.1 Typical research plan at the beginning of a research diary. The project was to design, pilot and validate a screening questionnaire for somatisation disorder in general practice. GP, general practitioner.

You will notice that the study has ended before a paper has been completed and accepted for publication. This is common and it is useful to add time after the end of the project to account for resubmission and editing of papers after peer review. It is wise to regard the end of the project as the successful publication of a paper.

Designing a protocol

This is an important exercise, even if you are not applying for a grant. Most grant-giving bodies, such as the Medical Research Council, the Wellcome Trust and the Department of Health, require protocols to be submitted in a particular form (usually these are provided in an electronic format). It is essential to look at these application forms closely, as they will give helpful guidance as to how a protocol should be set out. The general steps are listed in Box 1.1. Although you may be keen to get on with your project without going through this stage, it will save you time later and will be very helpful when you come to writing up your work. Your method section will be virtually written for you, as it has been described in your protocol. It is best to start with a first draft that includes as many ideas and alternative trial designs as possible, and then to discuss them with your supervisor and colleagues.

Applying to an ethics committee

Any research involving human participants is likely to need the approval of an ethics committee. In the UK this has recently been simplified by the development of an online version of a standard electronic application created by the Central Office for Research Ethics Committees (COREC). This can be easily accessed (http://www.corecform.org.uk) and first involves the registration of the research worker. Once you have registered with COREC you can fill in as many applications as you wish. This involves not only giving your e-mail address but also adding a password which ensures your information is secure.

Although there are always teething problems with new forms, the advantage of the online arrangement is that your application can be sent to any ethics committee in the UK and can be accessed by the appropriate personnel.

If your project is a multisite one (which is less likely for a project to be performed by a trainee) you apply to a multicentre research ethics committee and if it is on a single site you apply to a local research ethics committee. The forms give clear guidance on what information needs to be obtained, but it is important to recognise that all ethics committees require a set of answers to standard questions. Box 1.2 includes most of the information required, which applies no matter in which part of the world you are applying for ethical approval. Sometimes people think that in low- and middle-income

---

Box 1.1 The protocol: steps in planning a study

- Getting an idea
- General background reading and more formal literature searches
- Form a specific aim (hypothesis of study)
- Design a study protocol to attempt to falsify this hypothesis. This should include:
    - patient selection criteria
    - treatment schedules
    - methods of patient evaluation
    - study design
    - how participants will be randomised
    - patient consent
    - size of study
    - monitoring of study progress
    - forms and data handling
    - protocol deviations
    - statistical analysis
    - plans for administration/staff and finance
- Apply for ethical approval
- Run a pilot study
- Redesign study if necessary (different sample size, rate of recruitment)
- Contact ethics committee and inform them of changes
- Run main experiment
- Collect and analyse data
- Publish so as to inform and allow for replication.

---

countries that are generally less developed in terms of research potential, ethical hurdles will be easier to overcome. This is an unwise and unhelpful presupposition; a good study should be ethical and it is quite wrong to attempt to cut corners merely because you think you might get away with it. It is also fair to note that a good ethics application form also helps in the writing of a good protocol and should be done as early as possible in the investigation. This is also important because it often takes several months to obtain ethical approval and you do not want your project to be delayed any longer than necessary.

Box 1.2   Essential information to record in the application to the ethics committee

- Details of names of investigators and their affiliations.
- Dates for the beginning and end of the study.
- The primary purpose of the research.
- The principal research question (give this in as simple a form as possible as this really needs to be understood by everybody looking at the application).
- What are the secondary research questions? It is best to limit these to less than five, as they do not include some tertiary enquiries.
- Scientific justification for the research. This is the opportunity to describe your project in the context of previous work and state why it is appropriate at this time.
- A summary of the proposed research and its methodology. Again this should be in as simple a form as possible, preferably with an additional flow chart as this can often convey much more information than text alone.
- Is any treatment being withheld from patients as a consequence of the research? This is an important question, as clearly a valuable treatment should not normally be withheld from a patient just because they are taking part in a research investigation.
- Details of clinical interventions or procedures that are outside normal clinical care. Any intervention needs to be specified in reasonable detail, including its risks.
- Is any sensitive information being requested? Any questionnaires that deal with sensitive questions will need to be enclosed with the application.
- Duration of participation in the project. This should include follow-up as well as active treatment.
- Adverse effects of any research intervention. Please be open about these and their likely frequency.
- Potential benefit for participants. Again be honest here; many investigations are not of immediate benefit but only of longer-term benefit; this does not negate the research, but the immediate benefits should not be exaggerated.
- Adverse effects to researchers. These are not common in psychiatric settings but need to be considered.
- How will participants be identified and recruited? Be careful not to overstate the likely recruitment rate and be too restrictive about who is selected; one of the major problems in research is under-recruitment, and this causes many studies to founder.
- What are the main inclusion and exclusion criteria? Specify these accurately and unambiguously.
- Can informed consent be obtained? It is now common for informed consent to be obtained from all participants in research studies, and if the participant lacks capacity (e.g. has learning disability, dementia, etc.), a relative or independent third party should sign the consent form on behalf of the patient.
- Length of time the participant has to decide whether to take part in the research. One criticism of research workers is that they sometimes bully or bludgeon patients to take part in research and do not give them a chance to reflect on its purpose and whether they would like to take part; wherever possible a time interval between first approaching and recruiting patients is desirable.

continued

Box 1.2 *continued*

- Proposed feedback to patients who take part in a research project. Clearly if there are particular problems or benefits that are identified during the course of a study, there can be advantages in disclosing them to people who have already completed the project.
- Others to be informed about the project, including the patient's general practitioner (this is normally considered desirable).
- Payment for research participants. Small sums of money are now considered appropriate to reimburse participants for their travel expenses and time; provided these are modest they will not be misunderstood as bribes to take part in research.
- Arrangements for indemnity and compensation. These are normally accepted by the sponsor of any research project.
- Reporting of results of the study. Although this might be regarded as self-evident, clearly a well executed study that leads to no report or dissemination will be of no value to the scientific community and probably of no value to the patients who have taken part; good reporting and dissemination is therefore essential.
- How will the Data Protection Act 1998 be followed? It is important that personal and sensitive information is not communicated in any form without anonymisation, coding or other forms of encrypting; details of how these procedures will be carried out are normally required.
- How will confidentiality of personal data be ensured? This is an extension of the previous section.
- How will the data be analysed? Statistical help is almost always desirable with a research project and should be specified here.
- For how long will data from the study be stored? This is increasingly important, but as data storage becomes more difficult it is likely to lead to problems; ideally the original data should be kept for 15 years after they have been collected.
- Justification of the research, including the choice of primary and secondary outcomes and whether previous work has been carried out on the subject. This is an extension of the normal protocol and the questions are easily answered.
- Number of participants, including controls. It is often a good idea to state the upper and lower limits for a successful project, so that if recruitment is not as great as expected it could still be within acceptable limits.

Recruiting participants

One of the biggest problems in research is recruiting a sufficient number of participants. Obviously this is less of a problem with retrospective case studies, also called 'archival research'. Here the 'participants' have already been identified and one does not have to rely on new recruitment. Even under these circumstances it can be surprising how large the wastage can be. A computer printout from a case register of patients with a single diagnosis might reveal some who have been misdiagnosed and a few whose case notes do not seem to exist at all; there may be many other reasons why your previously clear-cut group of patients has to be whittled down to a smaller sample. This is before accounting for patients who have died and others who have moved away.

When conducting prospective research, most researchers find that appropriate patients seem to disappear just as the study is about to start. Lasagna's law predicts that the recruitment rate will fall by at least half at just the time your study starts. In general the best way to deal with this is to allow for such predictions in your research planning so that, for example, if your realistic prediction is that you can recruit 50 participants over 1 year, arrange your study so that your estimated prediction rate can be doubled either by lengthening your recruitment time or by widening your recruitment area.

Some researchers advertise for participants, and there is nothing wrong with this approach provided you are clear that you will get quite a different sample from that recruited via general practitioners or hospital referrals. Much research in the USA is done on this basis and it is often not made clear when the results are published how patients are recruited. This makes the interpretation of many such studies quite difficult, particularly in the area of depression, anxiety and eating disorders. In many studies, participants are college students who have been recruited via advertisements on campus, and who bear little similarity to a typical patient referred by a general practitioner in the UK National Health Service.

One effective way of recruiting participants is to offer a service: if, for example, you are looking for patients with chronic pain, offering some sort of assessment service or even a treatment programme is one way of ensuring a deluge of referrals.

Replication studies

Although it is usually desirable to try to carry out a piece of original research, especially for your first research project, replication studies are very important: it is only when a finding has been replicated in a number of different centres by different investigators that its significance can be properly assessed. There are a number of reasons for this. First, most investigators are not unbiased, and they embark on research projects because they have a particular idea which they think is correct. In other words, most investigators find what they hope or what they expect to find. It is always worth taking slightly more notice of those studies where a researcher appears to be genuinely surprised by the result obtained or where the results contradict the researcher's own favoured hypothesis.

Second, there is a marked publication bias. Studies with positive results tend to be reported and published much more frequently than those with negative results. It is quite possible for studies with a similar design to be carried out in a number of different centres, for the negative results never to see the light of day and for the one atypical positive result to be published. This is not usually a result of deliberate suppression of contradictory data but just the understandable desire that researchers and journals publish positive findings.

Finally, in any study involving human participants, one can never be sure how representative the sample is, and repeating the study on a different sample, perhaps in a different part of the country or a different setting, is always desirable.

The advantage for the trainee of replication studies is that there is an established method to follow. It is usually possible to contact the original researcher and indicate your desire to repeat the study in a different setting. Most researchers are delighted to collaborate with such endeavours. Do not therefore be ashamed of doing replication studies – they do not constitute second-class research and are vitally important for scientific advancement.

Coping with failure and how to prevent it

Very few research projects go as planned and many are never completed. If you do not get as far as collecting results, make every effort to write up the reasons in a form that is suitable for publication. Do not be too disheartened if you get a negative result. Indeed, when setting up the project it should be borne in mind that a negative result can be as important as a positive result. It has also been suggested that there should be special journals that publish only negative results or those studies that fail altogether. In fact, most journals will publish relevant negative research provided that it is of value to others, and some projects that turn out to be disastrous often provide the most powerful lessons.

There are many reasons why research projects fail that are outside the control of the researcher, but to minimise the chance of failure you should at least obey the following rules. First, have a clearly thought-out research design that you have put down on paper and discussed with others who have good critical faculties. Second, if possible try to arrange to have a supervisor. Third, design your study to collect as much information as you can at the beginning and as little as possible later. In other words, if you are following-up patients try to collect as many details as possible when you first see the patient and keep the amount of data you collect at follow-up interviews to a minimum. Fourth, try to write your project up as you go along even if it is only in note or diary form, as suggested earlier. This will aid you enormously when you come to the final write-up. Fifth, try to have some sort of fallback project instead of persisting with a failing main project. This will ensure that you will at least have a descriptive study or a literature review if the main project goes badly wrong.

Having said all this, projects most often fail at the beginning, before any data are obtained, and at the end, when all the data are collected but, for a variety of reasons, the project results are never analysed or written up. Clearly this is a terrible waste of time and effort, but it also has considerable ethical implications. If we carry out research which imparts at least some discomfort or risk to participants (most research involves some hazards), then we have an obligation to share the information with others so that the patients who originally took part or similar patients in the future might benefit. Even if the work is never published, it is useful to write a short summary so that patients who have taken part can be shown the value of the study. The study might benefit only the participating researchers, but if this makes them better practitioners the participants will certainly feel that their time has been well spent.

CHAPTER 2

Psychiatric research from the trainee's perspective

Neil Mayfield and Rebecca Tipper

At some point in their training, it is likely that most psychiatrists will have the opportunity to undertake research. For example, the current higher specialist training system in the UK explicitly states that doctors are 'expected to develop an understanding of research methodology and be encouraged to undertake research' (National Health Service Executive, 1998). Although profound changes in postgraduate medical education are being implemented in the UK as part of Modernising Medical Careers (Donaldson, 2002), it is clear that carrying out reserach will remain an integral part of competency-based curricula. Carrying out a research project is widely considered of central importance in the production of effective independent psychiatric practitioners.

Various possibilities exist for the trainee. First, for those with a consuming interest in research, it is possible to step off the ladder of clinical training and take up higher training in academic medicine with the intention of pursuing a career in research. Alternatively, a period can be taken out of clinical training for the purposes of taking up a research post for a defined period (often with the aim of acquiring a postgraduate degree such as a PhD or MD). Guidance for these two groups of doctors is provided by the short book by Murrell *et al* (1999). The present chapter is largely aimed at those trainees who are interested in a career in clinical psychiatry and who try to conduct research alongside other duties.

At present higher psychiatric trainees in the UK (specialist registrars) are allocated 1 day per week, which is supposed to be protected from other duties, for the purpose of undertaking research. The post-foundation training programmes which will replace the specialist registrar grade will continue to present opportunities for carrying out research, although their exact form remains to be seen. Foundation year trainees do not have protected research sessions but may have the option of doing an academic medicine block during the second foundation year. Similar short, dedicated research posts of this sort have previously been seen as a valuable training experience (Strydom & Higgins, 2004).

Given that most trainees will try their hand at research in some shape or form, the present chapter asks the following questions. What are likely to be the benefits of research to the trainee, their patients and the organisations for which they work? What preparations can be made to make the research experience as fruitful as possible? What difficulties might be encountered along the way? Can the benefits be obained in ways other than the trainee personally performing a research project?

What are the benefits to the trainee of research?

The benefits of a research project will differ from trainee to trainee. In theory at least, research could lead to a diverse range of positive outcomes, as listed in Box 2.1.

Many different skills can be acquired, including knowledge of specific computer packages, statistical tests or laboratory/clinical equipment. More generic and transferable skills include the appraisal of published literature and the effective presentation of data. Less tangible, but no less important, is intellectual stimulation and the deepening of understanding of psychiatric illness. More practically, the acquisition of a higher degree or a series of publications will improve the trainee's curriculum vitae and enhance future employment prospects (Mumford, 2000). It is important not to lose sight of the fact that the research, even if only a small project, could also benefit others – particularly patients – by leading to improvements in knowledge about a condition and its treatments. Particularly in an age of evidence-based practice, even the most committed clinician would have to accept that it is research that provides the theoretical base for logical clinical practice. An interesting personal account of the value of performing research during postgraduate medical training has been provided by Cullen (2002). Even a failed research project can be an enlightening experience, allowing useful insights to be gained (Vaidya, 2004).

However no project, no matter how well designed, could realistically be expected to provide all the benefits effects listed in Box 2.1. Different types of study will carry their own benefits; for example, different skills would probably be gained from a laboratory project than from a clinical study. There is therefore an argument for carrying out research in several different settings if time and opportunity allows.

Attempting research

The following two fictional vignettes are based on an amalgamation of real experiences – both positive and negative – of trainees who have attempted to get research projects off the ground. They offer two very different perspectives of conducting research as a trainee and illustrate some of the factors that can influence the success or failure of a study.

Box 2.1 Benefits to the trainee of doing research

- Gaining computer skills, e.g. using databases and spreadsheets
- Understanding statistics
- Improving ability to search the medical literature
- Acquiring skills in appraising published research
- Gaining knowledge of research methodology
- Improving writing and presentation skills
- Improving time management skills
- Gaining confidence in working independently
- Working as part of a team
- Acquiring ability to plan and implement projects
- Acquiring ability to supervise research projects of trainees
- Understanding illness at a more complex level
- Developing an area of special expertise
- Increasing interest in clinical work
- Moving into an academic career
- Obtaining publications or a higher degree
- Improving CV and increasing job prospects
- Increasing personal interest
- Advancement of knowledge and improvement of care.

Vignette 1

Trainee A joins a higher psychiatric training scheme in an area of the country with which he is unfamiliar. He has no previous research experience apart from conducting a small unpublished audit of physical examinations in acute wards. The scheme is in a geographically spread area, and there is consequently little peer support. He is interested in the effect of alcohol use on the attendance of general psychiatric patients at out-patient appointments. He takes a while to settle in and is working in a very busy acute unit, where his clinical duties (which he prefers) encroach on his research sessions (for clinical continuity, he takes 2 half-days). In view of this, he takes some time to design his project and only when he is about to start discovers that he needs ethical approval. He is unfamiliar with the local (or indeed any) ethics committees and is dismayed to be set back some months as he submits (and resubmits, owing to poor choice of rating scales and statistical ignorance) his proposal.

By the time he starts, he is losing interest, and has moved location to work in a sub-specialty. He also gets married and moves house. He completes a number of patient interviews but recruitment is much harder than he expected, particularly as he no longer has regular contact with staff who might help him with this. He has difficulty gaining access to a computer or training in IT skills at work, and has to enter all his data at home in the evenings, something he is unfamiliar with and finds laborious. He realises that he is unlikely to achieve the numbers he requires for a significant result and toys with the idea of writing it up descriptively, but never quite gets round to it. As a result of his excellent clinical work, he is offered a consultant post towards the end of his contract and decides that research is probably unnecessary for him. His work gathers dust on a shelf, and he comments to his own trainees that research is not really necessary for a general clinician and never stopped him getting a job.

Vignette 2

Trainee B joins the higher training scheme where she completed her foundation training, and has already completed a supervised master's research degree, from which she has gained a publication. She believes that these factors were highly relevant to obtaining her current post and, although having no wish for an academic career, she enjoyed her research and is keen to do more. She has similar interests to Trainee A and has already (prior to gaining her job) approached local senior academic staff for advice regarding designing a project. A fellow trainee has asked to join the project and is enthusiastic. By the time she starts the post, they have written a protocol and are ready to submit an application for ethical approval (something she has already done in the course of her master's degree). Few changes are required and they are able to pilot the project in a unit where she is known and liked by staff, who help with recruitment. She is expected to be away from clinical duties for a day a week for this purpose and experiences no difficulties in achieving this. She has a computer in her office and is able to get formal and informal advice regarding statistics and the use of databases from the local academic department. The results of the pilot study are promising and she has the opportunity to present her work while proceeding with the main project. She finishes gathering data a year before her training finishes and writes up the work with her co-trainee, who helps to maintain her enthusiasm for the project after Trainee B experiences some unexpected personal difficulties. Senior staff are again helpful in commenting on the final draft, and it is submitted, and accepted for publication just before she completes her training. Like Trainee A, she easily obtains a (non-academic) consultant post, and advises her trainees that this was, in part, a result of her enhanced curriculum vitae.

Difficulties doing research as a trainee

The experience of Trainee A exemplifies many of the pitfalls that beset the inexperienced researcher. Unfortunately, recent surveys of the experiences of research of psychiatric trainees have confirmed that problems are common (Vassilas *et al*, 2002; Petrie *et al*, 2003). The studies cited looked at the experiences of specialist registrars (previously called senior registrars) who are allocated 1 day per week for research which should be protected

19

from the clinical duties they perform at other times. In a survey of higher psychiatric trainees in the UK only 30% of respondents felt that allocated research time was used satisfactorily (Vassilas *et al*, 2002). Many experience problems with resources and supervision (Petrie *et al*, 2003). Two studies found that only roughly half of the specialist registrars in psychiatry had ever managed to secure a publication (Smart & Cottrell, 2000; Allsopp *et al*, 2002). Taken in combination, the surveys showed the specific difficulties described below (Trainee A was unfortunate to encounter them all).

Lack of time

This is particularly owing to the intrusion of clinical duties into research sessions and is especially acute for those who work part-time.

Inadequate supervision

Many trainees report difficulties accessing appropriate supervision and so have embarked on poorly planned projects that have little prospect of success. The importance of supervision is emphasised by a study of surgical trainees which showed that the degree of satisfaction with supervision was extremely strongly and positively correlated with subsequent beliefs about the value of research (McCue, 1994).

Inadequate training in research methods

Clearly an understanding of the principles of scientific research is a prerequisite for the performance of high-quality projects. In the UK attendance at a postgraduate educational course is mandatory to be eligible to take professional examinations in psychiatry. Although such courses would be expected to include teaching on research methodology, many trainees admit to having little confidence in their knowledge and skills in this area. The Royal College of Psychiatrists has recently emphasised the importance of an understanding of research methods and critical appraisal by introducing a paper specifically assessing this area in its membership examinations.

Problems accessing information technology and statistical support

All but the very smallest and simplest projects will require these resources. Trainees often have limited access to these, as demonstrated by the survey of Kotak & Butler (2001).

Low morale and lack of ideas

This may follow previous unsuccessful projects which have failed for the reasons outlined above.

Planning a successful project

The experience of Trainee B highlights the importance of adequate planning in the outcome of research. Aspects of research design are addressed in other chapters, so these general issues are not covered here. Instead, we concentrate on the factors that the trainee needs to take into account. There are several important questions that the trainee should ask at the very outset of the project.

Is this the right time for me to do this project?

Will I be able to devote adequate time to the study? Obviously, this is less of an issue for those taking up a full-time research post than for those trying to run a project alongside clinical duties. Intrusion of such duties is a common reason for failing to bring research projects to fruition. In some other branches of medicine, where there is severe competition to secure a limited number of training places, research publications and possession of higher degrees have become almost mandatory for career progression. This may result in the trainee having little option to 'pick and choose' when to do research. At present, this is not usually the case for psychiatry in the UK (although surveys have still shown 'CV building' to be a prominent motivation for carrying out research (Williams & Curran, 1998)). Hence for trainees in psychiatry there is likely to be more flexibility, with the result that the trainee is less likely to be saddled with uninspiring projects that are carried out with a feeling that they are necessary for advancement. In addition to clinical pressures, junior trainees will also have to contend with professional examinations. Needless to say, it is not prudent to consider starting research when examinations are looming. As a general principle, it is useful to estimate the probable timing of the whole project through all of the stages shown in Fig. 2.1 (being generous), as this can give some indication of its overall feasibility.

It is noteworthy that early exposure to research as a medical student has been linked to increased research interest and activity in the student's subsequent medical career (Segal *et al*, 1990). Many medical schools have now incorporated research into the curriculum, in the form of special study modules. If the project is right, it is not too early to start.

Am I asking an adequately focused question?

It is difficult to overstate the importance of being precise in defining the question you hope your research will answer. This is the foundation on which the study is based and if the aim of the research is vague or overly grandiose there is little prospect that the outcome will be satisfactory. It is best to try to answer as few questions as possible. Guidance on asking precise, structured questions is provided in other chapters and by Sackett *et al* (1998).

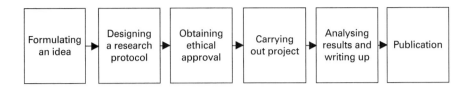

Fig. 2.1 Individual stages of a research project.

Can I answer the question with the resources at my disposal?

In addition to the availability of adequate time, it is also important to ensure that your project has adequate funding and supervision, that you possess the necessary skills and that you have material resources such as computer technology at your disposal. Trainees may be able to use a study leave budget to pay for courses to address any skills deficits. Good supervision is particularly important for the inexperienced researcher and time spent finding the right person will be rewarded by the quality of the finished study. Surveys of trainees show that lack of supervision is a common reason for failure of research projects. Weissberg (2002) has listed some useful questions to help in choosing an appropriate supervisor. Consultation with a statistician when designing the project is also extremely important, but again this resource may be difficult for the trainee to access. Even with all this support, it is wise to conduct a pilot study, as this can provide valuable information on the feasibility of the study.

What are my learning objectives?

It is useful to set clear learning objectives at the start of the project. This helps to clarify what you hope to gain from the research and highlights any training needs. Review of the objectives as research proceeds allows modifications to be made to help ensure that maximal benefit is derived with the limited time and resources.

Solutions to problems encountered

What can you do as a trainee if, despite your best efforts and attempts at planning, you encounter some of the problems mentioned previously (apart from abandoning the project like trainee A)? If you have managed to find a research supervisor, the logical first step is to discuss your difficulties with them. For those who find that clinical work encroaches upon research time, it may be possible to negotiate a more manageable timetable with the clinical trainer. It is ultimately in the interests of the trainers to have trainees who are able to fulfil their training requirements; this will prevent their training posts from becoming unpopular.

Aside from your supervisor, many trusts in the UK employ a research facilitator who can prove extremely helpful. Help may range from finding small amounts of funding from a trust research budget to providing information technology support or skills training. Budgets for study leave can also be used to fund courses that would address skills deficits.

An alternative approach to the problems of time constraints and lack of supervision is for trainees to form a local research group, preferably with input from an experienced researcher. The activities of such a group are described in Vignette 3. Not only can a local research group provide a forum for discussing ideas at an early stage, it also creates the opportunity for joint working with colleagues in similar positions, thus allowing pooling of time and resources.

Vignette 3 – A research group for trainees

At the time of joining the same higher training scheme, both the authors had some limited experience of research but were unsure of how to develop this over the next few years. As a result, both became involved in the inception and running of an informal research group. This has been entirely run by trainees, although there has been invaluable input from one consultant (in the role of research tutor).

The original purpose of the group was to provide mutual support (morale regarding research was low among many trainees at that time), to encourage trainees to work together on small projects rather than in isolation, to consider the possibility of projects undertaken by a large group of trainees and to organise occasional full-day sessions for review of projects and lectures by external speakers. All of these have succeeded to some extent and, although the problems that are described in this chapter continue to face trainees, this has proved a valuable resource and a forum to discuss such difficulties.

Problems have been experienced, notably with attempts to perform large-group projects. These have involved perceived uneven divisions of labour and contributions. Issues of authorship of publications have also caused awkwardness. Not everyone wished to attend such a group, some because they already had considerable research experience and some because they were less interested in research. This group has benefited from a core group of members, at least one of whom has substantial research experience. There are ongoing frustrations resulting from a lack of resources, including information technology and research training, and it is conceivable that such a group might ultimately have only a minimal impact on the research produced by trainees. However, it is a simple (and cheap) way of providing peer support and creating a cohesive group for trainees to look at the issues connected with performing research.

Other solutions

If it proves difficult to conduct a project using one allocated day each week, there is scope to save up the remaining days and take a 'block' of research time, say 3 months, during which one could devote all of the working week to the project. This may be particularly helpful for part-time trainees. An avenue that is relatively unexplored in psychiatry, but is becoming the norm in other branches of medicine, is to leave clinical work for several years and undertake research as part of studying for a higher degree, typically a PhD or MD. At least part of the time spent doing a higher degree can count towards the requirements of overall time spent in training before being eligible to take up consultant posts. Wider availability of this option is likely only to come with a change in the overall culture and attitude towards research within psychiatry.

A final, and perhaps controversial, solution to frustration with research is to decide not to do a project but to use the allotted time for other purposes which could satisfy some of the learning objectives of a research project (Ramchandani *et al*, 2001). For example, a trainee could devote sessions to developing an interest in evidence-based medicine, audit, clinical governance or teaching. Surprisingly, the issue of whether it is necessary to actually conduct a project to acquire some of the benefits listed in Box 2.1 has received little study, although there is some evidence to suggest that exposure to research is no guarantee of acquiring confidence in critical appraisal (Carey & Hall, 1999).

References

Allsopp, L., Allen, R., Fowler, L., *et al* (2002) Research in psychiatric higher specialist training: a survey of specialist registrars. *Psychiatric Bulletin*, **26**, 272–274.

Carey, S. & Hall, D. J. (1999) Psychiatrists' views of evidence-based psychiatric practice. *Psychiatric Bulletin*, **23**, 159–161.

Cullen, S. (2002) The value of research in the specialist registrar training program. *BMJ*, **325**, 103S.

Donaldson, L. (2002) *Unfinished Business: Proposals for Reform of the Senior House Officer Grade*. London: Department of Health.

Kotak, A. & Butler, R. (2001) Do trainees have adequate access to computers and computer software? *Psychiatric Bulletin*, **25**, 31–32.

McCue, J. (1994) Research in surgical training: the trainee's perspective. *Annals of the Royal College of Surgeons of England*, **76** (suppl. 3), 121–123.

Mumford, C. (2000) The *Medical Job Interview: Secrets for Success*. Oxford: Blackwell Science.

Murrell, G., Huang, C. & Ellis, H. (1999) Research *in Medicine: Planning a Project – Writing a Thesis*. Cambridge: Cambridge University Press.

National Health Service Executive (1998) A *Guide to Specialist Registrar Training*. London: Department of Health.

Petrie, R., Anderson, K., Hare, E., *et al* (2003) Research activity of specialist registrars. *Psychiatric Bulletin*, **28**, 180–182.

Ramchandani, P., Corby, C., Guest, L., *et al* (2001) The place and purpose of research training for specialist registrars: a view from the Collegiate Trainees' Committee (CTC) of the Royal College of Psychiatrists. *Irish Journal of Psychological Medicine*, **18**, 29–31.

Sackett, D. L., Richardson, W. S., Rosenberg, W., *et al* (1998) *Evidence-Based Medicine: How to Practice and Teach EBM*. Edinburgh: Churchill Livingstone.

Segal, S., Lloyd, T., Houts, P. S., *et al* (1990) The association between students' research involvement in medical school and their postgraduate medical activities. *Academic Medicine*, **65**, 530–533.

Smart, S. & Cottrell, D. (2000) A survey of training experiences and attitudes of higher specialist trainees in child and adolescent psychiatry. *Psychiatric Bulletin*, **24**, 302–304.

Strydom, A. & Higgins, N. (2004) Are dedicated research posts of value to psychiatry trainees? *Psychiatric Bulletin*, **28**, 260–263.

Vaidya, G. (2004) Lessons learned from a failed research project. *Psychiatric Bulletin*, **28**, 301–303.

Vassilas, C., Tadros, G. & Day, E. (2002) The research day: a suitable case for treatment. *Psychiatric Bulletin*, **26**, 313–314.

Weissberg, P. (2002) Research in clinical training. *BMJ*, **325**, 97S.

Williams, C. J. & Curran, S. (1998) Research by senior registrars in psychiatry. *Psychiatric Bulletin*, **22**, 102–104.

CHAPTER 3

Writing up research

Peter Tyrer and Chris Freeman

The trainee just beginning a research programme often has the understandable notion that the writing up of a research study is relatively easy. After all, the important part of the research is surely the development of the hypothesis and collection of data, followed by the analysis. After that, the optimistic trainee thinks that 'the paper will write itself'. Unfortunately, this notion could not be much further from the truth. Whereas a hundred years ago it would be perfectly in order to write up a fairly rambling account of a piece of work, including any number of whimsical musings, now the pressures of publication are such that every paragraph of text has to be fought for and writers who have the ability to precis the essentials are the most favoured.

It is important to start to write up research early. Far too late in the day, trainees decide it may be time to write up their projects and then realise all the disadvantages of doing this at a later stage. In fact, if a trainee has carried out a project correctly a large part of the research paper has already been written, because a good protocol gives the main reasons for carrying out the research and the methods to be employed. This protocol can often be used as a basis for the subsequent paper, so that the framework of the paper already exists. One of the other great advantages of this approach is that deviations from the protocol will be identified when the data are being analysed. By comparing the progress of the study with the original protocol it is easy to note any deviations from the original plan, allowing these to be noted in the final published version. This is particularly helpful when an unexpected finding emerges. There is a great temptation to suggest that your original protocol was looking for this unexpected finding all along, when in fact it was really a small ancillary part of the main investigation and quite unexpected. It takes a great deal of honesty to admit this in a published paper, but this really is the right way of presenting the finding if it was genuinely unexpected.

All significant deviations from the protocol can be identified by starting your writing early. Even if the deviations from the protocol are so great that the study has to be abandoned, this need not be a disaster. Research psychiatrists are nothing if not enterprising and it may be felt that the abandonment of the project has important lessons for us all and so publication of the findings still takes place (e.g. Blackwell & Shepherd, 1967; Cook *et al*, 1988). Even when a research programme has failed to deliver results worthy of report in any form, all is not lost. One of the major advantages of trainees doing research is that the subject is explored not only from the outside, in its more acceptable form, but also from the inside, so that the more subtle (and sometimes less attractive) aspects are exposed. This often enables an excellent review paper to be written, which, as Chapter 15 illustrates, can be a fundamental contribution to the literature that may even transcend the value of all the original papers on the subject.

The research paper

Potential authors will note that they are forced into a Procrustean system by journals, so that most original papers comprise four sections: an introduction; a method section; a results section; and discussion. Sometimes this template may be quite inappropriate, and this is recognised in sections of journals devoted to education and debate, editorial comment and points of view. However, we assume that the trainee wishes to write up the results of the research investigation and is not writing one of these other articles. It is worth discussing each of the sections of an original paper separately.

Introduction

Many who have not written a research paper before are flummoxed by this heading. What is it that is being introduced or, more pertinently, what is not? The introduction should prepare the reader for the essential information that follows, but should not be an introduction to the whole subject. If you wished to present ground-breaking information that the moon is made of green cheese you would not need to introduce the subject by describing the solar system and the moon's relationship to the earth. The reader knows all about the moon; what he wants to know is your evidence for its constituents. The reader of a specialist journal already has special knowledge and there is no need for the introduction to be a general tutorial. So give an introduction to the problem that you are addressing and do not deviate from this.

A recent review of the contents of papers in the *British Journal of Psychiatry* concluded that the introductions were the least satisfactory; they were over-long, rambling and often irrelevant, and it is now recommended that they do not exceed two paragraphs. In writing the introduction it is often best to imagine how you would present your findings to a group of your peers at a postgraduate meeting. You just need to say a few words to set the scene and explain why you have carried out the research. The introduction should be an expanded version of the ideas that led to the study and the objectives at the time the study was begun.

Method

A lot has to go into the method section and it should be written as concisely as possible. When writing it is a good idea to imagine that you are a new researcher wishing to replicate the study and wanting to know exactly how it was done. All the information should be present to allow such a replication. So if you are describing patients, you need to identify the population from which they came, the inclusion and exclusion criteria and how they were recruited. You will also need to describe the procedure for obtaining consent and confirm that ethical approval was obtained for the study. Any tests, treatment and more complex interventions need to be described clearly and succinctly. If this is not possible because of the space available, there is no harm in adding an additional sentence 'Further details of the exact methods can be obtained from the authors.' Sometimes the methodology is standard, but it may be quite complicated. In the latter instance it is appropriate to give a reference to a previous publication, but only if the procedure followed was exactly as described in the cited reference.

The method section should also include details of how the data were collected and how they were analysed. As noted in Chapter 8, it is best to procure statistical assistance early rather than late, and ideally this section of the paper should be written by the statistician. There is now abundant evidence that studies that are analysed by an independent statistician, preferably one placed at a reasonable geographical distance from the research site, are more likely to yield consistent results than those that are analysed 'in house'. There is an unfortunate tendency, now well established in the Cochrane Collaboration, to find early studies with small numbers that show much greater significance than later studies carried out with much larger numbers and with independent statistical analysis. The desperate need to produce a positive result at all costs in order to publish the results is also a major problem here. The ideal method section includes an analysis plan that was devised before any of the data were subjected to even the most primitive form of analysis. This avoids a common error of identifying a positive finding that was not predicted and then pretending that this was the main focus of the hypothesis. If a finding turns out to be highly significant but was not expected, this needs to be stated; it may be very important but it needs to be put in the context of the study.

Results

The results section is the meat of the paper. When writing this section the investigator should first confirm that everything that is included genuinely belongs there. It is a common mistake to include results in the method section and method in the results section. The method section should describe how data were collected but not give any figures; the results section should give those figures, as far as possible without comment.

Most of the tables and figures should appear in the results section. These are generally an efficient way of presenting data: one picture may be worth 1000 words and one table can be worth 500. However, it should also be borne in mind that pictures are expensive to reproduce and that there is no point in gaining space by producing a figure or table and then repeating the results in the text.

The use of computer packages (which are not always selected specifically for the analysis in question) in the analysis of data is now widespread and often yields a large quantity of data, which makes it difficult to decide what should be included. This is where the analysis plan comes in handy. Information that is not in the analysis plan could be left out of tables and perhaps commented upon in the text. Alternatively, many journals now offer the option of publishing additional tables or other relevant information as an online data supplement. Increasingly it is likely that published papers will not be as long as the electronic versions that can be accessed through the internet. The additional data available online might be of particular value for those performing systematic reviews when the scope of the review is wider than the subject of the paper. Too many results simply confuse the reader, but overselection of results for presentation can lead to bias. It is sometimes difficult to achieve the correct balance.

Discussion

The discussion is also a section that tends to be longer than necessary. The heading implies that the author has free rein to talk about anything that is relevant; the difficulty is in deciding what is relevant and what is not. Each sentence of the discussion section should be examined after this section is completed and the question asked 'Is this relevant to the aims and findings of the study?' If it is not, the sentence is probably redundant. There is always a danger that this section can allow the authors to venture into territory that they hold dear but that is nothing to do with the subject of the paper.

The discussion section could often be entitled 'Amplification and implication'. The amplification comes from discussing the findings in relationship to the original aims and hypotheses, and clearly this deserves comment of some sort, particularly if the results are not as expected. The implication comes from the interpretation of the findings in relation to other studies or to clinical practice. The implications might be considerable but it is wise not to be too bold in extrapolating from the results. Thus, for example, it would be premature to suggest from a randomised trial of 30 patients showing a significant benefit for an intervention that the intervention should be adopted widely throughout the country or even the world. All authors like to feel their work is important, but in presenting your findings in a research paper it is wise to be modest and cautious before reviewers make you so. If you subsequently show that your results were indeed right and have a major impact on science or clinical practice, then this modesty will only add to the stature of your work.

29

Publication of the paper

Although the essential elements of a paper can be written for any journal, there are major aspects of presentation that have to be taken into account before submitting the paper to a given journal. In short, the scientist has, even if only briefly, to become a salesperson. The intention of every author is to convince the editor that the paper being submitted could not be published in any other journal without a significant loss of impact and that the readers of the journal would be privileged to read it.

Who would be most interested in the findings?

This simple question is sometimes forgotten. It is natural that research workers would like the whole world to read about their findings after they have invested so much time and effort in their study, but the sad fact is that only a small minority of papers have genuine general interest and most are directed towards a small, specialised readership. When one considers that the average paper is cited only once in its scientific life it puts matters into perspective. It is often valuable to take advice from the more experienced investigator before deciding to which journal the paper should be submitted. There is a natural tendency for a trainee, with the great enthusiasm that follows the preparation of the paper, to decide that it is suitable only for the *British Medical Journal* or the *Lancet* and to send the paper accordingly to those journals. Although this may be perfectly reasonable, it is important to realise that the style of the paper as well as important issues such as the reference format might need to be altered for another journal. An experienced editor can detect without much difficulty a paper that has been submitted many times previously to other journals and there is a danger that the paper might never get published if it is sent too frequently to high-impact-factor journals only.

How many papers are needed?

The correct answer to this question is 'as few as possible'. There is a tendency for investigators to publish more papers than is necessary, a phenomenon commonly known as 'salami slicing'. In the long term this is counterproductive, as it adds needlessly to the world literature on the topic and often the good papers are hidden among the bad. There are many reasons why investigators publish too many papers. These include the natural wish to beef up a curriculum vitae with as many publications as possible, the wish to suitably acknowledge co-workers by giving them 'first author status' in subsidiary articles and to disseminate the information among as wide a readership as possible by publishing in different places. None of these can really be defended; numbers of publications are no substitute for quality, and although the additional citations may appear to be valuable at first, in the long term there is no major gain. Now that all established journals are readily available, at least in abstract form, on academic networks, the need to publish in several journals is becoming much less defensible.

However, there might be instances when several papers are necessary to describe one piece of work. These will usually concern large-scale studies that either have so many data that they cannot all be presented in one paper or studies where there are important differences in the data (e.g. of time scale, nature or measurement) that justify more than one publication. It is sometimes advantageous to publish these articles together in the same journal because their length can be reduced, but it is fair to say that editors are becoming less keen on this as pressure on journal space becomes greater.

Submission of the manuscript

Before the final manuscript is submitted to the journal of choice, it is advisable to show it to at least one colleague with more experience in the subject. Following many hours devoted to its preparation, it is chastening to have the paper dissected after what appears to be inadequate perusal, a feeling that is particularly common when a negative referee's report is received. Initial impressions count for a great deal and a badly written paper of excessive length creates a long-lasting negative impression long before its contents have been properly evaluated. A respected colleague should be able to identify such problems before the manuscript is submitted. Colleagues with knowledge of the literature will also be able to suggest the most appropriate journal for the paper, and this advice should be listened to very carefully.

There has been a major change in attitudes over the past 10 years towards choosing a journal. Authors are now asked to consider the 'impact factor' of the journal before making a submission. This factor, a measure of how many of the papers are cited in the literature in the 2 years after publication divided by the total number of papers published, has now become an accepted method of ranking the scientific importance of journals. This is generally but not universally applicable. Subjects that are important but are rarely studied are often cited much less than others that may have short-term attractions (e.g. a new drug) but in the long term disappear rapidly from the literature. So do not become too obsessed by impact factors; choose the journal that appears to be the best for your findings.

A checklist of important points that need close attention before a manuscript is submitted is given in Box 3.1. Some of these are self-evident and repetitious but need stressing over and over again. A good paper containing valuable information may often be rejected because it is not understandable or is presented clumsily. The converse, a poor paper that is presented well, is more likely to be published. Some of my more cynical colleagues have a motto that states, 'a determined author can get any rubbish published'. This is probably true, so if your paper is being rejected over and over again please ask yourself whether the presentation is at fault rather than the content.

Box 3.1 Points to check before submitting a manuscript to a journal

- **Length** Note the instructions to authors on length and make sure that you abide by these. It is often a good idea to give the word count on the first page (summary page) of the article even if this is not specifically requested by the editor.
- **Relevance** Ensure that all parts of the manuscript are linked in some way to the main aims and findings.
- **Summary/abstract** Again follow clearly the instructions to authors and note the format requested. This is especially important because often the abstract is the only part of the paper that will be quoted frequently. Hence ensure that the essentials are included there.
- **Format** Do not deviate from that given in the instructions to authors, even if you think the format spoils the paper. Under these circumstances you might be wise to submit to another journal.
- **References** Make sure that these are in the appropriate journal style and of the required number. Many journals now insist on a maximum of around 20 references. If this is the case, make sure you select the most appropriate ones.
- **Statistics** Observe the guidance on the presentation of statistics in the journal instructions. If statistical packages have been used it is advisable to reference them. Explain any unusual statistical tests and/or packages and the reasons for their use.
- **Duplication** Avoid repeating information in tables, figures and text. Look carefully for evidence of double publication if you have published previously. If in any doubt, send the other papers to the editor who will distribute them to the referees if they consider that it could constitute double publication.
- **Comprehension** Is the paper understandable? Ideally this can be assessed by giving it to someone who has no special knowledge of the subject but should still be able to understand the arguments.
- **Acknowledgements** Acknowledge those who deserve acknowledgement, usually those who have put themselves out in order to complete the research. Increasingly some journals are asking for the roles of each author to be defined. This is advisable to avoid 'gift authorship' (the attribution of authorship to someone who has played no part in the study but who may well write papers in which similar gift authorship is given).

When a manuscript has been through all its checks and revisions it is ready to be sent to the editor of the chosen journal, together with the required number of photocopies and signatures indicated in the instructions to authors. As part of the 'selling' task it is necessary to explain to the editor why you think your paper is suited to the journal. It is natural for all editors to feel that there is a particular reason for their journal being selected for submission and in most cases this will be true. If so, do not be shy about putting this into words, and if a little flattery creeps into the letter it will not do any harm. Although the editor relies on referees, they make the final decision about publication of the manuscript. If you have made an excellent case that the material in your paper would be out of place if published anywhere else, it may well sway the editor in your favour. It still surprises us (P.T. is Editor of the *British Journal of Psychiatry*) that authors often submit manuscripts with the barest minimum of accompanying information in the hope that their manuscript will somehow speak for itself. It may well do, but there is usually much to be gained by giving it a helping hand.

Very few papers (around 5%) are accepted by a peer-reviewed journal without revision. If you are asked to revise your paper, please do so as rapidly and as accurately as possible. Even if you feel all the referees' comments are wrong, biased, ignorant or ridiculous, please repeat to yourself the mantra 'the referee is the fount of all wisdom' before you angrily respond. It is important to do everything possible to please those referees, and the editor, in making your resubmission. This does not mean you cannot challenge some of the comments; if they run counter to an essential theme or understanding of your paper please explain why, but do it in an open-hearted and generous way. Always give an explanation of what changes have been made in your letter accompanying the revised manuscript.

It is very common for an editor to ask for a paper to be shortened, even though additional points raised by the reviewers may lead the author to expect a revised copy to be longer. Do not ignore such requests; most papers can be shortened successfully with effort. Recall Bernard Shaw's comment about a letter he had written: 'I am sorry this letter is so long; I did not have time to write a shorter one'. Also remember that some of the best papers are very short indeed. For example, Watson and Crick, writing in 1953, began a paper on an important topic quite modestly:

'we wish to suggest a structure for the salt of deoxyribose nucleic acid (D.N.A.). This structure has novel features which are of considerable biological interest.'

Less than 1000 words later their evidence was complete and one of the major biological mysteries of the 20th century had been solved. So do not feel a short paper is an inadequate one.

Sometimes it may be appropriate to appeal against a decision by a journal to reject your paper. Most appeals are unsuccessful, but if you feel that the referees or editor have completely failed to identify the important message of your paper this needs to be stated. This is particularly true with papers that are commonly described as 'ground-breakers', contributions that change perception across a whole area of research, when standard refereeing processes, which always have a tendency to become blinkered, fail to identify their significance. One, now well-known, researcher submitted her paper four times to the same journal arguing this case before the paper was accepted; it is now one of the most cited papers in the literature (Linehan *et al*, 1991). If you can make the case that other journals are not suitable for your paper this will also help appeal (although in this age of multiple journals this might be difficult).

After the paper has been accepted

The last stage of the publication process is the correction of proofs. These are important and should be checked very carefully. It is important to note that many journals employ copy-editors that will shorten or change sentences to produce a more telling effect (or to save space) and you must not alter this edited text back to your original. When checking the proofs please look carefully at the figures because any errors there will have a much greater impact than the odd word out of place in the text.

In the next few years researchers will hear a great deal about 'open access publication'. This follows the principle that any scientific work in the public arena should be accessible to all, not just the subscribers to a specialist journal. This is clearly desirable but there are many implications and much debate before it can be implemented fully. In particular it will lead to a system whereby authors will have to pay the publication costs (probably around £1500–£2000) once their papers are accepted for publication. Things are moving fast in this area, so please look carefully at comments in the major journals on this subject.

Finally, do not be tempted to brag about your paper too widely before it is published. Some journals impose a bar on any presentation of the results before publication, so please be careful not to say too much about your paper in advance. This does not mean that copies for restricted circulation cannot be sent to others who ask for details, but even here it is important to advise people not to publicise the results in advance of publication.

Some final pieces of advice are appropriate. Do not be afraid to go to others for help at any stage in the writing; do not be attracted by the idea of filling in gaps in your data with fictional data, as the exposure of fraud may lead to a permanent loss of career and reputation (Lock, 1995); and do not get disheartened by rejection. Regard rejection as part of the educational process of research, as it will come to everyone eventually and, although complete self-confidence in the quality of your work may seem to others to be delusional, it is very important in times of adversity to hold on to the beliefs that got you started on your research. Most good researchers are slightly egocentric; pioneers never have it easy for long.

References

Blackwell, B. & Shepherd, M. (1967) Early evaluation of psychotropic drugs in man. A trial that failed. *Lancet*, ii, 819–822.

Cook, C. C., Scannell, T. D. & Lipsedge, M. S. (1988) Another trial that failed. *Lancet*, i, 524–525.

Linehan, M. M., Armstrong, H. E., Suarez, A., *et al* (1991) Cognitive–behavioral treatment of chronically parasuicidal borderline patients. *Archives of General Psychiatry*, **48**, 1060–1064.

Lock, S. (1995). Lessons from the Pearce affair: handling scientific fraud. *BMJ*, 310, 1547.

Watson, J. D. & Crick, F. H. C. (1953). Molecular structure of nucleic acids. *Nature* 171, 737–738.

Part II

Different types of research

CHAPTER 4

Systematic reviews and meta-analysis

Matthew Hotopf

Most of this book is about primary research, which usually involves a researcher embarking on a new project where data are collected on project participants or patients. Primary research rarely tackles entirely new questions and should therefore be informed by what is already known about a topic. However, our knowledge of research that has gone before is often patchy. Secondary research, using systematic reviews, is the process by which all existing evidence is identified, summarised, synthesised and appraised. Its main function is to inform clinicians, researchers and patients on the best available evidence on a topic. A good systematic review is a useful exercise before embarking on new primary research, and some grant-giving bodies require evidence of systematic reviews before new research is funded.

In primary research there has been a long-understood need for using reproducible and unbiased methods. Until recently there has been little interest in applying the same principles to literature reviews. Narrative reviews – where an expert in the field summarises his or her knowledge – have been the norm and are still widespread. The process may involve some attempt to identify relevant primary research but may also make much of opinions based on clinical observation. There are times when such narrative reviews are entirely appropriate – opinions are not necessarily a bad thing and often allow the author and reader to clarify their thoughts and formulate hypotheses. However, most narrative reviews are presented as if they were unbiased, balanced descriptions of current knowledge, and there is sound evidence that this is far from the truth.

Rationale for performing systematic reviews

There are many reasons for performing systematic reviews (see Box 4.1). The need to distil a medical literature which continues to grow both in volume and complexity is obvious. However, the most compelling reason why reviews should be systematic is to avoid bias. Knipschild (1994) describes an elegant example centred on the widely held belief that vitamin

---

Box 4.1 Rationale for performing systematic reviews. Adapted from Mulrow (1994)

- To synthesise a massive medical literature
- To integrate critical pieces of biomedical information
- To use resources efficiently – primary research may not be required after systematic reviews have been performed
- To allow a better understanding of the generalisability of evidence
- To allow a better understanding of the consistency of relationships
- To explain data inconsistencies and conflicts in the data
- To increase power (via meta-analysis)
- To improve precision (via meta-analysis)
- To keep accurate and up to date.

C prevents the common cold, a view proposed by the Nobel Laureate Linus Pauling (1986), in his book *How to Live Longer and Feel Better*. Pauling performed a narrative review of around 30 trials of vitamin C and came to the firm conclusion that vitamin C was an effective means of preventing the common cold. However, he did not describe how he identified the trials he cited, most of which were 'positive' (i.e. finding an association between the consumption of vitamin C and the prevention of the common cold). Knipschild (1994) used an exhaustive literature search to identify 61 trials and found different results – most of the additional trials were negative and no benefit was found in those taking vitamin C. Thus the two reviews came to entirely different conclusions about the efficacy of vitamin C as a preventive agent against the common cold; this difference was a result of a number of negative studies which Pauling had failed to identify. This example demonstrates the potential for narrative reviews to be biased. It also demonstrates why many clinicians and researchers may be hostile to systematic reviews! By identifying the less visible research (which often consists of 'negative' studies), systematic reviews often give more conservative conclusions.

The reasons why narrative reviews tend to be biased are complex. It is probably rare for the reviewer consciously to discard good evidence that goes against their own views. It is more likely that they unconsciously pay greater attention to studies that support their views, in much the same way that observer bias may occur in primary research. Reviewers are also more likely simply to remember work which supports their ideas, and there is evidence that reviewers are more likely to cite studies that emanate from their own discipline and country (Joyce *et al*, 1998).

The past 20 years have seen an enormous expansion in our knowledge of the process of data synthesis. This has been a central component of evidence-

---

Box 4.2 Databases of the Cochrane Collaboration which are available via libraries and the internet (http://www.cochrane.org)

- The Cochrane Database of Systematic Reviews (CDSR), which is a database of all completed reviews and protocol reviews
- The Cochrane Controlled Trial Register (CCTR), which is a database of identified trials
- The Database of Abstracts of Reviews of Effectiveness (DARE), which is produced by the UK NHS Centre for Reviews and Dissemination
- The Cochrane Review Methodology Database, which is a database of research papers into the methodology of systematic reviews.

---

based medicine. The Cochrane Collaboration (http://www.cochrane.org) has been a key influence in this process (see Box 4.2). It is a non-profit-making organisation, with centres in Europe, Australasia and North and South America, which aims to assist researchers to perform systematic reviews and disseminate their results. The Collaboration also has review groups which focus on specific illnesses. In psychiatry these include the Schizophrenia Group and the Depression, Anxiety and Neurosis Group. Each group has several editors and one coordinating editor who assist researchers with new projects and ensure high-quality work. The Collaboration also produces software to assist meta-analysis and runs an annual conference, the International Cochrane Colloquium. The Database of Abstracts of Reviews of Effectiveness (DARE) is produced by the NHS Centre for Reviews and Dissemination, based in York, which as well as performing reviews, provides information on the methodology of systematic reviewing (http://www.york. ac.uk/inst/crd/). The QUOROM (Quality of Reporting of Meta-Analyses) group has collaborated to develop a set of guidelines for the reporting of systematic reviews. These guidelines are recommended reading for those embarking on such reviews (Moher *et al*, 1999).

Stages in performing systematic reviews

Formulating a question

As in primary research, the first step in performing systematic reviews is to formulate a question. Most systematic reviews have focused on treatment but any topic may be covered. It is just as legitimate to perform a systematic review to identify all prevalence studies of a condition as it is to review a specific medical treatment. However, the more nebulous the question, the more difficult systematic reviews are to perform – questions about specific diagnostic entities or treatments are much easier to answer. For the same reason, it is easier to perform systematic reviews on a single type of study. Probably the best known and most widely disseminated systematic reviews are those performed by the Cochrane Collaboration, which specifically address treatments and only include data from randomised controlled trials.

Developing a search strategy.

Over the past 20 years information has become more easily and widely available to doctors. Most doctors in the UK have access to a personal computer and most personal computers have access to search engines such as Medline or PsychInfo. Sources of information for systematic reviews are shown in Box 4.3.

The published literature should be easy to identify, but even sophisticated electronic databases have their problems. It was discovered from hand searches of major journals that even in the hands of expert literature searchers, a high proportion of trials would have been missed using electronic databases alone (Adams *et al*, 1994). The situation has gradually improved for randomised trials (McDonald *et al*, 1996) but there are potentially serious difficulties in identifying observational studies. It is also crucial that the searcher has a good understanding of the use of Medical Subject Headings (MeSH; Lowe & Barnett, 1994) in databases such as Medline. These constitute a controlled vocabulary used for indexing articles for Medline and provides a consistent means of retrieving information that may use different terminology for the same concepts. For example, apparently synonymous terms (DEPRESSION/ DEPRESSIVE DISORDER) have different meanings in Medline. However, there are many traps for the unwary or inexperienced searcher.

Electronic searches require skill and knowledge of the individual database. Searchers should develop a 'profile' of the type of studies they aim to identify in their searches, and these should mirror the inclusion and exclusion

---

Box 4.3   Sources of information for systematic reviews

- Electronic search engines (Medline, Bids, Cinahl, Cancerlit, PsychInfo)
- Cochrane Collaboration
- Previous systematic reviews, narrative reviews, textbooks, book chapters
- Hand searches of relevant journals
- References of references, and references of references of references
- Contact with known experts
- University libraries for 'grey literature'
- Pharmaceutical companies
- Government and non-government organisations
- The internet.

criteria to be used. It is worth considering the nature of an ideal target study – can it be identified by a specific disease, population, outcome, treatment, risk factor or study design? For each aspect of the target studies there may be many different possible search terms. Searching electronic databases for target studies is similar to screening populations for target illnesses: the searcher has to make a decision on how inclusive the search is to be. This has been called 'recall', where:

$$\text{Recall} \; = \; \frac{\text{Number of relevant citations retrieved}}{\text{Number of relevant citations in database}}$$

Recall is the equivalent of sensitivity in case-finding or screening studies and describes how many studies that might have been of interest were missed. Recall must be balanced against the possibility of identifying many 'false-positive' or irrelevant studies. This is referred to as precision, where:

$$\text{Precision} \; = \; \frac{\text{Number of relevant citations retrieved}}{\text{Total number of citations retrieved}}$$

Precision is the equivalent of specificity and reflects the degree to which the search turns up irrelevant studies. There is a play-off between recall and precision, and for the purposes of systematic reviews it is necessary to sacrifice precision for the sake of recall. We want our search strategies to identify all papers of possible interest, even though they may turn up hundreds of papers that are excluded.

Electronic literature searching is an iterative process whereby early results of the search are assessed and the search altered to either include or exclude further studies. The early searches may uncover many irrelevant studies and it may be possible to refine the search by adding a term that would automatically exclude such studies.

Hand searches are an important part of the literature searching required for systematic reviews. The rationale for hand-searching is that electronic searches may miss relevant studies even with skilled searchers (Adams *et al*, 1994). McManus *et al* (1998) found in a review that ultimately identified 135 eligible papers that hand-searching identified 31 unique papers, indicating that it was almost as important a source of papers as electronic searching, which identified 50 unique papers. The discovery that electronic searches may miss relevant papers led to the Cochrane Collaboration embarking on the Herculean task of identifying all randomised controlled trials in the medical literature. This task is ongoing, with over 14 000 citations already identified by the Depression, Anxiety and Neurosis Group alone. Although the efforts of the Cochrane Collaboration will make systematic reviews of randomised controlled trials easier to perform, hand-searching may still be necessary to ensure that the review is up to date. Hand-searching will also remain an important component of systematic reviews of observational studies.

Once some references have been identified, it is important to check their reference lists, as this may be a rich source of further studies and this process can be repeated through one or more iterations. An additional method is to contact experts in the field, and there is evidence that this can uncover further unique references which would not have been detected elsewhere (McManus *et al*, 1998).

Identifying published research is one thing, but identifying unpublished work, or work in the 'grey literature' (university theses, reports, etc), is even more complex and difficult. The main reason why unpublished work should be included is to avoid publication bias (see below). For pharmacological trials, one obvious source of unpublished work is the pharmaceutical companies that manufacture the compound. A recent systematic review was able to examine such data (Bech *et al*, 2000). It is therefore worth approaching organisations that might hold unpublished data and asking for access to this.

Developing inclusion and exclusion criteria

As in primary research, systematic reviews must focus on specific questions and the the primary research studies identified must be screened for suitability prior to inclusion. Developing inclusion and exclusion criteria is a vital part of this process. It is here that the advantages of focused research questions become obvious. After completing an exhaustive search, the reviewer may have several thousand potential references. Inclusion and exclusion criteria may be based on a number of different aspects of the study (see Box 4.4).

Study design

Most systematic reviews of treatments concentrate on randomised controlled trials, but in situations where there is very limited evidence, or where the treatment is not readily studied by a randomised controlled trial, it might be necessary or desirable to include non-experimental designs. When the question addressed is a specific one about aetiology, it might be reasonable to limit the studies included to case–control and cohort studies. Similarly,

---

Box 4.4 Aspects of studies to consider in devising inclusion/exclusion criteria

- Study design
- Population studied
- Treatments studied
- Outcomes assessed
- Risk factors studied.

systematic reviews can be performed on studies assessing prevalence (Hotopf *et al*, 2001; Fazel & Danesh, 2002), prognosis (Joyce *et al*, 1997; Altman, 2001) or screening (Deeks, 2001). In a review of the use of the Mental Health Act 1983 (Wall *et al*, 1999), we included a very wide range of studies, including randomised trials, cohort studies, case–control studies, cross-sectional studies, case reports, qualitative studies, and a range of opinion and polemic. In such situations it is necessary to consider the aims of the review and reflect them in the inclusion and exclusion criteria. Too rich a mix of information might make the review difficult to interpret.

The population studied

Primary research can include studies of disparate populations. For example, there are trials of antidepressants in children, adults and older adults. A reviewer might want to restrict the studies included to specific age-groups. Diagnostic groups are also important to consider – and reviewers have to decide whether to be 'splitters' or 'lumpers' – when deciding to restrict their review to narrow DSM categories or whether to reflect reality by taking a broader perspective.

Treatments studied

The choice of inclusion and exclusion criteria for studies of treatments should be obvious, but as randomised controlled trials accumulate, the reviewer is forced to be more explicit. There are now many systematic reviews comparing selective serotonin reuptake inhibitors (SSRIs) and tricyclics, and although there is substantial overlap, there are also differences in how SSRIs and tricyclics have been defined. 'Splitters' and 'lumpers' are likely to have different approaches when choosing the focus of their reviews – 'splitters' may focus on single drugs, whereas 'lumpers' may focus on whole classes of drugs (such as SSRIs), or even large groups (such as all antidepressants). Reviewers sometimes limit their studies to those that used drugs in dosages they believe are acceptable (Anderson & Tomenson, 1995). For psychotherapy trials, and trials into health service interventions, the definition of which treatment to include is even more complex. First, broadly similar approaches may be given a range of different names. Second, treatments may differ according to duration and frequency (the 'dose') but also according to the expertise of the therapist and how reproducible their interventions were.

Outcomes assessed

There are many potential outcomes of research. For example, in an ongoing systematic review assessing the prevalence of depression in patients with advanced cancer, we have identified over 40 studies that have used 13 different measures of depression, including single-item questions, questionnaires, and semi-structured or structured interviews generating DSM or ICD diagnoses. This range of outcomes may confuse readers, and it is sometimes necessary to restrict which outcomes are used. A systematic review (Thornley & Adams, 1998) of randomised trials in schizophrenia indicated that in 2000 studies, 640 different outcome measures had been used! These covered aspects of psychopathology, quality of life, service use, side-effects of treatment and so on. Good systematic reviews, like good randomised trials, should set out with a specific outcome of interest. When many alternative outcomes are available these can be presented as secondary analyses.

Risk factors studied

Reviews on aetiology may vary in terms of how the risk factor is defined. For example, obstetric complications may be defined in many different ways. The rates of complications may then differ markedly according to the measure used. The reviewer has to decide whether to exclude studies that fail to use validated measures. One solution may be to classify studies according to the way in which risk factors are defined and give more weight to studies that use validated measures.

Extracting data from studies

The extraction of data usually requires a pro forma which will capture the main points of interest in the individual study. As for data collection in primary research, it is often difficult to predict the scope of the information that will be required and pilot studies can be invaluable. Data may come in many different forms. Outcomes may be continuous, categorical or both. In trials involving people with depression it is common for outcome to be expressed both in binary form (remission/no remission) and as a mean score on a depression rating scale. When extracting data from studies, standard deviations should be noted as well as means, as these are necessary for meta-analysis of continuous outcomes.

The extraction of data is not always straightforward. In randomised trials it is common for results to be reported only for the participants who completed the trial, with dropouts ignored – this may cause bias (for example if one treatment is better tolerated than another). In order to avoid such problems it is good practice for the extraction of data to be performed by two independent reviewers. If there are disagreements between the reviewers, these can usually be resolved in consensus meetings. Data of interest to the reviewer are frequently missing from reports of randomised controlled trials. Under these circumstances the reviewer should contact the author of the original paper for further information. This may be impractical if the paper was published a long time ago.

Critical appraisal of studies

It is important to critically appraise studies once they have been identified and their results extracted (Hotopf *et al*, 1997). There are a number of rating scales available to assist the researcher to identify problems with randomised controlled trials or observational studies. Jüni *et al* (2001) have demonstrated that inadequate randomisation (in particular failure to generate allocation sequences randomly and failure to conceal allocation) and lack of masking each cause powerful biases. These biases tend to work in the direction of the active or new treatment. Many different quality rating scales are available and there is relatively poor agreement between them, as they place different emphasis on various aspects of study design and reporting (Jüni *et al*, 1999).

Summarising and synthesising data

Systematic reviews aim to distil complex information into a simpler form. This can be done statistically using meta-analysis. However, there are times when meta-analysis is not possible or desirable and the summary might then simply be a table, or series of tables, describing the studies that were included. When it is not possible to perform a meta-analysis, it can still be informative to arrange data so that median values for outcomes and their interquartile ranges can be determined.

Meta-analysis

Precision and power

Meta-analysis is the mathematical synthesis of data from several different studies. The main reason for performing meta-analysis is to improve the power and precision of individual studies. Many widely used treatments have been inadequately studied and one of the commonest problems is that trials tend to be too small. In our work on SSRIs and tricyclics, we found that a high proportion of trials were inadequately powered to detect very significant differences in treatment effect (Hotopf *et al*, 1997). Assuming that 60% of patients treated with a tricyclic improve within 6 weeks and that one wanted to detect a difference of 30% (i.e. SSRIs led to improvement in 90% of patients), over half the trials would have been unable to detect such a difference at 80% power and 95% confidence. A similar proportion of randomised controlled trials for schizophrenia have been found to be underpowered (Thornley & Adams, 1998). Meta-analysis aims to improve precision and power by taking the results from these small studies and combining them in a single analysis.

This section will mainly concentrate on meta-analysis of the results of randomised controlled trials. Although it is possible to use meta-analysis for observational data, there are theoretical reasons why this approach should be used cautiously. The main problem is that non-randomised studies are prone to selection bias and confounding, which randomisation should theoretically abolish. The effect of using randomisation for obervational studies may be to produce a more precise estimate of a biased parameter (Egger *et al*, 1998).

The statistics of meta-analysis

In meta-analysis, data from several studies are pooled in order to produce a single estimate of effect with 95% confidence intervals. This is done by weighting each study according to its sample size. The detailed statistics of meta-analysis are beyond the scope of this chapter, but there are a few principles that are worth considering.

The nature of the data

Data from randomised controlled trials are usually either binary (e.g. recovered/not recovered) or continuous (e.g. a score on a questionnaire). Software for meta-analysis can cope with either form of data. The minimum requirement for the analysis of binary data is to know the number of participants randomised to each treatment and the number with each outcome. Although this sounds straightforward, many randomised controlled trials do not use intention-to-treat analyses and it is often difficult to account for all the individuals randomised. Where follow-up is incomplete, the reviewer may make an arbitrary decision to assume that those who failed to complete the trial failed to recover. If data are continuous, the minimum information required for analysis is the final scores on the outcome measure with standard deviations. Again it is common for trials to report 'completer' analyses which ignore those who drop out from treatment, and the reviewer may not be able to determine what the values of a proper intention-to-treat analysis would have been.

Dichotomous variables

For dichotomous data the main output from the meta-analysis will be a risk ratio, or odds ratio, with 95% confidence intervals. Box 4.5 shows the calculation of risk ratios and odds ratios for data from a trial of antidepressants in which 100 patients were given treatment and outcome (remission of depression) was compared with 100 patients given placebo. In this example the odds ratio is considerably smaller than the risk ratio. Unless the outcome is very rare (in which case the odds ratio and risk ratio are similar), the odds ratio will always have a more extreme value than the risk ratio.

In a meta-analysis the computer program first calculates individual odds ratios or risk ratios for each component study and then summarises them as a single parameter, which is weighted for the size of the study. The risk difference is an additional parameter which gives an absolute, rather than a relative, marker of the difference between two treatments. The inverse of the risk difference is the number needed to treat, which indicates the number of individuals who would need to be treated to realise one good outcome that could be attributed to the treatment.

Continuous outcomes

Many outcomes in psychiatry and psychology are continuous. Continuous data provide more information than dichotomous outcomes but are often

Box 4.5 Calculation of risk ratios, odds ratios and risk difference for data from a trial in which 100 patients were given treatment and their outcome (remission of depression in 80 patients) was compared with that of 100 patients given placebo (remission in 30 patients)

- Risk of remission on treatment = 80/100 = 0.8
- Risk of remission on placebo = 30/100 = 0.3
- Risk ratio = 0.3/0.8 = 0.38
- Odds of remission on treatment = 80/20 = 4
- Odds of remission on placebo = 30/70 = 0.43
- Odds ratio = 0.43/4 = 0.11
- Risk difference = 0.5
- Number needed to treat = 1/risk difference = 1/0.5 = 2

harder to interpret. Meta-analysis is based on combining mean scores from several studies and it is therefore important that the data from the individual studies are not skewed. When data are skewed (which is often indicated by a standard deviation that is larger than the mean), it may be necessary to transform them (for example by working on a log scale). Alternatively the data can be dichotomised – that is, converted into a binary variable.

Assuming that the data are not skewed, there are two main methods for data synthesis of continuous data. The first applies only if the same scale for measurement of outcome has been used in many different studies. In this case the differences between the mean of each group can be pooled, giving a parameter called the weighted mean difference. This is simply the pooled average difference for all the studies using that scale. The second method applies to situations where several different scales have been used to measure the same outcome – as might happen with different questionnaires for depression (Box 4.6). In this case the standardised mean difference (SMD) is calculated for each study. This is the difference between means divided by the pooled standard deviation of participants' outcomes across the whole trial. The SMDs are then pooled statistically. It is difficult

Box 4.6 Meta-analysis of continuous data for trials using different scales to measure the same outcome

- Calculate means and standard deviations for treatment and control groups separately
- Calculate the standardised mean difference for each trial by dividing the difference in means by the pooled standard deviation for all participants' outcomes across the whole trial
- Pool the standardised mean differences for all trials.

to interpret an SMD on its own but it is possible to back-transform it to a familiar scale.

Fixed- and random-effects models

Meta-analysis can be performed with different underlying assumptions about the variability of the underlying effect. In fixed-effects models, there is an assumption that the studies all describe a similar underlying effect, and therefore only within-study variation is thought to influence the uncertainty of results. Random-effects models make no such assumption and allow for variation in the effects among the populations studied. Random-effects models are appropriate if there is significant heterogeneity (see below) among individual studies. Fixed-effects models produce somewhat narrower confidence intervals. Random-effects models give slightly more weight to smaller studies (because there will usually be more variation in effect sizes among smaller studies). Random-effects models may be more susceptible to publication bias.

Heterogeneity

There may be major differences in the effects of treatments or risk factors among the different populations in these studies. Alternatively, a reviewer may assume that a broad collection of treatments have the same underlying effect, whereas in fact they vary. This leads to heterogeneity in the results of the meta-analysis. Heterogeneity can be expressed in several ways but the simplest is to look at the visual output of the meta-analysis. If there is heterogeneity, then the trials appear to be widely spread around the centre. Statistical packages produce formal statistics for heterogeneity and if these show statistically significant heterogeneity, it is sensible to perform sensitivity analyses to investigate possible causes (Thompson, 1994). These may include different treatments used, different populations studied and differences in the underlying risk of the outcome (Thompson *et al*, 1997).

Problems in meta-analysis

Meta-analysis has its detractors (Eysenck, 1994; Feinstein, 1995) and in some circumstances has produced misleading results (Villar *et al*, 1995; DerSimonian & Levine, 1999). It is important to recognise the potential sources of bias, which are described below.

Publication bias

The most serious potential problem with meta-analysis occurs when the systematic review is incomplete. The most common reason for this is publication bias. It is widely recognised that 'negative' studies are less likely to be published than 'positive' ones. A follow-up study of ethics committee applications found that the most important predictor of research that had been approved by the committee not being published was a 'negative' result (Dickersin *et al*, 1992). This 'desk drawer' problem (where the negative study sits in the researcher's desk drawer, never to see the light of day) has the net effect of biasing the results in favour of the experimental treatment. One example of publication bias leading to a misleading finding was the use of magnesium in the management of acute myocardial infarction (Woods, 1995; Yusuf & Flather, 1995). A number of small- and medium-sized trials had indicated that this was an effective treatment and a meta-analysis confirmed this. However, a subsequent 'mega-trial' found no beneficial effect of magnesium. Similarly, a systematic review of St John's Wort for mild-to-moderate depression found that it was effective when compared with placebo (Linde *et al*, 1996), but a single, well-conducted large randomised trial failed to find such an effect (Hypericum Depression Trial Study Group, 2002). Such conflict between large well-conducted trials and meta-analyses are a cause for concern. Although systematic reviews and meta-analyses are sometimes considered the most rigourous of research methods, most clinical trialists would argue that a well-conducted definitive trial is more compelling than a meta-analysis, particularly because of the problem of publication bias. An assessment of publication bias in the Cochrane database suggested that it was a factor in 50% of meta-analyses and probably led to a misleading result in 10% (Sutton *et al*, 2000).

How can publication bias be detected? An elegant solution was proposed by Egger *et al* (1997*a*). The funnel plot (see Fig. 4.1) makes a simple assumption – large studies will be far less susceptible to publication bias than small ones. Researchers who have gone to the effort of randomising

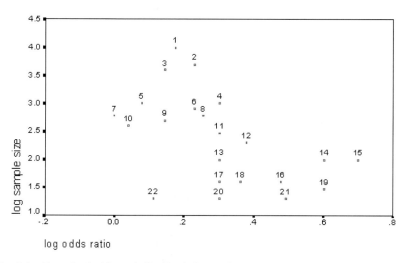

Fig. 4.1 Hypothetical funnel plot. Each data point represents an individual randomised trial. Trial 1 is the largest and estimates the odds ratio of a good outcome to be 1.5. Trials 2–10 are large and are evenly scattered around this value. Trials 11–22 are much smaller and are more scattered around larger effect sizes. There is an area in the lower left quadrant with only one trial (22). This represents possible publication bias, indicating that smaller 'negative' trials are less likely to be published.

hundreds of patients are unlikely to suppress their findings even if they are negative. In contrast, small trials may well be difficult to publish, especially if negative. If the effect size is plotted on a log scale against the sample size, one would expect a symmetrical pattern of studies with more spread in effect size for smaller studies. If a high number of small negative trials have remained unpublished, the funnel plot will no longer be symmetrical. There are now a number of formal statistical tests for assessment of asymmetry of the funnel plot (Sterne *et al*, 2001), but the visual assessment of data gives a good indication of the likelihood of publication bias.

There have been efforts to avoid publication bias in the medical literature. There has recently been an initiative offering investigators the opportunity to register unpublished randomised controlled trials. The Cochrane Collaboration also has a register of all new randomised trials.

Duplicate studies

Another form of bias occurs if the same results are published more than once. Dual publication is frowned upon but none the less happens. There are sometimes legitimate reasons why the results of a trial may be published more than once – investigators sometimes want to publish more-detailed analyses of specific outcomes separately from the main findings. However, it is not uncommon for investigators in a multicentre trial to publish the results of individual centres separately, in addition to the more orthodox report of the entire trial. Dual publication may be difficult to detect but often has important implications, as it tends to occur more for 'positive' results. In a systematic review of the anti-emetic ondansetron (Tramer *et al*, 1997), 28% of the data were duplicated and duplicated studies were more likely to favour the treatment. If the reviewer is not aware of this possibility, the result produced will tend to exaggerate the benefit of the new treatment. It is therefore important to consider the possibility of dual publication if two papers seem to include the same authors, using the same treatments on a similar population of patients.

Language bias

Finally, language bias may affect systematic reviews and meta-analyses. There is no evidence that papers published in foreign-language journals are inferior to those published in English-language journals (Moher *et al*, 1996). Researchers should take care to include studies from non-English-language journals. Because of American hegemony in the scientific world, English-language journals are frequently considered more prestigious by non-English-speaking researchers, who may be more inclined to publish their more 'positive' studies in English, leaving negative studies untranslated. There is evidence of such biases – one study (Egger *et al*, 1997*b*) showed that for research from German groups, 'positive' trials were nearly four times more likely to be published in English than 'negative' ones. This has a similar overall effect to publication bias – if only studies published in English are included, the review is likely to be biased in favour of the intervention.

Conclusions

Systematic reviews provide a method by which an often complex and confusing medical literature can be identified and summarised in a reproducible way. Meta-analysis provides a means of summarising these results statistically. Although meta-analysis has its detractors, and can suffer from publication bias, it is hard to argue against the importance of reproducible, unbiased systematic reviews. One of the main functions of systematic reviews is to inform us definitively of what we do not yet know – and as such they are a useful springboard into future research. They also sometimes tell us that enough is known about a topic for further research to be unnecessary.

References

Adams, C. E., Power, A., Frederick, K., *et al* (1994) An investigation of the adequacy of MEDLINE searches for randomized controlled trials (RCTs) of the effects of mental health care. *Psychological Medicine*, **24**, 741–748.

Altman, D. G. (2001) Systematic reviews in health care: Systematic reviews of evaluations of prognostic variables. *BMJ*, **323**, 224–228.

Anderson, I. M. & Tomenson, B. M. (1995) Treatment discontinuation with selective serotonin reuptake inhibitors compared with tricyclic antidepressants: a meta-analysis. *BMJ*, **310**, 1433–1438.

Bech, P., Cialdella, P., Haugh, M. C., *et al* (2000) Meta-analysis of randomised controlled trials of fluoxetine *v.* placebo and tricyclic antidepressants in the short-term treatment of major depression. *British Journal of Psychiatry*, **176**, 421–428.

Deeks, J. J. (2001) Systematic reviews in health care: Systematic reviews of evaluations of diagnostic and screening tests. *BMJ*, **323**, 157–162.

DerSimonian, R. & Levine, R. J. (1999) Resolving discrepancies betweeen meta-analysis and subsequent large controlled trials. *JAMA*, **282**, 664–670.

Dickersin, K., Min, Y. I. & Meinert, C. L. (1992) Factors influencing the publication of research results. Follow-up of applications submitted to two institutional review boards. *JAMA*, **267**, 374–378.

Egger, M., Davey Smith, G., Schneider, M., *et al* (1997*a*) Bias in meta-analysis detected by a simple, graphical test. *BMJ*, **315**, 629–634.

Egger, M., Zellweger-Zähner, T., Schneider, M., *et al* (1997*b*) Language bias in randomised controlled trials published in English and German. *Lancet*, **350**, 326–329.

Egger, M., Schneider, M. & Davey Smith, G. (1998) Spurious precision? Meta-analysis of observational studies. *BMJ*, **316**, 140–144.

Eysenck, H. J. (1994) Meta-analysis and its problems. *BMJ*, **309**, 789–792.

Fazel, S. & Danesh J. (2002) Serious mental disorder in 23000 prisoners: a systematic review of 62 surveys. *Lancet*, **359**, 545–550.

Feinstein, A. R. (1995) Meta-analysis: statistical alchemy for the 21st century. *Journal of Clinical Epidemiology*, **48**, 71–79.

Hotopf, M., Lewis, G. & Normand, C. (1997) Putting trials on trial: the costs and consequences of small trials in depression: a systematic review of methodology. *Journal of Epidemiology and Community Health*, **51**, 354–358.

Hotopf, M., Ly, K. L., Chidey, J., *et al* (2001) Depression in advanced disease – a systematic review. 1. Prevalence and case finding. *Palliative Medicine*, **16**, 81–97.

Hypericum Depression Trial Study Group (2002) Effect of *Hypericum perforatum* (St John's Wort) in major depressive disorder: a randomized controlled trial. *JAMA*, **287**, 1807 –1814.

Joyce, J., Hotopf, M. & Wessely, S. (1997) The prognosis of chronic fatigue and chronic fatigue syndrome: a systematic review. *QJM*, **90**, 223–233.

Joyce, J., Rabe-Hesketh, S. & Wessely, S. (1998) Reviewing the reviews: the example of chronic fatigue syndrome. *JAMA*, **280**, 264–266.

Jüni, P., Witschi, A., Bloch, R., *et al* (1999) The hazards of scoring the quality of clinical trials for meta-analysis. *JAMA*, **282**, 1054–1060.

Jüni, P., Altman, D. G. & Egger, M (2001) Systematic reviews in health care: assessing the quality of controlled clinical trials. *BMJ*, **323**, 42–46.

Knipschild, P. (1994) Systematic reviews: some examples. *BMJ*, **309**, 719–721.

Linde, K., Ramirez, G., Mulrow, C. D., *et al* (1996) St John's wort for depression: an overview and meta-analysis of randomised clinical trials. *BMJ*, **313**, 253–258.

Lowe, H. J. & Barnett, G. O. (1994) Understanding and using the Medical Subject Headings (MeSH) vocabulary to perform literature searches. *JAMA*, **271**, 1103–1108.

McDonald, S. J., Lefebvre, C. & Clarke, M. J. (1996) Identifying reports of controlled trials in the *BMJ* and the *Lancet*. *BMJ*, **313**, 1116–1117.

McManus, R. J., Wilson, S., Delaney, B. C., *et al* (1998) Review of the usefulness of contacting other experts when conducting a literature serach for systematic reviews. *BMJ*, **317**, 1562–1563.

Moher, D., Fortin, P., Jadad, A. R., *et al* (1996) Completeness of reporting of trials published in languages other than English: implications for conduct and reporting of systematic reviews. *Lancet*, **347**, 363–366.

Moher, D., Cook, D. J., Eastwood, S., *et al* (1999) Improving the quality of reports of meta-analyses of randomised controlled trials: the QUOROM statement. *Lancet*, **354**, 1896–1900.

Mulrow, C. D. (1994) Systematic reviews: rationale for systematic reviews. *BMJ*, **309**, 597–599.

Pauling, L. (1986) *How to Live Longer and Feel Better*. New York: Freeman.

Sterne, J. A. C., Egger, M. & Smith, G. D. (2001) Systematic reviews in health care: investigating and dealing with publication and other biases in meta-analysis. *BMJ*, **323**, 101–105.

Sutton, A. J., Duval, S. J., Tweedie, R. L., *et al* (2000) Empirical assessment of effect of publication bias on meta-analyses. *BMJ*, **320**, 1574–1577.

Thompson, S. G. (1994) Why sources of heterogeneity in meta-analysis should be investigated. *BMJ*, **309**, 1351–1355.

Thompson, S. G., Smith, T. C. & Sharp, S. J. (1997) Investigating underlying risk as a source of heterogeneity in meta-analysis. *Statistics in Medicine*, **16**, 2741–2758.

Thornley, B. & Adams, C. (1998) Content and quality of 2000 controlled trials in schizophrenia over 50 years. *BMJ*, **317**, 1181–1184.

Tramér, M. R., Reynolds, D. J., Moore, R. A., *et al* (1997) Impact of covert duplicate publication on meta-analysis: a case study. *BMJ*, **315**, 635–640.

Villar, J., Carroli, G. & Belizan, J. M. (1995) Predictive ability of meta-analyses of randomised controlled trials. *Lancet*, **345**, 772–776.

Wall, S., Buchanan, A., Fahy, T., *et al* (1999) *A Systematic Review of Data Pertaining to the Mental Health Act (1983)*. London: Department of Health.

Woods, K. L. (1995) Mega-trials and management of acute myocardial infarction. *Lancet*, **346**, 611–614.

Yusuf, S. & Flather, M. (1995) Magnesium in acute myocardial infarction. *BMJ*, **310**, 751–752.

CHAPTER 5

Epidemiology

Mike Crawford

The term epidemiology is derived from two Greek words *epi* – meaning upon or among – and *demos* – meaning the people. Epidemiology is the study of illness and health-related problems among groups of people. It is a quantitative approach to understanding the frequency, distribution and determinants of illnesses and the effects of interventions aimed at reducing their occurrence, ameliorating their effects and improving health.

Epidemiological methods underpin most clinical research including:

- descriptive studies examining how common health-related problems are
- analytical studies which seek to identify factors that give rise to illnesses
- experimental studies such as clinical trials which examine the effectiveness of interventions aimed at improving health.

Because epidemiological studies investigate the health of populations they have the potential to improve public health. This potential can be illustrated by studies conducted over the past 50 years which have tracked a rise in the number of people dying from lung cancer, identified smoking as an important risk factor for lung cancer and demonstrated reductions in death rates from lung cancer in places where public health measures have been taken to reduce smoking (Doll & Hill, 1950; Tyczynski *et al*, 2003).

Attempts to study the health of populations face several potential challenges which need to be considered when planning an epidemiological study or critically appraising a paper based on a completed project. Three of the most important factors are:

- validity – the need to ensure that findings offer a true reflection of reality rather then an artefact resulting from the way a study was conducted
- precision – the need to ensure that the study findings are not simply the result of chance
- generalisability – the need to obtain results which are applicable to the population as a whole, and not just the sample of people who were involved in the study.

Although these factors complicate all epidemiological studies, those in the field of psychiatry have to overcome additional challenges because of the difficulty of reliably measuring mental states and quantifying risk factors for mental disorders. Most forms of illness encountered in a general medical setting can be divided into communicable and non-communicable diseases. The former are strongly associated with the presence or absence of infectious agents and the latter are generally associated with reliable pathological indices. In contrast, most mental disorders do not have reliable biological correlates and deciding whether someone has a mental health problem generally relies on clinical judgement. Measuring risk factors for illnesses is never easy but in psychiatry, factors that may be important in the aetiology of mental distress, such as the level of social support or experiences of adversity or loss, are particularly hard to measure (see Chapters 10 and 11).

The application of epidemiological methods

Epidemiological methods can be used to address a range of important clinical questions concerning health-related problems – which are usually referred to as *outcomes* – and potential risk and protective factors – referred to as *exposures*. Risk factors for health problems may be *proximal* (near to) or *distal* (far from) the onset of a disorder. Although proximal factors are often easier to measure, distal risk factors, particularly those that influence social and environmental conditions, may have a greater impact on public health (McMichael, 1999). Epidemiological studies usually involve obtaining information from a *sample* of participants who take part in a project and using these data to make judgements about the whole *population* that the study sample comes from. Epidemiological research is based on the assumption that it is possible to learn about health problems in whole populations by studying samples of people derived from these populations.

Three types of question that epidemiological studies often try to answer are described below.

How common is a health-related problem?

An important starting point for determining the importance of a health problem is to work out its frequency. Measures of the frequency of an outcome require information about the number of people with the illness or disorder (the numerator) as a proportion all the people in the study (the denominator). There are two main measures of the frequency of an outcome – prevalence and incidence (Box 5.1).

In order to calculate the number of new cases of an illness in a population it is important that all those included are disease free at the start of a study. The incidence *risk* is a simple measure reflecting the number of new cases of the disorder divided by the number of people in the sample being studied. The incidence *rate* is calculated by dividing the number of new cases of the

---

Box 5.1 Measures of the frequency of a health-related problem within a population

Prevalence – the proportion of people in a defined population who have an outcome at a defined point in time i.e. existing cases;

Incidence – a measure of the number of new cases of an illness in a defined illness-free population over a defined period of time.

---

disorder by the amount of 'person-time at risk'. The person-time at risk differs from the total population because it takes account of the fact that once someone has become unwell they are no longer able to become a new 'case'. If the incidence is low, then the risk and rate will be almost the same, but if the incidence is high, the rate will provide a more accurate estimate of the likelihood of a person developing the illness.

Information on the frequency of a health problem can come either from a survey, in which data are collected from specific groups of people, or from ongoing systems for surveillance whereby the number of people making contact with healthcare services or dying from a particular health-related problem are monitored over time in a particular area or country. The validity of data on changes in the frequency of an illness or disorder depends on the comparability of data collected in different areas or at different time periods. Changes in the definition or diagnosis of a disorder can lead to apparent differences in its incidence that do not in fact exist.

Changes in the prevalence of a condition do not necessarily mean that the incidence of a condition is increasing. Prevalence will also increase if the population changes and new people who already have the disorder enter the area. Prevalence will also increase if treatments mean that people with a particular disorder live longer. For instance, the prevalence of some cancers are increasing, not because the incidence is rising but because interventions are prolonging the life expectancy of people with these disorders.

What are the important risk and protective factors for a particular disorder?

Having determined the frequency of a disorder, it is important to try to identify factors that may give rise to it. A first stage in this process is to examine differences in the frequency of a disorder in different populations or among individuals in the same population who are exposed to different factors.

Differences in prevalence or incidence among people who are exposed and not exposed to a potential risk factor can be calculated by simply subtracting one from the other to derive a prevalence or rate difference. Alternatively differences can be expressed in terms of a ratio, which provides a measure of the relative risk of a disorder among people who are and are not exposed to a potential risk factor. As part of a national cross-sectional survey of the mental health of people in Britain, Jenkins *et al* (1998) examined the relative prevalence of neurosis among those who are unemployed compared with those who are employed. The prevalence among the employed was 11.8% compared with 25.9% among the unemployed. The difference in prevalence was therefore 14.1% and the prevalence ratio for unemployment was 259/118 = 2.19. In other words people who were unemployed were more than twice as likely to have neurosis. A prevalence ratio below 1.0 indicates that the outcome is less common in the exposed group.

In order to calculate a prevalence or rate ratio, information about the frequency of an outcome from a sample of the general population is required. In case–control studies (see below) such data are not available. Instead information on level of exposure is collected from those with a disorder and a control sample of people selected on the basis of not having the disorder. However, an estimate of the relative importance of the exposure factor can still be obtained by calculating an odds ratio.

The odds of a condition is the number of people who have a disease divided by the number who do not at a particular point in time:

$$\text{Odds ratio} = \frac{\text{Odds of the outcome in the exposed group}}{\text{Odds of outcome in the non-exposed group}}$$

In a study examining risk factors for neuroleptic malignant syndrome (NMS) among people admitted to psychiatric units Sachdev *et al* (1997) compared hospital records of 25 people who had developed NMS over a 5-year period with those of 50 matched controls. Because they did not have detailed data on all people admitted to hospital during this period they could not calculate the rate ratio for NMS among people with different risk factors. However, they were able to compare the prevalence of potential risk factors among people with NMS and controls and found that 6 of the 25 who had NMS were dehydrated at the time they were given antipsychotics compared with 4 of the controls. The odds ratio for dehydration was therefore:

$$\frac{6/19}{4/46} = \frac{0.32}{0.087} = 3.68$$

For rare conditions the odds ratio and the rate ratio will be similar. Hence data from case–control studies of rare disorders can still be used to estimate rate ratios for different exposures.

Although rate ratios and odds ratios provide a sound basis for estimating the likelihood of a disorder in exposed and non-exposed individuals, they do not provide information about the relative importance of exposures for public health. This is because the impact of an exposure on a population depends not only on the relative risk of the exposure but also on how prevalent it is within a given population. Hence, although the relative risk of a homicide being committed by someone with schizophrenia has been estimated to be 4.2, the relatively low prevalence of schizophrenia (about 5 per 1000 population) means that people with schizophrenia make a small contribution to overall levels of homicide within a community.

The impact of a risk factor within a population can be estimated by calculating the population attributable risk fraction (PAF):

$$PAF = \frac{p\,(RR-1)}{p\,(RR-1)+1}$$

Where p is the proportion exposed in a population. In relation to schizophrenia and homicide;

$$PAF = \frac{0.005\,(4.2-1)}{0.005\,(4.2-1)+1} = 0.016$$

In other words homicide by people with schizophrenia contributes to 1.6% of all incidents of homicide occurring in Britain.

Another measure of the strength of association between a risk factor and an outcome is the standardised mortality ratio (SMR). Standardised mortality ratios allow comparisons to be made between a sample and the whole population when factors other than the exposure of interest differ between the two. For instance, age is obviously an important factor to consider when comparing death rates in two groups, because the older the sample the higher the death rate will be. Age may therefore be partly responsible for apparent differences in death rates between a study sample and the general population. Standardised mortality ratios can take account of differences in age and are calculated using the formula:

$$SMR = \frac{observed\ deaths}{expected\ deaths} \times 100$$

Details of how to calculate the expected number of deaths can be found in Mausner & Kramer (1985). The most commonly used method, called *indirect standardisation*, involves applying rates of death from the general population to the age distribution found in the study sample. This allows calculation of the number of deaths expected in the sample if they had the same rate of mortality as the general population. If the rate of death in the sample is the same as the rate expected in a population, then the SMR will be 100 (as this is the result of dividing any number by itself and multiplying this by 100).

Hence, studies examining the rate of death among people with schizophrenia have concluded that it is more than twice the rate among the general population. However, because clinical samples of people with schizophrenia are often younger than the general population, they underestimate the extent of the association between schizophrenia and premature mortality, and the SMR for schizophrenia has been estimated to be 300 (Brown *et al*, 2000).

Standardisation does not need to be confined to age; it can be used to take account of other variables that may affect the level of mortality and have different distributions in the sample and the population of interest.

Investigating the impact of interventions

Differences in outcomes in experimental studies provide an indication of the impact of different interventions. For instance in the randomised trial of psychological treatment for depression by Dowrick *et al* (2000) the prevalence of depression at the end of the 6-month follow-up was 41% among those randomised to problem-solving therapy and 57% among controls. The risk reduction was therefore 13%. It has been argued that interpreting findings from clinical trials is made easier by calculating a number needed to treat (NNT). The NNT is the number of people who would need to be treated in order to prevent an additional person being ill. It is calculated from the formula:

$$\text{NNT} = \frac{1}{\text{Risk reduction}}$$

The NNT for problem-solving therapy for depression based on this study was therefore $1/13 = 6.25$. In other words 6 people had to be provided with problem solving-therapy in order to prevent an additional person being depressed.

Study design

When planning an epidemiological study it is important to select the study design best suited to addressing the study aims. As different designs have different strengths and weaknesses, it is also helpful to check what design was used when critically appraising a research paper, as this can help direct you to potential problems. Epidemiological studies can be divided into those that use 'area-level' (or aggregate) data or individual-level data and those that are observational or experimental (see Fig. 5.1).

Aggregate-level studies

Aggregate-level studies use outcome data from entire populations to track changes in the level of health-related problems in different areas or different time periods. If aggregate data on exposure variables are also available, then correlations between exposure and outcome variables can be explored. Aggregate-level epidemiological studies have the potential to explore the effect that environmental factors have on health-related problems. Also called 'ecological' studies, this design can enable the impact of social processes to be explored. The potential of such studies has long been recognised. For instance, in the second half of the 19th century Emile Durkheim conducted a series of seminal analyses which examined the social conditions which give rise to suicide.

However, it is important that findings from aggregate-level studies are not used to draw inferences about risk factors that increase the likelihood of illness among individuals (an error often referred to as the 'ecological

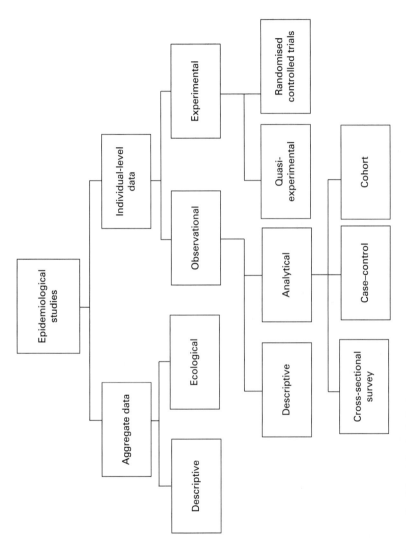

Fig. 5.1 Different types of epidemiological study.

fallacy'). Another problem with ecological studies is that data on potential confounding factors may not be available.

Individual-level studies

Cross-sectional survey

The simplest form of individual-level analytical study is the cross-sectional survey in which data on exposures and outcomes are gathered simultaneously from a study sample. The main advantage of cross-sectional studies is that they are relatively quick to perform and therefore relatively inexpensive. The main problems are bias and reverse causality (Box 5.2).

None the less cross-sectional surveys have been widely used to gather data on the frequency of health outcomes and generate hypotheses regarding potential risk and protective factors.

Case–control study

Cross-sectional surveys provide an effective means of investigating rare disorders. For instance, Creutzfeldt–Jakob disease has a community prevalence of less than one in a million and even large community surveys would fail to collect much information on people with this condition. Case–control studies provide an effective way of examining rare conditions because they sample people known to have the condition and a group of 'controls' free of the condition. In case–control studies participants are selected on the basis of whether they have or do not have an outcome. Because there is no need to follow-up the sample, case–control studies are relatively inexpensive. The main challenges when conducting a case–control study are:

- researcher and recall bias (because researchers and participants know the outcome status of the sample)
- sampling bias (if controls differ from the population from which the patients are derived).

The greatest challenge when conducting a case–control study is to obtain data from an unbiased sample of controls. Controls need to provide a valid measure of the prevalence of exposures in the population from which the patients came. If cases are restricted in some way, controls should therefore be similarly restricted.

Case–control studies provide relatively weak evidence for causation because measures of exposure are made when patients are already ill.

Cohort study

In cohort studies participants are selected on the basis that they are, or are not, exposed to potential risk factors. Cohort studies aim to select a disease-free sample and follow them with the aim of identifying the impact that different exposures have on the likelihood of developing an illness. Because it is possible to recruit a disease-free sample at the start of the study, cohort studies usually provide a more robust form of evidence to support temporal associations than other types of analytical study.

Box 5.2   Main problems with cross-sectional surveys

Bias – researchers may know the exposure status of participants when they are collecting outcome data

Reverse causality – it may be difficult to find out if exposures predate outcomes or vice versa.

However, because they rely on following a sample of people they are relatively time consuming and expensive. This is especially true for conditions that have long latency periods, that is when the period between being exposed to a risk factor and experiencing an illness is long (e.g. obstetric complications and schizophrenia). Loss to follow-up can result in bias, not least because people who are most difficult to follow-up may also be those who have developed the condition (outcome) of interest.

One way to get around problems associated with a long follow-up period is to try to identify old records that provide accurate information about exposures. In the study by Dalman *et al* (1999) information on obstetric complications from the 1970s was used as the basis for a 'historical cohort study'. In the 1990s researchers examined hospital records for evidence of whether members of the cohort had subsequently received in-patient treatment for schizophrenia. This study is still a cohort study because participants were selected on the basis of their exposure. In historical cohort studies it is important that those assessing outcome status are unaware of the exposure status of participants if problems of researcher bias found in other types of observational study are to be avoided.

Experimental studies

Experimental studies are those in which researchers manipulate exposures. Changing the experiences of participants places additional ethical obligations on researchers. The main advantage of experimental studies over observational studies is their potential for limiting the effects of confounding factors on associations between exposures and outcomes. Although known confounders can be measured in observational studies, and their effects explored through multivariate analysis, experimental studies provide an opportunity to control for both known and unknown confounders if large randomised trials are conducted. If participants are allocated to different exposures by chance, then all confounding factors should be equally distributed between the groups so long as studies are large. Small randomised trials do not offer this advantage because the smaller the study the greater the possibility that confounding factors will not be equally distributed between the groups.

The possibility of interviewer and recall bias are not necessarily reduced in randomised trials. Although the use of placebos in drug trials reduces the likelihood of bias, side-effects from many drug treatments which are generally absent in those taking placebos mean that participants and clinicians may not be masked to allocation status. It is even harder to mask researchers and participants in trials of psychosocial interventions. The use of active control treatments, such as supportive counselling, in trials of specific psychological treatments may help researchers to remain masked to which arm of a trial participants are in, but it is often not possible to mask participants to their allocation status and additional steps need to be taken to mask researchers if interview bias is to be avoided (see below).

Which is the best study design?

There is no study design that is intrinsically superior to any other. The most appropriate study design depends on the aims of the study. Although cohort studies are generally better at minimising interviewer and recall bias than other types of observational studies and large randomised trials have the potential to minimise the impact of confounding factors, a cross-sectional design is superior if the aim of the study is to establish the prevalence of a health-related problem. Because participants are selected on the basis of outcomes, case–control studies are often the most effective for examining the aetiology of rare conditions.

The strengths and weaknesses of different study designs are summarised in Table 5.1. In addition to methodological considerations, logistical considerations, such as the availability of time and other resources, also have an impact on the choice of study design.

Alternative explanations

Analytical epidemiological studies all aim to establish valid associations between exposures and outcomes. Before considering if an association between an exposure and an outcome is valid it is important to consider the possibility of 'alternative explanations' for the apparent association. Consideration of these factors before a study starts can help ensure that an appropriate study design is selected. Alternative explanations should also be considered when critically appraising a research paper based on the findings of an epidemiological study.

Chance

If a study sets out with the question 'Do doctors in Britain drink more alcohol than the general population?', a definitive answer could be achieved by obtaining a 100% response to a national survey (of all doctors and the entire population of Britain). Clearly such a large survey will not be conducted. Logistical and ethical considerations mean that most studies

Table 5.1 Strengths and weaknesses of different study designs

Design	Main uses	Strengths	Weaknesses
Descriptive aggregate-level studies	Monitoring changes in levels of illness in populations	Relatively cheap and quick	Reliant on the quality of routine data collected Difficult to account for changes in the classification of disorders
Ecological studies	Examining the effect of social conditions on health outcomes Generating hypotheses on the aetiology of health-related problems	Relatively cheap Relatively quick	Reliant on the quality of routine data Data on important confounding factors may not be available May not provide a valid indication of risk factors relevant to individuals
Cross-sectional surveys	Quantifying the prevalence of a condition Generating hypotheses on the aetiology of health-related problems	Relatively cheap and quick Can explore multiple outcomes and exposures at the same time	Researcher bias Recall bias Difficulty in establishing temporal associations Not suitable for rare conditions
Case–control studies	Exploring the aetiology of rare conditions and those with a long latency period	Relatively quick Can explore multiple exposures at the same time	Researcher bias Recall bias Selection bias (especially in selection of control group) Not suitable for rare exposures
Cohort studies	Examining impact of rare exposures Establish temporal relationships between exposures and outcomes	Minimise bias Easier to establish temporal associations	Relatively expensive and time consuming Selection bias Loss to follow-up, especially if long latency period – unless historical data on exposure are available May not be suitable for rare outcomes
Experimental studies	To evaluate effectiveness of interventions	If large: they minimise the impact of confounding Easier to establish temporal associations	Ethical considerations limit their use It may not be possible to mask researchers and participants, increasing the potential for researcher and recall bias

rely on collecting data from a sample of people and using the information gained to try to draw inferences about the population as a whole. However, any study that attempts to draw conclusions based on data collected from a sample of the population runs the risk that findings are the result of chance. Hence, in the study of the drinking habits of doctors it is possible that levels of consumption among doctors were higher than among the general population because of random variation; that is, by chance, doctors who were asked to take part in the study drank more heavily than those in the population from which they were selected.

Two factors determine the likelihood that chance is responsible for apparent association: the size of the sample and the degree of variation in the exposures and outcomes being studied. Clearly, the larger the sample the less likely that chance will be responsible for an apparent association. If there is less variation in the population, then the likelihood that chance is responsible for an apparent finding is also reduced.

Hence in the study of doctors drinking habits, chance is less likely to play a part in determining study findings if data were collected from a sample of thousands of doctors than in a study involving hundreds of people. If there are very large differences in drinking habits among doctors, a larger sample of doctors would need to be included in order to obtain an accurate estimate of their mean consumption, than if nearly all doctors drank about the same amount of alcohol.

The only way to rule out the possibility that chance plays a part in determining study findings is to collect data from the whole population. If a sample has to be used, as is nearly always the case, then statistical methods can be used to quantify the possibility that chance has affected the study findings. The main approach that is used to determine the probability that chance is responsible for an apparent association is either to calculate the *P* value (the probability that chance could have led to the study findings) or to calculate confidence intervals which provide an estimate of the range of values that are likely to be present in the whole population given the findings from the sample (for further details see Chapter 8).

When planning an epidemiological study, estimates of the degree of variation present in a population can be used to determine the sample size required for the study. Small studies may have insufficient power to test study hypotheses. Such studies may be unethical because they inconvenience participants with no prospect of adding to medical knowledge. Calculation of the necessary sample size is therefore a prerequisite of any epidemiological study.

Bias

Bias is the name given to *systematic errors* that can occur in epidemiological studies. Such errors can give rise to false-positive or false-negative findings. When planning a study it is important to consider possible sources of bias and take steps to avoid them. The three main sources of bias in epidemiological studies derive from the way that study participants are selected (selection bias), errors in the information provided by participants (recall bias) and in the way that researchers collect information from participants (researcher bias).

Selection bias

Selection bias is the result of choosing a study sample that is not representative of the whole population being investigated. To avoid selection bias it is important to decide what the study population is and then select a representative sample of that population. How should the study sample be selected for a study to estimate the prevalence of dementia in a local community? Interviews conducted among a consecutive sample of people who are admitted to hospital wards will clearly provide a biased sample, because people admitted to hospitals are more likely to have cognitive impairment. Bias could also be introduced if researchers contacted people in neighbouring streets because housing is organised in a non-random way and some areas have larger numbers of older people and may contain residential units specifically for people with dementia.

The best approach would be to draw up a list of all people living in a particular area and use this list, called a *sampling* frame, to randomly select a sample of the entire community. Unfortunately such lists are not readily available. In Britain it is estimated that 96% of people are registered with a general practitioner (GP), so GP lists may provide a fairly robust basis for a sampling frame for a study of dementia. The same is not true, however, for other study outcomes such as a study seeking to estimate the prevalence of drug misuse, where an important minority of people with such problems may be homeless or in prison. Estimates based on those registered with GP practices will underestimate the scale of the disorder. A gold-standard approach for estimating the prevalence of a disorder is to draw up a sampling frame based on a door-to-door survey of all households. However, although such studies are conducted (e.g. Jenkins *et al*, 1998), they are generally beyond the means of a small research team.

Close attention must be paid to deciding how to compile a sample for an analytical study. For instance, how should controls be selected for a case–control study exploring the role of substance misuse problems in suicides among young people? Cases of suicide could be identified by contacting local coroners' courts serving a given population and interviews with relatives and friends could be used to establish levels of substance misuse; but how could controls be found for the study? One possibility would be to obtain data from the relatives of other young people whose deaths had been dealt with by the coroner. However, this could provide a biased sample because levels of substance misuse may also be higher among those who had died in accidents or secondary to medical problems associated with drug misuse. Controls in a case–control study should provide an accurate estimate of the prevalence of the exposure *among the population from which the cases were derived.* In this example, a better estimate of levels of substance misuse might be obtained by interviewing relatives of young people registered with the same GPs as those dying by suicide.

In a cohort study the sample of non-exposed people should be as similar as possible to the exposed sample in all respects other than the exposure of interest. In an investigation of whether social support has an impact on relapse rates of people with bipolar affective disorder, those who have high levels of social support would need to be selected in the same way and in the same settings as those with poor social support.

Loss to follow-up

Loss to follow-up in cohort studies can create bias because the relationship between exposure and outcome variables may be different in those who are and are not followed-up. Although statistical methods can be used to estimate the impact of missing data, the only way to avoid this form of bias is to make every effort to avoid loss to follow-up. Means of avoiding this include obtaining reliable contact information at the start of a study, gaining informed consent to obtain contact details of relatives or friends if initial attempts to contact participants are unsuccessful, limiting the length of the follow-up period, and maintaining regular contact with participants during the course of the study.

Recall bias

Recall bias results from people with a health-related problem remembering or reporting details of exposures differently to those that do not have these problems, or from people who have been exposed to a risk factor reporting information on health outcomes in a different way to those who were not exposed. For instance, in a cross-sectional survey or case–control study examining risk factors for chronic fatigue, people with symptoms of chronic fatigue may be more likely to recall having had symptoms of a recent viral infection than controls. This is because people who develop an illness often wonder about the 'causes' of their condition, and people who remain well are more likely to forget incidents that do not lead to adverse outcomes. Cohort studies have the potential to reduce this problem by selecting people who are well at the start of the study. However, people who have been selected because of their exposure status may be more likely to report symptoms of an illness if they believe that the exposure may have a toxic effect.

Researcher bias

Researcher bias refers to systematic differences in the way that information is collected from different groups of people. In cross-sectional surveys and case–control studies, interviewers may pay greater attention to obtaining information on exposure status from those who are unwell. In cohort studies, interviewers may be more inclined to rate someone as having symptoms of a disorder if they know that they were exposed to a potential risk factor. Although researcher bias is particularly a problem during interviews, other assessments of outcome status may also be influenced by knowledge the researchers have of a person's exposure status. For instance, studies comparing ventricular enlargement in people with schizophrenia and controls reported larger differences when researchers knew whether participants did or did not have psychoses (Van Horn & McManus, 1992).

Experimental evaluations of complex interventions are just as likely to encounter problems with researcher bias as observational studies. Ways of reducing the effect of researcher bias are shown in Box 5.3.

Confounding

Confounding factors also provide alternative explanations for apparent associations between exposures and outcomes. In order to be a confounder a factor has to *alter the likelihood of an outcome and be associated with the exposure*. So in a case–control study examining whether abnormalities on the electroencephalogram (EEG) are more frequent among people with depression, exposure to medication could act as a confounder, as antidepressants alter the EEG and are obviously more likely to be taken by people with depression. Approaches for reducing the possibility that confounding factors explain associations between exposures and outcomes are given below.

- **Randomisation** – if the sample size is large, this will ensure that all confounding factors are equally distributed between the exposed and the non-exposed
- **Restriction** – the effects of a confounding factor can be removed by recruiting a sample who have not been exposed to this factor (for instance by comparing EEG abnormalities among people who have and who do not have depression and excluding participants who have been exposed to antidepressants)

Box 5.3 Means of reducing researcher bias

Developing clear protocols for data collection that seek to ensure that methods for collecting data do not differ between study participants

Using routine data or self-report measures to assess study outcomes

Masking researchers by methods such as ensuring that people collecting follow-up data were not involved in collecting exposure data, and attempting to make those assessing exposure status in case–control studies unaware of outcome status

Use of placebos in clinical trials.

- **Matching** – by ensuring that potential confounders are equally distributed among participants during the recruitment phase of a study. For instance, because gender is an important risk factor for depression, and men and women have different patterns of employment, a decision might be made to recruit equal numbers of men and women in a cohort study examining the effects of unemployment on the subsequent incidence of depression
- **Statistical analysis** – if accurate data on potential confounding factors are collected at the start of a study, attempts can be made to account for their effects using methods such as stratification or multivariate analysis.

Establishing causality

The aim of analytical epidemiological studies is to establish risk and protective factors for disorders. However, establishing that apparent associations between exposures and outcomes are valid (not a result of chance, bias or confounding) is not in itself sufficient to have confidence that one *causes* the other. For instance, it has repeatedly been demonstrated that levels of depression are increased among people who have physical illnesses but this valid association does not demonstrate that depression is caused by physical illness. Indeed, studies have shown that people with depression are more likely to develop physical illnesses and that *reverse causality* explains at least part of this association. In some instances, reverse causality is implausible (e.g. where genetic factors are thought to give rise to a disorder); however, in other instances the best approach to examining the possibility of reverse causality is to conduct a cohort study among people known to be disease free at the start of the study.

When studies are based on samples of the population, the likelihood that chance is responsible for an apparent affect can be estimated (see above), but it cannot be ruled out. Most epidemiological studies use a 5% level of statistical significance. This means that associations are considered valid if there is less than a 5% chance that they could have arisen through chance. However, this means that 1 in 20 studies that report 'valid' findings are reporting chance associations, so inferring causality from the results of a single study is problematic. It has been argued that causality can not be established unless valid associations between risk factors and outcomes are repeatedly demonstrated.

In 1965 the epidemiologist Bradford Hill laid down the following criteria to judge whether valid associations based on findings from epidemiological studies provide good evidence for causality.

- Strength of association (the stronger the association the more likely it is to be causal)
- Consistency of association (similar findings from different studies)

- Specificity of association (a specific exposure linked with a specific outcome)
- Temporal sequence of association
- Biological gradient (being able to demonstrate that the greater the exposure the greater the likelihood of the disorder)
- Plausibility (the association is supported by theory)
- Coherence of association (the association does not conflict with other established knowledge)
- Experiment (evidence that removing the risk factor reduces the likelihood of the disorder)
- Analogy (other similar causal relationships exist).

These criteria continue to provide a helpful basis on which to judge whether associations are causal. In recent years the value of experimentation has been emphasised because the potential that large randomised trials have for taking account of known and unknown confounders has been increasingly recognised.

Planning an epidemiological study

When planning a high-quality epidemiological study consideration should be given to the following factors.

- Review previously published literature.
- State clear aims and a single null hypothesis and agree a plan for analysis of data. This helps to maintain the focus of a study and avoid the potential for false-positive findings as a result of chance.
- Conduct a sample size calculation to ensure that the study has sufficient statistical power to examine the study hypothesis.
- Consider the representativeness of the sample and avoid selection bias. Ensure that study participants reflect the make-up of the study population. Ensure that controls or non-exposed participants are selected on the same basis as exposed participants in every respect other than the variables being studied.
- Use appropriate, validating instruments for assessing exposures and outcomes (see Chapter 11).
- Ensure that observer bias is minimised. Take steps to reduce the impact of recall and researcher bias.
- Try to ensure a high rate of follow-up and consider effects of non-response. Every effort should be made to maximise follow-up rates – loss to follow-up of more than 15–25% of participants would severely hamper the interpretation of study findings.
- Measure and account for confounders. Check previously published reports for evidence of possible confounders and plan the sampling strategy and data analysis to try to account for these.

- Take care when entering data. Making mistakes when handling data leads to 'random error', which will decrease the likelihood of demonstrating positive findings. Some computer packages allow data to be 'double entered', allowing errors to be identified and corrected.
- Consider all relevant ethical aspects of the study. Ethical matters go beyond the statutory requirement to obtain ethics committee approval. It is essential to ensure that the sample size is not larger or smaller than required to address the study aims, that potential participants are recruited in a fair and even-handed manner, that data are collected and participants followed-up in a way that minimises inconvenience, and that data are handled, stored and presented in an appropriate manner.
- Consider the limitations of the study design and their implications for the conclusions. When preparing a study report make sure that weakness in the study design are acknowledged and that the implications of these are taken into consideration when formulating the conclusions.

Conclusions

Epidemiological methods underpin most quantitative clinical research in psychiatry and familiarity with these methods can improve the quality of such studies. By starting any new study with a clear statement of the study aims and accompanying hypotheses it should be possible to ensure that an appropriate study design is selected. An awareness of sources of systematic error most commonly found in different types of study can reduce the likelihood of generating biased data. Steps taken to avoid or account for the effects of confounding factors and the use of appropriate statistical methods can also help to ensure that study findings are valid and reliable.

References

Brown, S., Barraclough, B. & Inskip, H. (2000) Causes of the excess mortality of schizophrenia. *British Journal of Psychiatry*, **177**, 212–217.

Dalman, C., Allebeck, P., Cullberg, J., *et al* (1999) Obstetric complications and the risk of schizophrenia: a longitudinal study of a national birth cohort. *Archives of General Psychiatry*, **56**, 234–240.

Doll, R. & Hill, A. B. (1950) Smoking and carcinoma of the lung: a preliminary report. *BMJ*, ii, 739–748.

Dowrick, C., Dunn, G., Ayuso-Mateos, J. L., *et al* (2000) Problem solving treatment and group psychoeducation for depression: multicentre randomised controlled trial. Outcomes of Depression International Network (ODIN) Group. *BMJ*, **321**, 1450–1454.

Durkheim, E. (1952) *Suicide: A Study in Sociology*. London: Routledge & Keegan Paul (original work published in 1897).

Hill, A. B. (1965) The environment and disease: association or causation? *Proceedings of the Royal Society of Medicine (London)*, **58**, 295–300.

Jenkins, R., Bebbington, P., Brugha, T. S., *et al* (1998) British psychiatric morbidity survey. *British Journal of Psychiatry*, **173**, 4–7.

Mausner, J. S. & Kramer, S. (1985) *Epidemiology: An Introductory Text*. Philadelphia: Saunders.

McMichael, A. J. (1999) Prisoners of the proximate: loosening the constraints on epidemiology in an age of change. *American Journal of Epidemiology*, **149**, 887–897.

Sachdev, P., Mason, C. & Hadzi-Pavlovic, D. (1997) Case–control study of neuroleptic malignant syndrome. *American Journal of Psychiatry*, **154**, 1156–1158.

Tyczynski, J. E., Bray, F. & Parkin, D. M. (2003) Lung cancer in Europe in 2000: epidemiology, prevention, and early detection. *Lancet Oncology*, **4**, 45–55.

Van Horn, J. D. & McManus, I. C. (1992) Ventricular enlargement in schizophrenia. A meta-analysis of studies of the ventricle: brain ratio (VBR). *British Journal of Psychiatry*, **160**, 687–697.

CHAPTER 6

Qualitative research methods in psychiatry

Deborah Rutter

This chapter will try to convince the reader of the value of qualitative research techniques in psychiatric practice and research. Why should a reader need convincing? First, qualitative methods have always been assessed in comparison with quantitative methods, including the 'gold standard', the randomised controlled trial. This is a misleading comparison because the two paradigms are appropriate to different types of enquiry and may well be entirely complementary, rather than competing. Second, clinicians use qualitative interviewing methods every day in clinical work with patients, but may not realise that they do so. Collecting a patient's history relies on the clinician's ability to draw out information from a patient and then reorganise the data to meet diagnostic criteria and develop an acceptable care and treatment plan. Diagnostic interviews such as those used for personality disorder (Hare, 1991; Tyrer & Cicchetti, 2000) are quite explicit about the need for the interviewer to elicit from the patient everyday examples of behaviour that will illustrate particular traits. Qualitative research skills are then frequently used in psychiatry and with purposeful planning can contribute much to formal research in the field.

What is qualitative research? A brief overview

The essential features of qualitative research are described in Box 6.1. Qualitative research concerns the subjective meaning people give to their experience. Evidence of meaning comes from analysing what people say or by observing what they do. Qualitative methods are particularly useful in complex health and social care systems to clarify 'hidden' processes such as clinical decision-making and procedures. What actually happens (within an organisation or to a patient during their treatment) can be directly observed and compared with what participants say happens (Mays & Pope, 1995a). Although qualitative researchers are not seeking an 'objective truth' or seeking to prove a hypothesis, they may be able to bring together all the 'partial' (meaning both biased and incomplete) accounts of different contributors in a way that offers either predictions of organisational

---

> **Box 6.1**   Essential features of qualitative research
>
> - It is concerned with what, how and why research questions, rather than the how often and how many type of question (Buston *et al*, 1998)
> - It is linked to methods that do not predetermine the form or content of the data (though the data are likely to be verbal).

outcomes (Ferlie, 2001) or suggestions for interventions that may move particular objectives forward.

In psychiatry and psychology, qualitative research is most commonly practised through semi-structured interviewing. The researcher interviews a selected sample of individuals about their own experiences or views of a situation or a treatment. Interviewees are not steered towards a limited number of set options or structured responses, because the researcher does not know in advance what people are likely to say. Such interviews do, however, guide respondents to talk about particular topic areas, which is why they are not 'unstructured' interviews.

Qualitative research studies have a developmental 'feel', taking a very open-ended stance as to what is relevant at the beginning and gradually homing in on key factors or aspects of the investigation as it becomes apparent what these are. Research protocols summarising the plan for the study and the samples of people who will be involved may therefore be amended as the qualitative study proceeds. The initial protocol may build in an interim analysis of preliminary findings, after which the plan for subsequent work will be finalised. So the protocol is not followed nearly as rigidly as, for example, in a randomised controlled trial.

How does qualitative research differ from quantitative research?

This section compares qualitative and quantitative research methods to illustrate some of the key differences (Table 6.1).

Quantitative research usually follows a predetermined experimental design that tests one or more hypotheses. Ideally the analysis plan for the results should be predetermined and should not (unless adverse events occur) change over the lifetime of the research project. Setting up a quantitative experiment will almost always require some amendment to usual clinical practice (Hotopf *et al*, 1999), particularly if the intervention is a complex one (Campbell *et al*, 2000). For example, Scott *et al* (2000) described a controlled trial in which patients with residual symptoms of major depression were randomised either to standard clinical management or to clinical management plus 18 sessions of cognitive therapy. Randomisation interferes with the

Table 6.1 Key differences between quantitative and qualitative approaches to research

	Quantitative approach, following scientific method	Qualitative approach
Aim/purpose of research	Tests (proves/disproves) a predetermined hypothesis	Exploratory, flexible: no initial hypothesis
Relationship of data to theory	Deductive (by reason): data are collected to support/disprove a proposed theory (the hypothesis)	Inductive: theories 'emerge' as the data are analysed, to be supported, refined or overturned by subsequent data
Methodological plan	Predetermined, experimental design: should not deviate from protocol	Has predetermined aims to explore specified areas of enquiry: design and methods may adapt to changing focus
Outcome variables	Tries to isolate one/two variables as primary outcome measures	Range of variables: often not clear which are most important to outcomes. How the variables interact may be a key aspect of study
Measurement of outcomes	Measurable/quantifiable outcomes	Outcomes not predictable, rarely quantifiable
Setting	Setting is likely to be artificial in some sense (e.g. in the way participants are referred)	More likely to take place in naturalistic setting (unless supports a trial in artificial setting)
Can study be replicated?	Should be replicable, with similar findings. Different findings from repeated studies may be inexplicable	May be replicable in similar settings: findings may be dissimilar because of differences in context. Comparison of different findings can be instructive
Are results generalisable?	Claims to be generalisable to like contexts	May be generalisable to like contexts, but identifying similar contexts may be problematic

usual practice in which psychiatrists tailor their prescription according to their knowledge of individual patients. It is likely (although not discussed in the report) that cognitive therapy was made available at short notice solely for the purpose of this study (to avoid waiting lists), so again the setting was not naturalistic. Outcomes from such a trial are normally scores illustrating change in symptoms of depression, social adjustment or other measures. Results are analysed taking into consideration sources of bias and the possibility that misleading conclusions have arisen purely by chance. Quantitative techniques are used when the outcomes to be measured are known and there are instruments, such as validated questionnaires, available to measure those outcomes.

Therefore a good quantitative study requires a good background knowledge of the health intervention. In the example above (Scott *et al*, 2000), both treatments and the means of delivering them within the context of the study were well understood and considered to be widely acceptable to patients. If the researchers had suspected variation in the way these treatments were delivered and received by patients, qualitative methods could have been used to explore these in preparation for the trial. Once a trial is under way a qualitative researcher might investigate the subjective experience of the patients and staff involved in the trial to consider their views of the different treatments. In the study of Scott *et al* (2000) such qualitative research might have helped to explain why differences between the two arms at follow-up were so minor that they 'may not be clinically significant'.

Because of its potential for methodological flexibility and sensitivity to contextual factors, a qualitative study is unlikely to be entirely replicable, but the findings may be generalisable to other similar contexts. Qualitative research should investigate and describe the setting of the study, emphasising the relationship between different factors and how they appear to influence each other. In any meta-analysis of findings from different settings this will help to explain why results from superficially similar settings vary.

'The aim of a good qualitative study is to access the phenomena of interest from the perspective of the subject(s); to describe what is going on; and to emphasize the importance of both context and process.' (Buston *et al*, 1998)

When are qualitative methods appropriate and useful in psychiatric research?

This section presupposes a preference, wherever possible, for the use of the 'gold standard' of health services research (Campbell *et al*, 2000), the randomised controlled trial.

Although quantitative and qualitative research methods are presented here as contrasting approaches (Table 6.1), it is relatively common for both approaches to be utilised – either simultaneously or at different stages – in a research project (Weaver *et al*, 1996; Barbour, 1999; Crawford *et al*, 2002). Examples of studies where qualitative methods have contributed to the implementation of quantitative research are described below.

Addressing shortcomings before evaluation

Qualitative research is useful when existing policy, protocol or treatment is dysfunctional in some way, the reasons why and/or the best way of amending the situation are uncertain, and the service wants to address shortcomings before engaging with evaluation. We hoped to implement a formal randomised controlled trial of residential therapeutic community treatment for people with personality disorder. However, practitioners

75

reported that referrals from general psychiatry and psychology were alarmingly low. A small qualitative investigation of practitioners working in community settings in the regional catchment areas was organised to investigate the reasons behind these low rates of patient referral. This qualitative study showed poor understanding of this type of treatment, particularly among younger consultants, and the need for services to offer more flexible models of treatment (part-time, day care), with some revision of admissions criteria and punitive sanctions and better integration with other service providers (community psychiatry, probation, etc). Increasing the number of referrals will impact not only on the viability of the treatment itself but also on the viability of evaluating that intervention.

Supplementing formal quantitative research

Qualitative research can supplement a more formal quantitative research design by helping to explain the findings or generalisability of an investigation. In a study of 400 patients with severe mental illness (Tyrer *et al*, 1995), patients were randomised either to intensive supervision by nominated keyworkers (according to the newly implemented care programme approach) or to standard follow-up by services. The results of the trial showed that patients who were closely monitored were less likely to lose touch with services but, at variance with the hypothesis, had more and longer hospital admissions. The authors were unable to explain why this might be as there was no complementary qualitative exploration of process. In a subsequent trial investigating outcomes from different models of care management, a substantial qualitative component was built into the study. Although the trial collapsed prematurely, the qualitative work was able to explain why preliminary findings showed no significant difference in outcomes for patients: the features identified as essential to integrated working between health and social care staff (such as joint allocation systems, role flexibility and improved access to funding by team managers) were unaffected by the new arrangements. Barbour (1999) suggests that adding qualitative explanatory aspects to trials may help to dispel the 'positive publication bias', in which trials with significant findings are far more likely to be published than those supporting the null hypothesis (Dickersin & Min, 1993).

Qualitative research can also be an important supplement to quantitative research by clarifying the *context* of the study and whether its findings are likely to be generalisable. Services that offer superficially similar treatments may have very different outcomes. Qualitative investigation of the context and process in different services can help to explain why. Gilbody & Whitty (2002) argued convincingly that new mental health services and new ways of organising and delivering them 'often can be offered only at the level of hospital or general practice', so that randomisation by cluster (the general practice, the specialist clinic) rather than by individual patient is necessary. To reduce the intrinsic differences between and within such clusters (the intraclass correlation coefficient which estimates the potential for biased results), Gilbody & Whitty suggested matching clusters in pairs according to known variables thought to be associated with outcomes, with one of each matched pair randomised to the intervention and control arms respectively. Qualitative as well as quantitative methods can be used to identify appropriate matching variables.

Obtaining information before the design of a quantitative study or to formulate policy

Qualitative research is useful when too little is known about a health problem, a treatment or policy intervention, or about how patients and professionals make decisions, to design or extend a structured quantitative enquiry or to formulate appropriate policy to address need. In the field of addiction, Wiltshire *et al* (2001) undertook qualitative research among smokers randomly selected from the lists of general practitioners (GPs) in socially deprived areas. Smokers were not passively responding to price increases designed to reduce consumption but were engaged in cigarette and tobacco smuggling, which most respondents regarded with approval. The study concluded that health promotion strategists could not necessarily assume that health-based reasons for giving up smoking would be reinforced by economic incentives. There might also be active opposition from local people benefiting from the illegal trade. This study illustrates the success that qualitative researchers may have in collecting anonymous but detailed data about illegal, stigmatised or 'shameful' activities. Qualitative studies carried out by colleagues with clientele from sexual health clinics at St Mary's Hospital, Paddington, have explored such sensitive issues as the use of condoms by working prostitutes and whether, when and how patients of genito-urinary clinics tell sexual partners that they have a diagnosis of genital herpes. Interviews were undertaken by psychologists and researchers who were independent of the clinic; guarantees of confidentiality were given to the respondents.

Feasibility studies

Qualitative research is used in feasibility studies, when it is unclear whether a particular research design will be acceptable to patients or to clinicians, or whether clinicians will have the skills, motivation and expertise to recruit patients to such a trial. Donovan *et al* (2002) conducted qualitative research with both patients and professional 'recruiters' to a controversial trial of screening for prostate cancer. They uncovered uncertainty and disparity among professionals in the way they communicated the trial design to patients, which in turn influenced patients' views of the potential disadvantages of taking part. Snowden *et al* (1997) retrospectively interviewed parents who had consented to enrol their critically ill newborn babies in a neonatal trial and found that many did not comprehend the concept of equipoise or randomisation (and so by implication did not give informed consent). The cost of setting up randomised controlled trials, and the huge waste entailed if such trials are abandoned because they cannot recruit sufficient numbers to generate a significant result with any confidence, justifies preliminary investment in a brief qualitative investigation of the feasibility of using a particular quantitative method. This may be particularly pertinent in research with psychiatric patients, where capacity to give informed consent may affect levels of participation.

Gaining information about patient motivation

Qualitative research can be useful when patient motivation is essential to the outcome of a treatment or management intervention but little is known about patients' attitudes and activities and how these might be influenced. Eagles *et al* (2003) carried out a small qualitative study of patients' views on suicide prevention. The study was divided into two parts. In preliminary, in-depth tape-recorded interviews, 12 psychiatric patients were asked to reflect on what they had or might have found helpful at times when they had felt suicidal and what they had experienced as unhelpful. These interviews were analysed in order to construct a topic guide (see Table 6.2) for a second version of the semi-structured interview, this time informed by patients' views, which was used for a second round of interviewing of 59 patients.

Gaining information on the views of different stakeholders

Qualitative research has a role to play when the issue being explored is likely to be perceived very differently by different stakeholders, with important consequences for policy and practice. Investigating user involvement in two London mental health trusts, we carried out qualitative interviews with patients, managers, clinical staff and voluntary sector personnel (Rutter *et al*, 2004). Our analysis showed a range of views about the efficacy of user involvement; we organised these views according to the different types of respondents. Service users were generally more frustrated and disappointed by the effects of user involvement than managers, and nurses were mindful of their own lack of influence over trust management. We concluded that user involvement will not achieve its alleged potential unless and until service users see more concrete outcomes, managers are more forthright about the limits of patient involvement, and nurses have a means of promoting their own views on desirable health service change.

Getting started: practical aspects of qualitative research

Although there is insufficient space to provide comprehensive guidance on how to carry out qualitative research (see Bowling, 1997; Ritchie & Lewis, 2003; Silverman, 2005 for useful guides), there are a number of key requirements that must be addressed at the planning stage of the study. Table 6.2 summarises these requirements. It is recommended whatever the study size or purpose that plans be reviewed with an experienced qualitative researcher.

Qualitative research should have very clear aims from the outset. What questions are you trying to answer or what areas of social experience are you trying to understand or explore? Your interview questions (and topic guides) can change over the course of the study, but research aims must be consistent and will need to be pitched at the right level of abstraction: not so broad that you may never be able to fulfil them within the constraints of time and resources, but not too detailed, since the *process* of doing qualitative research will open up areas of interest that you had not realised were important. As in all research, the resources available will be a key influence on the study plan.

Your sampling strategy should specify the numbers of people you aim to involve in the investigation, the different types of people you will involve, and how you will access them. The numbers of people in your sample and the amount of data you aim to collect will depend very much on time and resources. Qualitative interviews with very small numbers of patients may be very informative: unlike quantitative research designs, there is no direct relationship between numbers in the sample and the validity of, and confidence in, findings. However, one person's view on a topic cannot inform us about the range of views, so sensible sample sizes – commensurate with resources – should be specified. It is probable that the sample will be broken down into different types of people (e.g. patients, nurses, doctors), who will have different perspectives on your topic and require different topic guides. It is important not to plan to collect huge amounts of data which you do not have the expertise or resources to analyse. Remember that analysis is often the most demanding task and collecting more data will compound rather than reduce those demands.

You will need ethics committee approval for the research if you plan to interview National Health Service (NHS) patients and/or staff. Information will be needed on how confidentiality will be assured, whether quotes will be used anonymously and what will happen to tapes (if recorded) and transcripts. Consent forms will also be needed. Employees will need to know that information given will not be relayed to their colleagues and managers. When working with psychiatric patients, interviewees will need an explicit strategy, which should be included in the information, for dealing with disclosure of intent to cause harm to self or others. Qualitative interviews can rouse unexpected emotions, for example when relevant experience is linked to associated traumatic events. An interviewer should be competent (from experience gained in research or clinical practice) to deal with such expressions and should be prepared to help the respondent deal with their distress.

Accessing willing interviewees may not be a problem: if the information sheet succeeds in explaining that the interview is informal and 'safe', and

Table 6.2 Key requirements that must be addressed at the planning stage of qualitative research

Requirement	What to do
Clear purpose/aims to research	Ask yourself and colleagues, what exactly are your research questions? What will you want informants to tell you about?
Justification for methodology	Is qualitative research the best means of exploring these questions?
Resources to carry out the study	Who will collect and analyse the data? Do they have time? Do you have a tape recorder, funds for transcribing, funds for travel?
Plan your sampling strategy	How many interviews or groups can you 'afford'? Are there particular types of people you should include? How will you access them?
Topic guide	Draft your topic guide or guides (to submit to funders, ethics committee, etc). Include a list of areas you aim to cover in order to address the study aims. Novices should include non-leading questions to introduce the topic areas. Pre-planned prompts to encourage people to elaborate can be useful if respondents give very succinct answers.
Ethics committee approval	This is a technical requirement (for work with patients or staff). Draft an information sheet and consent form for participants. Are there particular ethical issues? Are you obliged to report any particular interviewee statements (such as intention to harm self), and if so, has the participant been explicitly warned? Could participants become upset? If so, how will interviewers support them?
Confidentiality or anonymity?	Can you guarantee that no one not present at the interview will ever know what was said (confidentiality)? Or do you envisage including unattributed quotations (anonymity)? Quotes will be unusable if they suggest the source (even if you consider them uncontroversial): the consent form should ask permission to use quotes, and should state that taking part will have no effect on patient care (patients) or on employment (staff).
Interview arrangements	How are the participants approached? Are the arrangements for interview safe, private and convenient for all parties (including paranoid patients)? Can you offer refreshments and travel expenses?
Recording the interview/focus group	If manually recorded, the record will not be verbatim but can be a summary of key points. A verbatim account requires a good tape recorder and considerable time to transcribe recordings.
Data protection	Data could be on paper, on recorded tape cassettes, or on computer. How are these stored and protected? Are files anonymised? When will data be destroyed? Have participants given informed consent to storage, use and destruction of data from their interviews?
Analysis	Has the project got an experienced analyst to undertake or supervise the analysis? The more data generated, the more demanding of experience this task becomes. Could you afford a parallel analysis; if so, does the 'weight' of the project justify such a safeguard?

why you think their views on the topic are important, you may find that you can even recruit a random sample from a large potential pool (e.g. of patients), although a self-selected sample of people who meet your criteria is more common. A purposive sample is one in which particular types of people are deliberately targeted to ensure that major divisions within the group of interest are reflected in the study. It is important that any invitation to be interviewed that requires knowledge of patients' names and addresses is sent on your behalf by a person who is entitled to have that information, such as a GP or consultant. As an external researcher you would then supply unaddressed letters to the practice or clinic, with an invitation to the patient to reply directly to yourself disclosing their name and address, which would constitute a part of the patient's consent to participate. If you are conducting research internally as a member of staff, you may find, especially if your research concerns the patients' views of the service, that patients are reluctant to talk frankly to you. Information sheets must state precisely who will have access to interview notes and transcripts. Transport and childcare costs should always be reimbursed to interviewees. Conducting the interview in a place of mutual convenience and safety is important, and the comfort of the person may require you to provide refreshments, breaks, etc.

A tape or digital recorder is the best means of recording the interview, although its use requires time or money to type up transcripts. A study exploring complex decision-making processes may require verbatim accounts, so interviews must be recorded. However, a study exploring fairly routine processes may not need full transcripts. A compromise might be to conduct interviews with two researchers: one responsible for guiding the interview, the other solely taking notes. Interviewees must consent to the recording of interviews: if you are interviewing paranoid patients or others who might feel that recording may compromise them in some way, you should be prepared to take handwritten notes.

You must approach the interview with a topic guide, which is a flexible 'agenda' for the interview which outlines (according to your current knowledge) areas that you need to cover to address the aims of the research. It is a good idea to include a few 'structured' questions in the opening stages of the interview (record gender, age, perhaps job title or relationship to the organisation or area you are researching) so that you can describe your sample and analyse your material according to different types of respondent. It is the responsibility of the interviewer to lead the interview: researchers with limited experience can give themselves confidence by drafting questions or remarks which can be used to introduce each area to the interviewee. The use of unclear, leading or 'multiple' questions in an interview is a common pitfall (in surveys and structured assessments, as well as qualitative interviews) which may invalidate findings. A question should never 'hint' at an expected or desired answer. Questions should be 'open-ended', that is the interviewee's response is, *as far as possible*, not influenced by the implied attitudes, expectations or moral judgements of the questioner. Compare, for example, 'Do you think your current care plan is rather limited and dominated by medication?' (an example of two questions combined, both leading the interviewee to make a negative judgment) with 'How do you feel about your current care plan?' (open-ended question). The use of non-technical language and short words is usually appropriate with patients who may speak other languages better than English. 'Tell me what you thought when you first came into hospital' is more appropriate than 'Describe your impressions of in-patient care'. However, when interviewing specialised staff it is possible that they will expect you to have a grasp of common technical terms: if any used are outside your knowledge, be prepared to humbly ask for definitions.

Although the interviewer can depart substantially from the guide, it is important to make judgements *as the interview progresses* about whether the conversation is addressing the aims of the research. An interviewee who has departed from relevant areas needs to be directed by the interviewer, who should show sensitivity and diplomacy. However, informants often refer in passing to points of interest. The interviewer may want to return later to these points and it is helpful to jot down keywords as an aide-memoire for clarification at a later opportune moment. There is nothing designed to alienate interviewees more than the impression that they are not being listened to, but if the plot is lost, apologising and asking for a recap of something they have already told you may reinforce the impression that you value everything they have said. There are many pitfalls associated with this form of data collection but most can be overcome with experience and 'reflexive' practice, that is by being aware of your mistakes and shortcomings and considering how to overcome them.

Although you should plan to interview a specific number and range of people, you may decide in the course of the study to stop interviewing shortly after you begin to recognise that you are getting the same information from the same type of respondent. This is known as 'saturation' (and will probably be reached at different points within a single study for different types of respondent). However, it is important that you do not confuse saturation with the use of a 'stale' and restrictive topic guide, which requires rethinking.

Qualitative research with focus groups will also need ethics committee approval and will involve the same sampling techniques, topic guides, etc as interviews, but focus groups enable the researcher to expand the range of views explored on a single occasion and can generate both illuminating discussion and even qualified consensus (e.g. if the purpose of the group is to make recommendations about how a particular problem may be tackled). However, running a focus group of maybe six people is not an easy alternative to interviewing, as the researcher (who should be assisted at a focus group) will also need to retain some notion of the differences between these people and to 'referee' contributions, so that the less assertive participants are not excluded by the more assertive. Participants of a focus group should all have a similar relationship to the phenomena or experiences in question (e.g. all doctors or all patients of the same service) or the discussion will be too diffuse to be productive. The (London-based) National Centre for Social Research offers training in qualitative interviews and focus groups (http://www.natcen.ac.uk; see also Ritchie & Lewis, 2003)

Analysis of qualitative data

The term 'grounded theory' (Strauss & Corbin, 1994) has become almost synonymous with qualitative data analysis. 'Grounded theory' is inductively derived from the study of the phenomena it concerns; that is, from the data. The researcher begins with an area of study, collects the data and generates meanings, knowledge and understanding by reference *to the data itself*, rather than to any preconceived theory that they seek to verify. The methodology of grounded theory has done much to improve the status of qualitative research in health services, as it proposes the systematic application of an analytical framework, takes into account all the data and enables the findings and conclusions to be traced back to primary data (interview transcripts in most cases).

The analysis of qualitative data is possibly that part of the research process that is given the least attention in planning the study, perhaps because it is assumed that computer software will do the job. Sadly, computers do not understand meaning. Computer analysis of data uses sorting and collating packages, which enable the researcher to practice grounded theory by sorting data 'bytes' (paragraphs from transcribed interview text, bits of information) into categories, which should initially be broad but can later be broken down into more specific categories. The computer package (from which there are several to choose, including the widely used NVivo 7: get a free trial and/or purchase it at http://www.qsrinternational.com) facilitates this process by allowing a 'tree-like' framework to be built up as the analysis progresses, with passages of highlighted text sent rapidly into identified 'nodes', along with identification from the interview header, so that they can be traced back to source. In a small study, a similar framework can be built up using the copy and paste facilities of a word-processing programme. The analysis can be organised in the form of a tabular grid (with each informant's data occupying one column and themes arising from the interviews becoming row 'headings' as they arise), but as each interview is a unique collection of themes, many grid spaces will be blank.

The first-sort phase of the analysis before the theoretical implications begin to emerge can seem long and tedious, and it is a good rule never to collect more data than you can comfortably analyse. It is also helpful to conduct an analytical review of data collected at some midpoint in the study, both in order to assess the data in relation to the aims of the study and to reflect on the emerging themes and issues while there is still the opportunity to amend or supplement topic guides and samples.

Language-based primary data such as interview transcripts can be subjected to infinite degrees of meticulous content analysis. A study considering the consultations in which a positive HIV diagnosis was communicated to patients analysed (with some justification and generous funding) every grunt, cough and hum, and constructed a means of recording body language from the video data used. However, health services researchers should consider the aims of their research, and the audience and uses to which it will be put, before investing in analysis of such detail.

The analysis and synthesis of different types of qualitative data are demanded in a variety of research and policy contexts, including public inquiries which use qualitative techniques to combine largely qualitative witness evidence and expert views to arrive at their conclusions. As a result guidance on synthesising the findings of qualitative research studies has been published (Dixon-Woods & Fitzpatrick, 2001; Mays *et al*, 2001; Paterson *et al*, 2001) with the aim of making available systematically developed, integrated bodies of knowledge about specific phenomena. Unlike the quantitative systematic review (NHS Centre for Reviews & Dissemination, 2001), which seeks primarily to determine the efficacy of health technologies, qualitative studies may provide useful accounts of context and process even when the scientific rigour of the conclusions is in doubt (Sandelowski *et al*, 1997).

The qualitative research report

There are no rules about what constitute key findings in qualitative research but the issues that should be addressed in a report of the findings are described in Box 6.2.

The aims of the research should be stated clearly. The prevalence or prominence of particular views should also be stated. Although it is beyond the scope of qualitative research to estimate the prevalence of particular views *outside* the sample interviewed, it is appropriate to give an idea of prevalence *within* the sample (e.g. '13 of the 20 respondents felt that ...') (Barbour, 1999). The consequences of the views expressed for the service, policy or field of enquiry should also be discussed.

Factors that might influence the views of the respondents should be discussed. For example, qualitative interviews of psychiatric patients living in the community about unmet need may need to draw distinctions between interviewees within the sample according to living circumstances. If the relevance of this factor has been anticipated, topic guides for interviews should have prompted some discussion of living circumstances; if not, and no systematic information is available about these characteristics of the sample, a hypothetical association may be discussed in the study report.

If the analysis is advancing 'theories' or hypotheses (for further testing), or even describing how a system works, it will be important to discuss data that do not fit.

Box 6.2   Issues that should be addressed in a qualitative research report

- The stated aims of the research
- The prevalence of particular views within the sample
- Factors that might influence the views of the respondents
- Discussion of data that do not fit
- Consequences of views expressed for the service or field of enquiry.

What are the shortcomings of qualitative research and how might they be minimised?

All types of research can be badly planned, employ inappropriate methods, have poor sampling strategies, weak linkage of conclusions with findings and/or can discount data that fail to fit the research hypothesis or emerging theory. Qualitative research is susceptible to all these faults, but there are additional common 'quality' or bias problems frequently linked to qualitative methods, some of which can be addressed to some extent, and some of which will remain (Mays & Pope, 1995*b*, 2000; Murphy *et al*, 1998). Table 6.3 summarises some of these.

Qualitative researchers – especially those who work in relative isolation – are themselves a source of bias if they make all the choices, and this is a very good reason for sharing qualitative work, especially at the planning and analysis stage, with others. 'Reflexive' research practice means that researchers continuously assess the effect of strategies they adopt upon the findings.

Questioning the validity of findings will refer the researcher back to the aims and methods of the study. Did the study focus on its stated aims? Did the sampling strategy reflect the different types of people using the service or health technology under scrutiny? Is there any reason informants might wish to mislead researchers? Conducting interviews with offenders with severe personality disorder for a Home Office study, the researcher might be unwise to take every expression of dissatisfaction at full face value. If the informant's experience is sufficiently extreme, the researcher may seek some corroboration (triangulation) from other sources or will report the experience as uncorroborated but possibly accurate. 'Triangulation' describes the use of different sources and types of data to corroborate findings. Jones *et al* (2001), studying the use of new drugs by GPs, compared actual prescribing records with statements about prescribing made by GPs and found them to be largely consistent. Triangulation can 'support a finding by showing that independent measures of it agree with it, or at least, do not contradict it' (Miles & Huberman, 1994, p. 266).

Table 6.3 Alleged shortcomings of qualitative research

Alleged problem	Strategies for overcoming problem
Bias inherent in research team's choices	Consulting with commissioners and experts (e.g. convening steering group) Not taking decisions in isolation Constructing parallel independent topic guides Conducting parallel independent analyses
Validity of the findings	Purposive sampling strategy, considering how all relevant groups can be included Reflexivity in conducting interviews: is the interviewer leading informants? Listen to a sample of tapes Consider motives informants have for misleading Continuously update topic guide Conduct interim analysis to consider 'gaps' in data Triangulation: use of other methods/data sources to test findings and conclusions Consider feeding back your preliminary findings to your informants: do they recognise your conclusions?
Generalisability of the findings	Be specific about research context Express doubts about generalisability
Subjectivity	Is there an objective 'truth'?

Randomised controlled trials are only the gold standard (Campbell *et al*, 2000) in health services research because they *minimise*, rather than eliminate, that part of the bias in outcomes that relates to differences between individual patients. When considering whether findings are generalisable, randomised controlled trials remain subject to contextual bias (Hotopf *et al*, 1999). One strength that qualitative research may have in relation to the issue of generalisability is that, from its roots in social science, it is particularly sensitive to context generally and to the links between different aspects of social phenomena. A qualitative researcher investigating the use of illegal drugs on psychiatric in-patient wards will not rely on the measurement of primary and secondary variables (such as self-reported use by patients, supplemented by hair and urine analysis) but may initially list potential areas of interest as patients' and staff views/experience of using different types of drugs, security and visiting procedures on the ward and in the hospital generally, smoking facilities, average length of stay and impact on patients' benefits, staff morale and continuity of care, use of agency staff, policy directives within the trust, etc (the list is very broad).

Qualitative studies may well make explicit the particular characteristics of the research setting. This may raise doubts about the generalisability of the key findings to other, dissimilar contexts, but minimising or failing to report the peculiarities of a trial setting, as quantitative reports often do, does not mean they have not had an impact on the findings. A popular measure of the comparative efficacy of psychiatric interventions (used in Tyrer *et al*, 1995) is the number of days spent in hospital by patients. However, it is well known that unpopular patients who abuse other people or defecate on the floor are likely to be discharged before those that are less troublesome. Moreover, using such a measure in a region where 'move-on' supported accommodation is in short supply will also cast doubts upon the validity and generalisability of findings. Difficulties with validity and generalisability will be less prominent in all types of research if reporting is (a) specific about the context of the research, describing it well; (b) explicit about the *clinical* significance (and not just the statistical significance) of findings; and (c) honest about possible reasons why results may not be generalisable (part of reflexivity).

Finally, qualitative data are often considered 'subjective' and therefore not useful within a scientific discourse. One influential theme of *social* science discourse is that *all* human experience is subjective: that each person's understanding, and actions taken in consequence, are potentially unique, although there will be many areas of similarity (without which we could hardly expect to make social relationships). We know from cross-cultural discussions of disease and health (Rack, 1982; Helman, 1994) that a patient's ethnicity, customs and expectations of the (Western) medical profession all influence their experience of their health problems, as well as experience of treatment. A clinical psychiatrist or psychologist who tries to treat patients without accounting for their *subjective* cognitive and psychological processes, their phobias, delusions and attitudes, will not have much success. Assessment of health technology is focusing more upon the evaluation of technologies as they are experienced and distorted by patients, with more interest in the pragmatic trial (Schwartz & Lellouch, 1967; Hotopf *et al*, 1999). If patients find it difficult to continue their allocated treatment in a masked randomised controlled trial, what use will the treatment be in a real setting, however efficacious it may prove for particular symptoms? In psychiatry and psychology, where patients must often be persuaded to adhere to treatment, subjective states are what we deal with.

Conclusion

This account of qualitative research in psychiatry has clearly neglected debates about the epistemological status of qualitative data (well covered in Murphy *et al*, 1998) but is intended to be an accessible and practical account, which may encourage readers to consider promoting and carrying out such investigations. As always, chosen methodology will depend upon the aims of any investigation and is a technical judgement. However, as the emphasis on user involvement in health services design and delivery increases (Department of Health, 2002) and patients become less willing to leave the planning of health services and policies to professionals (Barnes, 1999), there would seem to be a need for research that addresses not just formal clinical outcomes but also the context and processes of NHS services, and of the research agenda itself. Qualitative research has the capacity to democratise health services research by expanding our perceptions of what matters.

References

Barbour, R. (1999) The case for combining qualitative and quantitative approaches to health service research. *Journal of Health Services Research and Policy*, **4**, 39–43.

Barnes, M. (1999) *Public Expectations: From Paternalism to Partnership, Changing Relationships in Health and Health Services.* London: Nuffield Trust/Judge Institute of Management Studies.

Bowling, A. (1997) *Research Methods in Health.* Buckingham: Open University Press.

Buston, K., Parry-Jones, W., Livingston, M., *et al* (1998) Qualitative research. *British Journal of Psychiatry*, **172**, 197–199.

Campbell, M., Fitzpatrick, R., Haines, A., *et al* (2000) Framework for design and evaluation of complex interventions to improve health. *BMJ*, **321**, 694–696.

Crawford, M. J., Weaver T., Rutter D., *et al* (2002) Evaluating new treatments in psychiatry: the potential value of combining qualitative and quantitative research methods. *International Review of Psychiatry*, **14**, 6–11.

Department of Health (2002) *Improvement, Expansion and Reform: The Next 3 years: Priorities and Planning Framework 2003–2006.* London: Department of Health.

Dickersin, K. & Min, Y. I. (1993) Publication bias: the problem that won't go away. *Annals of the New York Academy of Sciences*, **703**, 135–148.

Dixon-Woods, M. & Fitzpatrick, R. (2001) Qualitative research in systematic reviews. *BMJ*, **323**, 765–766.

Donovan, J., Mills, N., Smith, M., *et al* (2002) Improving design and conduct of randomized trials by embedding them in qualitative research: ProtecT (prostate testing for cancer and treatment) study. *BMJ*, **325**, 766–770.

Eagles, J. M., Carson, D. P., Begg, A., *et al* (2003) Suicide prevention: A study of patients' views. *British Journal of Psychiatry*, **182**, 261–265.

Ferlie, E. (2001) Organisational studies. In *Studying the Organisation and Delivery of Health Services: Research Methods* (eds N. Fulop, P. Allen, A. Clarke, *et al*), pp. 24–39. London: Routledge.

Gilbody, S. & Whitty, P. (2002) Improving the delivery and organisation of mental health services: beyond the conventional randomised controlled trial. *British Journal of Psychiatry*, **180**, 13–18.

Hare, R. D. (1991) *The Hare Psychopathy Checklist–Revised.* Toronto: Multi Health Systems.

Helman, C. G. (1994) *Culture, Health and Illness: An Introduction for Health Professionals.* Oxford: Butterworth Heinemann.

Hotopf, M., Churchill, R. & Lewis, G. (1999) Pragmatic randomised controlled trials in psychiatry. *British Journal of Psychiatry*, **175**, 217–223.

Jones, M., Greenfield, S. & Bradley, C. (2001) Prescribing new drugs: qualitative study of influences of consultants and general practitioners. *BMJ*, **323**, 378–381.

Mays, N. & Pope, C. (1995a) Qualitative research: Observational methods in health care settings. *BMJ*, **311**, 182–184.

Mays, N. & Pope C. (1995b) Rigour and qualitative research. *BMJ*, **311**, 109–112.

Mays, N. & Pope, C. (2000) Assessing quality in qualitative research. *BMJ*, **320**, 50–52.

Mays, N., Roberts, E. & Popay, J. (2001) Synthesising research evidence. In *Studying the Organisation and Delivery of Health Services: Research Methods* (eds N. Fulop, P. Allen, A. Clarke, *et al*), pp. 188–220. London: Routledge.

Miles, M. B. & Huberman, A. M. (1994) *Qualitative Data Analysis.* Newbury Park, CA: Sage Publications.

Murphy, E., Dingwall, R., Greatbatch, D., *et al* (1998) *Qualitative Research Methods in Health Technology Assessment: A Review of the Literature* (Health Technology Assessment), Vol. 2, no. 16. Southampton: NHS Health Technology Assessmant Programme.

NHS Centre for Reviews & Dissemination (2001) *Undertaking Systematic Reviews of Research on Effectiveness: CRD's Guidance for Carrying Out or Commissioning Reviews* (2nd edn). York: CRD. http://www.york.ac.uk/inst/crd/pdf/crd4_ph2.pdf

Paterson, B. L., Thorne, S. E., Canam, C., *et al* (2001) *Meta-Study of Qualitative Health Research*. London: Sage Publications.

Rack, P. (1982) *Race, Culture and Mental Disorder*. London: Tavistock.

Ritchie, J. & Lewis, J. (eds) (2003) *Qualitative Research Practice. A Guide for Social Science Students and Researchers*. London: Sage Publications.

Rutter, D., Manley, C., Weaver, T., *et al* (2004) Patients or partners? Case studies of user involvement in the planning and delivery of adult mental health services in London. *Social Science and Medicine.*

Sandelowski, M., Docherty, S. & Emden, C. (1997) Qualitative meta-synthesis: issues and techniques. *Research in Nursing and Health*, **20**, 365–371.

Schwartz, D. & Lellouch, J. (1967) Explanatory and pragmatic attitudes in therapeutical trials. *Journal of Chronic Disability*, **20**, 637–648.

Scott, J., Teasdale, J. D., Paykel, E. S., *et al* (2000) Effects of cognitive therapy on psychological symptoms and social functioning in residual depression. *British Journal of Psychiatry*, **177**, 440–446.

Silverman, D. (2005) *Doing Qualitative Research* (2nd edn). London: Sage Publications.

Snowden, C., Garcia, J. & Elbourne, D. (1997) Making sense of randomization: Responses of parents of critically ill babies to random allocation of treatment in a clinical trial. *Social Science and Medicine*, **45**, 1337–1355.

Strauss, A. & Corbin, J. (1994) *Grounded Theory Methodology*. In *Handbook of Qualitative Research* (eds N. Denzin & Y. Lincoln). Thousand Oaks, CA: Sage Publications.

Tyrer, P. & Cicchetti, D. (2000) Personality assessment schedule. In *Personality Disorders: Diagnosis, Management and Course* (ed. P. Tyrer), pp. 51–71. Oxford: Butterworth-Heinemann.

Tyrer, P., Morgan, J., Van Horn, E., *et al* (1995) A randomized controlled study of close monitoring of vulnerable psychiatric patients. *Lancet*, **345**, 756–759.

Weaver, T., Renton, A., Tyrer, P., *et al* (1996) Combining qualitative data with randomised controlled trials is often useful. *BMJ*, **313**, 629.

Wiltshire, S., Bancroft, A., Amos, A., *et al* (2001) 'They're doing people a service': Qualitative study of smoking, smuggling and social deprivation. *BMJ*, **323**, 203–207.

CHAPTER 7

Research with single or few patients

David F. Peck

There is a long tradition in medicine in general, and in psychiatry in particular, of intensive investigations of single patients. Although studies of single patients have often set the scene for important advances, they are sometimes regarded with suspicion; however, there is not necessarily an incompatibility between research studies on small samples (often called small N designs) and scientific acceptability. The seminal publication on small N research is the book by Barlow & Hersen (1973), which brought together a series of *experimental* designs that could be applied to single patients or small groups of patients. Although many of the experimental designs for single patients have evolved from within behavioural psychology, these methods are generally applicable across the whole field of mental health. Moreover, they are increasingly used in areas such as medical education (Bryson-Brockman & Roll, 1996), physical rehabilitation (Simmons *et al*, 1998), paediatric pharmacology (Carlson *et al*, 1999), speech and language therapy (Millard, 1998) and psychiatric nursing (Ricketts, 1998).

There are several varieties of experimental design that are appropriate for use with small numbers of patients. There are no standard procedures but rather a series of experimental manipulations all designed to demonstrate a functional relationship between two variables, such as treatment and outcome. Typically, this involves systematically altering one variable and observing its effects on the other. Precisely how this relationship is demonstrated will depend on each clinical situation. As long as this basic logic is followed, it is for the clinical researcher to use whatever design is considered appropriate. Nevertheless, for practical purposes experimental designs with small samples tend to be discussed under two broad headings: ABAB designs and multiple baseline designs. With the former, single patients or single groups of patients may be used, whereas the latter can be appropriate for either single or up to about ten patients (all with a similar problem). The examples given below illustrate the kinds of designs that have been used and the problems for which they were deemed appropriate. One of the main attractions of the small N approach is that a great deal of creativity and ingenuity is required in devising an experimental design appropriate for specific clinical purposes.

ABAB approaches

The standard ABAB design

This design involves frequent measurement of the patient's problems before, during and after treatment. The period before treatment (baseline or 'A' phase) should contain at least two measurement points but preferably more. Ideally, baseline measurements should continue until a reasonable degree of stability has been achieved. At that point, a treatment (B) is introduced and the effect on the problem is measured at several time points. When a change has been observed, treatment is discontinued but the problem continues to be measured. If the treatment is responsible for improvements, there should be a deterioration at this point. This is the second A or second baseline period. Treatment is then reinstated (second B period) and again an improvement is anticipated. Additional A and B phases can be added, but sequences longer than ABABABAB are unlikely to be practicable. If there is a clear and consistent relationship between when the treatment is applied and when the clinical problem improves, one may conclude that the treatment is probably responsible for the change (Box 7.1). Certainly alternative explanations of any change become increasingly unlikely as the sequence of A and B phases extends. However, if improvements occur during A phases (or if there is a deterioration in B phases), this conclusion would be more equivocal. Thus a clear systematic relationship should be demonstrated between the application of treatment and improvement in the patient's problem. The length of the treatment and baseline periods will depend on how quickly the treatment is expected to produce any changes; generally the A and B periods should be of comparable length. A further example of an ABAB study design is shown in Box 7.2.

Box 7.1 Example of a standard ABAB design with a single patient

A man with multiple disabilities and minimal movements was taught to control the amount of environmental stimulation he received by using chin movements linked to a microswitch. After a baseline period (A), chin movements affected the stimulation only during the intervention (B) phase. A steady increase in chin movements was observed.

Lancioni *et al* (2004)

Box 7.2 Example of an ABAB design with 100 participants who were treated as a single 'unit'

The participants were provided with dawn simulators during the winter to overcome the effects of lack of light on sleep quality. Sleep was rated during two A phases (no simulation) and two B phases (with simulation), each phase lasting for 2 weeks. Sleep quality was significantly better during the simulation phases.

Leppamaki *et al* (2003)

The AB design

This is a more basic and less convincing form of the ABAB design because the relationship between the application of treatment and improvement is observed on one occasion only; thus other factors could account for the change in the patient's condition. This design might seem to offer few advantages over the gathering of routine clinical data but much more information can be gained because of the frequency and systematic nature of the measurements. This design is useful when there are good reasons why it would be undesirable to withdraw the treatment and thereby risk deterioration, for example when a patient's condition could be considered dangerous to themselves or to others. An example of a study using the AB design is given in Box 7.3.

Variants of ABAB designs

Researchers may devise any number of variants of the basic ABAB design. The design has been used to compare different treatment regimes. Hellekson *et al* (1986) investigated the effectiveness of phototherapy in the treatment of seasonal affective disorder. After obtaining initial assessments of depression,

---

Box 7.3 Example of a study using an AB design

Naloxone was given to a 21-year-old woman with epilepsy for the treatment of self-harm. In a double-blind AB trial, a placebo (saline) was given in the first session, followed by three sessions in which naloxone was administered. Improvements were observed in event-related potentials, a memory task, anxiety levels, and frequency of self-harm during these B phases. The authors concluded that naloxone was responsible for improvements because no improvement was observed during the placebo period (phase A).

Sandman *et al* (1987)

---

phototherapy was given to six people at three different times of the day in a different order. Between each session there was a period of no treatment (the A phase). Depression improved in all participants during phototherapy but this improvement was reversed when treatment was withdrawn. There was, however, no difference between the times of day. This study is particularly interesting because it reports a systematic replication using the same method with six participants, thus adding credibility to the effectiveness of the treatment.

The alternating treatments design

This design may be used to compare the effects of two or more treatments on one individual. It comprises rapid and, as far as possible, random alternation of all treatments, with an interval between (Box 7.4).

Questions of interference and carry-over effects across treatments may arise but some possible solutions have been suggested. These include restricting the study design to the investigation of problems that can easily be reversed, using treatments that have little or no carry-over effect and using some form of design or cue that is unique to each treatment and relevant to the patient.

Technical problems in ABAB designs

Many of the ABAB designs might seem attractive to the practising clinician, who may consider it straightforward to incorporate these research designs into clinical practice because they would not interfere with clinical routines. In reality, clinicians may find that the designs are difficult to implement. There may be reservations concerning the desirability of withdrawing an effective treatment in the A phase; it may prove difficult to establish a stable baseline; the outcome may not reversed when treatment is withdrawn, particularly if the treatment is potent; the treatment effects may continue for

---

Box 7.4   Example of a study using an alternating treatments design

Means of behavioural modification were investigated in two 3-year-old children with learning disabilities. The first child exhibited poor attention, inadequate self-care, odd social behaviour and self-harm. Four methods were used, each with a different cue: interruption, differential reinforcement of other behaviour, visual screening and extinction. Extinction was the most effective but differences between treatments were not apparent when there was only a minute between treatments. Differences were more clear-cut when the interval between treatments was longer. Similar findings were reported with the second child, whose main problems were non-adherence and aggression.

McGonigle *et al* (1987)

a long time after the treatment has stopped, and hence even if the outcome variable is in principle reversible, there may be a long interval between stopping the treatment and the observed change.

For these and other reasons, clinicians may prefer to use the simpler but less powerful AB design. Although this design cannot unequivocally demonstrate that the treatment has been effective in a single patient, if the same systematic approach subsequently gives similar results with several patients with similar problems, the evidence in favour of treatment efficacy would be compelling. Within the constraints of the clinic, this might be the most achievable level of experimental sophistication.

Multiple baseline approaches

In multiple baseline designs, several problems are investigated simultaneously during a baseline period; subsequently one problem is treated but the other problems continue to be assessed. After a further period a second problem is treated and all the other problems continue to be assessed. After a further period treatment is applied to a third problem (randomly determined) and again all the problems are assessed. Treatment is applied sequentially for each problem in this way until all the problems have been treated. Thus each problem has a different duration of baseline assessment, which helps to control for 'spontaneous' change. It may be concluded that the treatment has been effective if an improvement is observed for each problem soon after the treatment has been applied; if no improvement is observed, or if one or more of the problems improves before the institution of treatment, then it cannot be concluded that the treatment is definitely responsible for any improvement. This description applies to the multiple baseline design across problems; there are also the multiple baseline design across patients (the same problem is tackled but with different patients) and multiple baseline design across settings (the same problem is tackled in the same patient but in different settings).

Multiple baseline across problems

Ducker & Moonen (1986) wished to promote the development of expressive communication in children with severe learning disabilities who had no meaningful expressive verbal or non-verbal vocabulary. Manual signs were used as the medium of communication: those for 'scissors', 'mirror' and 'marbles'. The frequency of use for each sign before training was observed for six sessions for 'scissors', after which the expressive communication training was started; the frequency of use for 'mirror' was observed for nine baseline sessions before treatment was initiated, and for 'marbles' there were 14 baseline sessions. There were no observations of the appearance of the three signs before the treatment was initiated, but after each treatment there were marked increases in the relevant signs. This is a particularly interesting study because it also incorporated an ABAB component.

Multiple baseline across participants

In this design, several patients with a similar problem are treated, again after different baseline periods and with frequent measurements for all participants throughout the study. For rare conditions it is unlikely that all potential participants would be available at the outset of the study and it is not be feasible or ethical to delay treatment for some patients until five or six with a similar problem have been referred. Under these circumstances it is possible to carry out a 'non-current' multiple baseline study, in which the lengths of the baseline periods are specified in advance for as many patients as are expected to participate, and one of these durations is randomly selected as each patient is referred, thereby controlling for spontaneous change. An example of a multiple baseline design across participants is given in Box 7.5.

Multiple baseline across settings

In this design treatment is applied to a particular problem with a single patient, in one particular setting; the same problem is also assessed in different settings but without treatment. Some time after, the treatment is applied in the second setting and so on until treatment has been applied across all the settings. This design is used infrequently used since it assumes that the improvement in one setting will not also occur in the other settings involved. There may be few clinical problems where this pertains.

This study design was used by Odom *et al* (1985). Three boys with learning disabilities were taught to increase the frequency of social interactions, such as demonstrating affection, sharing things with other children and helping children. These social interactions were initiated by other children without learning disabilities who had previously been trained to do this by teachers. The training took place across three classroom settings in sequential order. A marked improvement in social interaction was observed but only when it was applied in each setting individually.

Box 7.5 Example of a multiple baseline design across participants

Five patients with driving phobia were treated at intervals, using virtual reality simulations over eight sessions. Three showed marked improvement after treatment was introduced, one showed moderate improvement and one did not improve. Improvements were not noted before the treatment was introduced. The authors suggested that the results were sufficiently promising to warrant larger-scale trials.

Wald & Taylor (2003)

Technical problems with multiple baseline designs

If the problem improves before the treatment is due to start, this will undermine the logic of the design and obscure clear-cut conclusions; it is important that any improvement should not occur in other clients, other problems, or other settings before treatment is initiated. Furthermore, the therapist must know in advance whether there will be any generalisation, before deciding if a multiple baseline design will be appropriate; such information may not be available. Generalisation would seem to be particularly likely across problems and across settings since the changes are occurring in the same individual and for the same problem. Further difficulties arise if the time to respond after treatment begins is long and/or variable.

Implementation problems in small N designs

Researchers often report difficulties in adhering strictly to the design as originally planned. This reduces the confidence with which conclusions about treatment efficacy can be drawn. This may in part account for the decrease in the number of studies with small N designs published in the mental health literature. Publication of such studies in the journal *Behaviour Research and Therapy* has declined from at least 10 per annum in the 1980s to about 2 or 3 in the 2000s, despite a doubling of the number of pages per issue over that period (further information available from the author on request).

Several studies have reported practical problems in implementing ABAB designs. Jones & Baker (1988) were unable to assess self-harm directly because of 'the possibility of physical damage occurring during the baseline', and the design had to be modified because the therapist 'was finding it difficult to continue to monitor the response latencies'; furthermore the improvement unexpectedly deteriorated at the end of the second B phase. Lieberman *et al* (1976), in an evaluation of numerous clients of a community behaviour therapy service, were able to fully implement single-case designs (mainly ABAB) with only one-third of the clients.

As regards multiple baseline designs, Carr & Wilson (1983) had only two baseline observations in their 'across-settings' study, in part because staff 'were too busy to observe reliably'. Marshall & Peck (1986) were unable to keep to the predetermined number of baseline sessions because of the death of a participant's relative. Charlop & Walsh (1986) attempted a complex 'across-setting' design but the improvement occurred prematurely across the settings.

Recommendations

Experience with small N designs has enabled researchers to pinpoint the designs that are useful in providing interpretable data, those that are not unduly time-consuming and those which have fewer ethical problems and are less prone to problems of patient adherence. The suggestions below represent compromises between ideal experimental rigour and practical constraints. As Hayes (1981) declared:

'If time series designs are to be opened up to the practising clinician, we must abandon the notion that only the purest designs are of value. It is the integrity and progress of the overall enterprise that is critical, not the purity of a single study standing alone'.

In most cases, simple AB designs will probably suffice. That is, the problem should be assessed on at least two occasions before treatment and continue to be assessed throughout the treatment and follow-up sessions. This can provide convincing evidence of change, particularly when more than one outcome variable is used and when the problem is of long duration despite previous treatments.

In addition, the alternating treatments design can be usefully employed when two or more treatments are to be compared, although there is a danger of carry-over effects and other forms of interference. Finally, one might also consider the non-current multiple baseline across-participants design.

If further patients are referred with the same problem, the clinician can build up a series of patients using the same small N design. Each new patient would add credibility to the notion of treatment efficacy (assuming similar results were obtained). If similar results were not obtained, enough detailed information might be available to generate hypotheses about the differences in outcome. For example, Peck (1977) reported the successful treatment of a woman with blepharospasm (or spasmodic winking) using electromyogram (EMG) feedback. Patients with the same problem who were subsequently treated had a mixed outcome. However, enough patients were assessed to suggest that EMG feedback is more useful for patients with clonic rather than tonic spasms. If small N designs were routinely adopted in clinical work, similar interesting and testable hypotheses would be generated across a variety of clinical conditions.

In short, despite reservations about the scientific worth of simple AB designs, they will probably serve most of the needs of clinical researchers when using small N designs. Because the logic behind more complex designs is often transgressed, one often finds oneself with an AB series anyway, irrespective of the original intentions. If a clinician decides that a more convincing design is required or if more complex questions are asked, the multiple baseline across participants (particularly the non-current version) and the alternating treatments designs can be considered. However, the clinician should remain cautious about whether the additional complexity is warranted.

Finally, Elliott (2002) has outlined an interesting combination of quantitative and qualitative methods designed to clarify the causal links between process and outcome in dynamic psychotherapy, with a strong focus on investigating alternative explanations of patient change. The approach bears much resemblance to the small N approaches outlined here, and merits wider consideration by clinical researchers.

Interpretation of changes in small N designs

It is traditional in group experimental studies to use inferential statistics, such as *t*-tests and analysis of variance, to help researchers to decide whether a treatment has been effective. It has been argued that in small N research, because each participant is assessed frequently and intensively, treatment effects are normally quite clear-cut and statistical techniques to help in decision-making are not necessary. Moreover, it is argued that if statistical analysis is needed to identify an effect, then the effect must be quite small and the treatment may be insufficiently powerful for practical clinical purposes.

To some research workers such notions may be appealing. Others have argued that visual inspection of results alone can lead to major errors, and that statistical analysis is vital to assess treatment effects properly. Under most circumstances the same conclusions are reached using statistical analysis or visual inspection of the data. However, there are some circumstances, particularly where there is a trend in the baseline, where discrepancies may occur. Hence, some form of statistical analysis is usually required.

Unfortunately the data from the simplest of experimental designs (AB designs) require complex statistical procedures for analysis (time series analysis) because small N data typically violate a basic assumption of traditional statistical tests, that of independent data points. Time series methods require sophisticated computer programs and a large number of observations, typically over 50. Such analyses are unlikely to appeal to most clinical researchers. However, a new approach to statistical inference has come to the fore in recent years. These 'randomisation tests' are relatively assumption free and seem to be ideally suited to analysing data from small N research. This topic cannot be discussed in detail here but an excellent reference is Todman & Dugard (2001).

Conclusions

Clinical research designs with small samples appear to have many advantages: few patients are required; matched control groups are not necessary; scientifically acceptable research may be fitted into everyday practice; and inferential statistics may (although this is not advised) be avoided. However, there are several pitfalls with the use of these designs and enthusiasm should be tempered with caution.

It is worth reiterating that a 'cookbook' approach to small N research is not appropriate. The design should be tailored according to the circumstances of the particular patients and problems. As Hayes (1981) has argued, one should maintain 'an attitude of investigative play' rather than slavish adherence to a standard design.

Some of the authors of publications mentioned in this chapter (e.g. Hellekson *et al*, 1986) did not refer to their studies as small N designs. They devised an experimental method to answer specific clinical research questions and the resulting design happened to follow the same kind of logic.

Small N designs should not be considered simply as alternatives to large-scale group studies but rather complementary to them. Although a randomised controlled trial is regarded as the 'gold standard', no single study and no single methodological approach can answer all the important questions that arise when investigating the effectiveness of treatment. Different methods are needed to address all the relevant questions and small N designs have a key part to play in a multi-method approach. Moreover, interesting hypotheses may emerge from a small N study that would warrant a large-scale trial and data from patients in a large trial can be examined individually, giving a more precise picture of variation in response to treatment.

Small N designs constitute a coherent strategy for clinical research, a coherence that has led to increased scientific acceptability. Psychiatric research and clinical practice would gain much from a more widespread use of this approach.

References

Barlow, D. & Hersen, M. (1973) Single case experimental designs: uses in applied clinical research. *Archives of General Psychiatry*, **29**, 319–325.

Bryson-Brockman, W. & Roll, D. (1996) Single case experimental designs in medical education: an innovative research method. *Journal of Academic Medicine*, **71**, 78–85.

Carlson, J. S., Kratochwill, T. R., & Johnston, H. F. (1999) Sertraline treatment of 5 children diagnosed with selective mutism: a single case research trial. *Journal of Child and Adolescent Psychopharmacology*, **9**, 293–306.

Carr, S. & Wilson, B. (1983) Promotion of pressure relief exercising in a spinal injury patient: a multiple base-line across settings design. *Behavioural Psychotherapy*, **11**, 329–336.

Charlop, M. H. & Walsh, M. E. (1986) Increasing autistic children's spontaneous verbalisations of affection: an assessment of time delay and peer modelling procedures. *Journal of Applied Behavior Analysis*, **19**, 307–314.

Ducker, P. C. & Moonen, X. M. (1986) The effect of procedures on spontaneous signing with Down's syndrome children. *Journal of Mental Deficiency Research*, **30**, 355–364.

Elliott, R. (2002) Hermeneutic single case efficacy design. *Psychotherapy Research*, **12**, 1–21.

Hayes, S. C. (1981) Single case experimental design and empirical clinical practice. *Journal of Consulting and Clinical Psychology*, **49**, 193–211.

Hellekson, C. J., Kline, J. A. & Rosenthal, N. E. (1986) Phototherapy for seasonal affective disorder in Alaska. *American Journal of Psychiatry*, **143**, 1035–1037.

Jones, R. S. P. & Baker, L. V. J. (1988) The differential reinforcement of incompatible responses in the reduction of self-injurious behaviour: a pilot study. *Behavioural Psychotherapy*, **16**, 323–328.

Lancioni, G. E., O'Reilly, M. F., Sigafoos, J., *et al* (2004) Enabling a person with multiple disabilities and minor motor behaviour to control environmental stimulation with chin movements. *Disabilities Rehabilitation*, **26**, 1291–1294.

Leppamaki, S., Meesters, Y., Haukka, J., *et al* (2003) Effect of simulated dawn on quality of sleep – a community based trial. *BMC Psychiatry*, **3**, 14.

Lieberman, R., King, L. W. & Deris, W. J. (1976) Behaviour analysis and therapy in community mental health. In *Handbook of Behavior Modification and Behavior Therapy* (ed. H. Leitenberg). Englewood-Cliffs: Prentice-Hall.

Marshall, M. J. & Peck, D. F. (1986) Facial expression training in blind adolescents using EMG feedback: a multiple base-line study. *Behaviour Research and Therapy*, **24**, 429–435.

McGonigle, J. J., Rojahn, S., Dixon, J., *et al* (1987) Multiple treatment interference in the alternating treatments design as a function of the intercomponent interval length. *Journal of Applied Behavior Analysis*, **20**, 171–178.

Millard, S. K. (1998) The value of single case research. *International Journal of Language and Communication Disorders*, **33**, 370–373.

Odom, S. L., Hoyson, M., Jamieson, B., *et al* (1985) Increasing handicapped preschoolers' peer/social interactions: cross setting and component analysis. *Journal of Applied Behavior Analysis*, **18**, 3–16.

Peck, D. F. (1977) The use of EMG feedback in the treatment of a severe case of blepharospasm . *Biofeedback and Self-regulation*, **2**, 273–277.

Ricketts, T. (1998) Single case research in mental health. *Nursing Times*, **94**, 52–55.

Sandman, C. A., Barron, J. L., Crinella, F. M., *et al* (1987) Influence of naloxone on brain and behavior of a self-injurious woman. *Biological Psychiatry*, **22**, 899–906.

Simmons, R. W., Smith, K., Erez, E., *et al* (1998) Balance retraining in a hemiparetic patient using center of gravity biofeedback: a single case study. *Perceptual and Motor Skills*, **87**, 603–609.

Todman, J. B. & Dugard, P. (2001) *Single Case and Small N Experimental Designs: A Practical Guide to Randomisation Tests*. Mahwah: Erlbaum.

Wald, J. & Taylor, S. (2003) Preliminary research on the efficacy of virtual reality exposure therapy to treat driving phobia. *Cyberpsychology and Behavior*, **6**, 459–465.

Part III

Tools

CHAPTER 8

Statistical aspects of clinical trials in psychiatry

Tony Johnson

Since its inception in the 1940s, the randomised clinical trial has become the principal method of comparing the efficacy of all forms of medical treatment and care of hospital in-patients, out-patients and patients in the community. One of its founders, Bradford Hill, described the clinical trial as:

'a carefully, and ethically, designed experiment with the aim of answering some precisely framed question. In its most rigorous form it demands equivalent groups of patients concurrently treated in different ways. These groups are constructed by the random allocation of patients to one or other treatment. In some instances patients may form their own controls, different treatments being applied to them in random order and the effect compared. In principle the method is applicable with any disease and any treatment.' (Hill, 1955).

The distinction between this form of assessment and epidemiological studies is the objective and efficient prospective comparison of concurrent, randomly allocated treatments.

Many clinical trials are conducted each year within all specialties of medicine, and these exhibit a range of designs from very simple to highly complex, from tiny to enormous, and from short term to long term, with methods of analysis that vary from the crude to the sophisticated. The past 50 years have seen many developments, as researchers have tackled the problems of design, conduct and analysis of clinical trials, in attempts to tailor them to the study of specific diseases, methods of assessment and patient management. Today there are several comprehensive and readable texts devoted to the methodology of clinical trials; these are illustrated by examples drawn from the medical literature (see References and Further reading). There are good reasons for having a text specific to each subspecialty of medicine, so that the problems of actually carrying out clinical trials can be exhibited and discussed as close as possible to their clinical context. This has happened rarely (Buyse *et al*, 1984; Guiloff, 2001; Girling *et al*, 2003), and only recently in psychiatry (Everitt & Wessely, 2004), although a multidisciplinary textbook on clinical trials devotes five chapters to this specialty and covers Alzheimer's disease, anxiety disorders, cognitive behaviour and depression (Machin *et al*, 2004).

The burgeoning methods of clinical trials have led to some standardisation of terminology to provide a broad classification of the types of trial, the information collected, and the way in which it is handled in the analysis. The purpose of this chapter is to present some of the basic terminology and methods of clinical trials as simply as possible, with illustrations drawn from general psychiatry. In one chapter it is not possible to enter into highly specific details; for these, as well as the arguments for and against various practices and procedures, the reader should consult the list of references at the end of this chapter.

The protocol

We begin with the protocol, the construction of which is the first major milestone that must be passed if any clinical trial is to be organised and carried out successfully. The protocol is a complete manual that provides a full specification of the clinical trial, from a statement of its objectives to the writing of the final report. It embraces every aspect of the management and assessment of patients, including copies of forms and rating instruments, together with instructions for their completion and scoring, a summary of the data collected, and the methods for computerisation and analysis. Some of the key features that should be included in the protocol are listed in Box 8.1.

The protocol for a specific clinical trial will not necessarily incorporate all these items, and the order of presentation may be changed. Some investigators use both a protocol and an operators' manual (see Meinert, 1986).

Of these features, a few will be singled out for discussion in this chapter. However, the third (objectives) merits special attention, for many clinical trials in psychiatry are overambitious and attempt to resolve too many, often diverse issues simultaneously. The inevitable result is that inadequate information is obtained about many of them, and investigators are forced to perform rescue operations on selected and perhaps biased data. The primary objective of a clinical trial is the estimation of the difference(s) between the randomised treatments on some chosen measure of efficacy or cost-effectiveness, and this should never be lost sight of. The temptation to investigate secondary objectives on an 'available' sample of patients must be curtailed. Searches for prognostic factors, identification of the characteristics of 'responders' and 'non-responders', breakdown of drugs into metabolites and other biochemistry, development of rating scales and assessments of associations between them, relationships with brain scans, and so on, are better left to other studies, and perhaps more efficient techniques of investigation. Remember Bradford Hill's 'precisely framed question' and attempt to answer it (and little else) as simply and as quickly as possible.

Clinical trials conducted at just one hospital, one clinic or in one practice by a single investigator are termed single-centre trials; by contrast

Box 8.1 Key features of the protocol

- Title, abbreviated title and acronym
- International Standard Randomised Controlled Trial Number (ISRCTN)
- Objectives: primary aims, secondary aims
- Background and rationale
- Medical coordinator – contact details and responsibilities
- Statistical coordinator – contact details and responsibilities
- Local coordinators – contact details and responsibilities
- Other specialists – responsibilities
- Trial office – contact details and staff, including responsibilities
- Period of recruitment (starting and finishing dates) and follow-up
- Baseline information (demographic, psychiatric history, current illness/condition, assessments)
- Inclusion and exclusion criteria
- Consent procedures and audit
- Patient registration
- Trial design (stratification, masking, sample size, safety clause)
- Randomisation
- Administration of treatments
- Safety monitoring
- Methods of patient follow-up
- Assessments and frequency
- Discharge from trial on completion
- Deviations from protocol
- Deaths – post-mortem reports and certificates
- Data handling – data flow, computerisation and summarisation
- Statistical power
- Overview of data summarisation and analysis
- Audit – centres, procedures, data
- Progress reports
- Committees – trial steering committee, trial management committee, data monitoring and ethics committee – membership and responsibilities
- Publications – policy and authorship
- Submission to ethics committees
- Patients' and relatives' information sheets
- Patients' consent forms
- Standardised assessments – instructions for completion and scoring
- Trial forms
- Flow chart for patients
- Flow chart for forms
- Participating centres and local coordinators
- Standard operating procedures.

multicentre trials recruit patients from two, or usually more, sometimes many more, settings. However, the distinction between the two is not always clear and may be confused when patients at just one hospital are entered by several independent physicians or clinics. The protocol must list the principal investigator as well as the collaborating centres, together with the names of the co-coordinating physicians. The number of hospitals/clinics should be justified by sensible estimates of the rates of patient recruitment and the choice of sample size, the latter determined objectively, for example by a power calculation.

The statistical co-coordinator

All clinical trials should be carried out in conjunction with a statistical co-coordinator (aided by a trial manager and data manager), whose functions include those listed in Box 8.2.

These details must appear in the protocol. Ideally it should be possible for an independent team of investigators to take over the organisation and running of a clinical trial to the extent of completing and publishing it as planned, after reading and studying the protocol alone.

The pilot study

Since the conduct of any clinical trial is a very complicated exercise in the management of patients, it is sensible to ensure that important logistic elements in the protocol have been tested adequately before the trial commences. Such testing is often carried out within a pilot study, especially to check the design of forms, the recruitment of patients, indistinguishability of treatments in a masked design, and handling of the data. However, the objectives of a pilot study should not be too ambitious; for example, pilot studies are not suitable for the design of rating instruments – this constitutes a research project in itself!

A pilot study would have identified the problems encountered by Blackwell & Shepherd (1967), who recruited only eight patients out of 518 admitted to the two participating centres. Cook *et al* (1988) encountered problems

---

Box 8.2   Functions of the statistical co-coordinator

- Selection of clinical trial design
- Selection of response (outcome) variables
- Determination of sample size
- Estimation of recruitment rates and number of participating centres
- Design of clinical trial forms
- Design and analysis of pilot studies
- Determination of method of randomisation
- Implementation of selected randomisation scheme
- Checking and computerisation of clinical trial data
- Validation of clinical trial data (audit)
- Preparation of the trial analysis strategy
- Analysis of data
- Summarisation of data and analysis.

---

of organisation, management, conception of treatment and finance. Both reports are highly instructive and worthy of detailed study.

Recruitment rates

The principal difficulty encountered in the design of most trials is the accurate estimation of recruitment rates, even when a pilot study is conducted. Indeed, it is often said ruefully by clinical researchers that if you wish to reduce the impact of a disorder you need only set up a clinical trial of its treatment; all the suitable patients will then disappear! In view of this it is sensible to incorporate a clause within the protocol that allows the abandonment of the trial if the recruitment of patients over an initial specified period is below a designated target.

Sample

Patients entered in a clinical trial form a sample selected from some much larger population. The characteristics of both the population and the sample, as well as the method of selection, must be defined precisely so that the results from the clinical trial can be used in making decisions about the care of future patients. Strictly speaking, the sample should be selected randomly from a defined population, but this is rarely possible in clinical trials for ethical reasons. Consequently it is impossible to establish the specific nature of the population represented by the chosen sample, and necessary to make some broad, although not necessarily unreasonable, assumptions in generalising the results of the clinical trial. Standardised instruments, such as the Brief Psychiatric Rating Scale (Overall & Gorham, 1962) and the Hamilton Rating Scale for Depression (Hamilton, 1967) and Anxiety (Hamilton, 1959), as well as diagnostic instruments such as DSM–IV and the Present State Examination (Wing *et al*, 1974), are useful for characterising patients entered in a clinical trial and may serve in the selection of a reasonably homogeneous sample of patients. The inverse process of deciding whether the results from a trial can guide treatment of a particular patient is a less structured process requiring clinical intuition and judgement.

Entry criteria

The sample and population are specified in terms of inclusion and exclusion criteria, known collectively as entry criteria, that determine the patients who should be considered for entry to the trial, as well as those who are actually entered. There is no specific rule for choosing whether a criterion is inclusive (for example, selecting patients in the age range 20–65 years) or exclusive (leaving out patients less than 20 or older than 65 years). In practice it is convenient to establish the broad category of patients intended to be treated by the inclusion criteria and to use the exclusion criteria to establish contra-indications; examples appear in Table 8.1. The exclusion criteria must embrace patients for whom the caring psychiatrist has a preferred treatment as well as patients who do not consent to randomisation. Patients in either of these two categories inevitably introduce some nebulosity into the entry criteria, since it is extremely difficult to quantify the reasons for a preferred treatment, and virtually impossible to establish the personal reasons for rejecting randomisation. The best that can be achieved is to report the numbers of such patients, as suggested by the CONSORT Statement (Moher *et al*, 2001). Consent to follow-up (not included in the original publications) is now particularly important. The other inclusion and exclusion criteria should be specified precisely using recognised definitions and established instruments.

Data

The information about patients considered for entry into a clinical trial may be divided into several categories: first, the basic demographic data that describe the broad characteristics of the sample, for example gender, age, social class and residence; second, the medical history that summarises relevant aspects of previous diseases and treatments; third, clinical details of the illness or condition that led to consideration for entry to the trial; fourth, monitoring information about the treatment of patients in a trial; and finally, information on the progress of the disease or condition that will form the basis for the comparison of treatments.

Variables

To the statistician, any item of information or characteristic that may vary from one patient to another, or within a patient, from one time to another, is termed a variable. Variables can be subdivided into different types, each of which requires specific methods of summarisation and analysis. The principal types are:
- continuous (e.g. age), which can take any value within a limited range;
- binary (dichotomous), such as gender (male, female) and patient status (in-patient/out-patient), which can take only one of two values;
- categorical (polychotomous), such as hospital of treatment or diagnostic group;
- ordinal, such as age-group or response to treatment (worse, none, improved), where there is a natural ordering of the categories;
- time to event, such as interval from randomisation to either depressive relapse or end of observation period when there is no relapse. These data comprise both the time to event *and* an indicator of whether the event has occurred or not.

Variables can sometimes be changed from one category to another by recoding, thus enabling alternative methods of summarisation and statistical

Table 8.1 Examples of entry criteria for clinical trials

Inclusion criteria	Exclusion criteria
Depression in women in general practice (Corney, 1987)	
Women aged 18–45 years	Major physical ill health
Referred by one of six designated general practitioners	Already under treatment by social worker
	Preferred treatment
Acute depression in previous 3 months or chronic depression intensified in previous 3 months	
Score of 2 or more on Clinical Interview Schedule	
Consent to randomisation and follow-up	
Unipolar depresssion in in-patients and out-patients (Glen et al, 1984)	
Aged 25–65 years	History of mania
Attending/referred to nine designated centres	Contraindication to randomised treatment
Diagnosis of primary depressive illness (defined) lasting at least 1 month	
Consent to randomisation and follow-up	
Confusion in the elderly (Baines et al, 1987)	
Resident at specific local authority home for the elderly	Severe communication problem
Confused	Preferred treatment
Moderate/severe impairment of cognitive function (Clifton Assessment Procedures for the Elderly)	
Consent to randomisation and follow-up	
Out-patients with schizophrenia (Johnson et al, 1987)	
Consecutive out-patients at specific centre, diagnosed with schizophrenia and satisfying Feighner criteria	Organic brain disease
	Physical illness
	Alcohol or substance misuse
Total score of less than 4 on the Brief Psychiatric Rating Scale	Below normal IQ
	Additional mental illness
Maintained on low doses of flupenthixol decanoate for previous year and stable dose not exceeding 40 mg per 2 weeks over past 6 months	Preferred treatment
Consent to randomisation and follow-up	
Melancholia and dysthymic disorder in out-patients (Vallejo et al, 1987)	
Unmedicated psychiatric out-patients attending specific clinics	Severe physical disorder
	Ongoing medical treatment
Aged 18–63 years	Pregnancy
Major depressive disorder with melancholia or dysthymic disorder (DSM–III)	Psychopathic/sociopathic disorder
	Briquet's syndrome
	Alcohol/drug misuse
Hamilton Rating Scale for Depression score of more than 16	Psychotic illness
Consent to randomisation and follow-up	Bipolar, obsessive–compulsive, somatoform, panic, eating, or phobic disorder (DSM–III)

continued

Table 8.1 *continued*

Inclusion criteria	Exclusion criteria
Persistent generalised anxiety (Butler et al, 1987)	
Referrals from specific general practitioners or psychiatric out-patient clinics	Satisfies Research Diagnostic Criteria for phobic, obsessive–compulsive, or major depressive disorder
Generalised anxiety disorder with or without panic disorder as defined by Research Diagnostic Criteria	Chronic anxiety with no period of 1 month in past 2 years of symptoms
Score of 7 or more on Leeds Anxiety Scale	Preferred treatment
Current episode of anxiety lasted at least 6 months	
Consent to randomisation	

Adapted from the papers quoted; not all of them give 'consent to randomisation and follow-up' among the inclusion criteria or 'preferred treatment' among the exclusion criteria.

modelling. For example, rating scales such as the Hamilton Rating Scale for Depression (Hamilton, 1967) can be analysed as continuous variables using the actual (or perhaps transformed) score, as an ordinal variable by recoding into groups (less than 10, 11–19, 20–29 or at least 30) or as a binary variable by defining a cut-off point (less than 15, at least 15).

As well as subdividing variables by types as above, it is convenient in clinical trials to subdivide them according to their status in the analysis. Data about patients collected before randomisation (which is usually taken as the time of entry to a clinical trial), as well as the allocated treatment itself, are called baseline variables; other collective nouns, such as concomitant and independent variables, covariates and covariables, are sometimes used, although some of these have specialised interpretations in the context of statistical analysis. Data collected to assess adherence to treatment, such as tablet counts and blood or serum concentrations, are called monitoring variables, whereas the measures used to assess the effects of treatment, including side-effects, are referred to as response or outcome variables; monitoring and response variables collectively may be called follow-up variables.

Masking

In many clinical trials of treatment, particularly for psychiatric patients, in whom there is some subjectivity in both disease definition and quantification of response, it is necessary to make the assessment of response as objective as possible. In practice this is helped by masking the assessor to the identity of the allocated treatment. Trials in which one assessor (patient or clinician) is masked are called single blind; when both are masked they are double blind. When the results from laboratory assays are reported to the managing physicians in standardised (or coded) units, thus not revealing the identity of the treatment, the trial may be termed triple blind. However, triple blindness may also be used to refer to other aspects of masking, for example not revealing the identity of treatment to the data analysts. Clinical trials where there is no attempt to disguise the nature or form of treatment, either to the patient or to the managing physicians, are termed open studies.

Forms and computers

Information about patients entered into clinical trials is either recorded on specially designed paper forms and later transferred to a computer for storage and analysis (see Chapter 9), or is entered into a computer directly, often using a database that provides an on-screen form image. Each step of the process of eliciting, recording and transferring information may introduce inaccuracies (errors and miscodings) into the data actually analysed, and no amount of checking and rechecking will eliminate all of the errors. The best practice is to simplify each step.

Forms should be designed primarily to aid patient assessment and accurate recording, and secondarily to enable easy transfer of information to a computer; there are a number of principles that should be observed (Wright & Haybittle, 1979; Gore, 1981a; Meinert, 1986). Perhaps the most important are that separate forms should be used for each source of information (one for baseline clinical interview, another for standardised ratings, a third for baseline biochemistry and laboratory assays, and yet others for follow-up information); they should have a unified (same print style), and above all simple, format (not too many items per page), with data entry towards one side, usually the right. The layout of forms for clinical interview should follow the natural order of information retrieval and patient assessment, and standard rating instruments borrowed from external sources should be recast in the style and format of other study forms. Transfer of data to computer (as well as summarisation and analysis) is aided by structuring the form to provide a standardised response to each question and by the liberal use of boxes, either for the recording of numerical information or to be ticked; the boxes should not be too small (at least 8-mm square) and should be aligned both horizontally and vertically.

It should be possible, to transfer information directly from the forms to a computer. This can be achieved with a computer database (for example, DataEase, Epi Info and SPSS Data Entry Station), which may provide an on-screen image of the form itself, or by direct entry to a standard computer file or database (Compact, Excel, Access, Oracle). Before using any database on a personal computer, make sure that the data can be output in a standard (text) file, since this may be required during analysis. Such files should be structured so that they provide a usable manual record; this is achieved by the insertion of a blank field between blocks of data (at least one blank for every 10–15 characters) rather than entering data across every column of the record.

It is not always appreciated that it is unnecessary to convert all information to numerical digits (0–9) in computer records; alphanumeric characters (letters as well as numbers) can be used, are visually informative and help limit coding errors, for example using 'SCH' for schizophrenia, 'ANX' for anxiety, and so on, instead of recoding to numbers such as 01, 02, etc. The recoding can be performed by the computer. Data should be stored in a basic form (date of birth, date of previous admission) rather than a derived form (age, period from last admission) that is subject to the inaccuracies of mental arithmetic; leave the calculations to the computer! Unstructured data, especially unsolicited comments and anecdotal information, should not be entered into a computer file; if desired, its presence on forms can be flagged by an indicator in the computer record. (A blank field for no comment and 1 to denote some comment.) Personal data (name and/or address) that could lead to easy identification of patients from a terminal or printed output should not be entered into the computer; use an identity number in the computer record and keep a master list of names and identity numbers in a secure place.

The ubiquity of personal computers has made their operation familiar to most. However, data summarisation and analysis still pose many problems especially as computer packages (see Chapter 9) enable most users to produce enormous on-screen and paper outputs, much of which will be but vaguely comprehensible to the uninitiated. Older software packages are reliable and still popular but may lack the versatility of more recent packages.

One of the worst problems resulting from the easy availability of fast, cheap computation is the belief that computers can fairly easily summarise and analyse almost unlimited volumes of data, much of it of quite dubious quality. Many clinical trials attempt to collect far too much information, and researchers discover only at the end that their data do not serve the purposes of the study, or that the structure of the data is too complex to provide a convincing analysis. Most would appreciate intuitively that it is difficult to place much reliance on statements about the interrelationships between 100 different items of information collected from just ten individuals, yet in many clinical trials the ratio of variables to patients may still be on this scale. It is sometimes advised that the ratio of patients to variables should exceed five, ten or the actual number of variables. The origin of such rules is obscure and recent recommendations suggest that the number of patients should be at least eight times the number of variables plus fifty (Tabachnick & Fidell, 2001); a more complicated version of this rule also takes account of effect sizes (Green, 1991). It should be remembered that the total score from a rating scale will count as one variable but the analysis of each component item (item analysis) counts as many variables as items.

Stratification

Quite often it is known before the start of a clinical trial that some of the baseline variables influence response to treatment. For example, neurotic and endogenous subtypes of depression affect the response to antidepressants, whereas the interval from onset of schizophrenia to randomisation is related to the recurrence of psychotic symptoms. Such variables are called prognostic variables or prognostic factors.

In any clinical trial it would be unfortunate if a majority of patients with good prognosis were concentrated in one treatment group. Simple comparisons of response between the treatment groups would then be biased by the imbalance of the prognostic factor. One of the purposes of randomisation is to guard against such imbalance and the bias it produces. Since even with randomisation it is possible that there will be some imbalance, investigators often prefer to ensure that the bias from known prognostic factors is minimised by pre-stratification, that is, stratification before randomisation. Essentially patients are split into groups ('strata') defined by the levels (or some combination of levels) of an important prognostic (stratifying) variable; assignment to treatment is then carried out randomly within each stratum. More than one stratifying variable can be chosen, although there is no point in selecting more than three or four. In multicentre trials it is standard practice to pre-stratify patients according to centre, partly because it is likely that patients at one centre will have a different prognosis from those at another and partly to avoid the awkwardness and suspicion that results from treatment imbalances within centres.

As an alternative to pre-stratification, the comparison of treatments can always be adjusted in the analysis for any variable considered of prognostic importance (given sufficient patients in the trial) provided it has been recorded as a baseline variable; this technique is known as post-stratification. In view of this facility some statisticians recommend that large clinical trials should be performed without pre-stratification. However, both pre- and post-stratification are frequently used in the same trial.

Randomisation

It has been acknowledged for many years that the only satisfactory method for assigning treatments in a clinical trial is by randomisation. Today no other method is acceptable, for reasons that are well presented in many textbooks. Here we are concerned not with reasons for randomisation but with just two of the many ways by which the process may be carried out, namely the 'sealed-envelope' technique and the method of minimisation. Whichever method is chosen, it should be set up in consultation with a statistical coordinator who can not only maintain it but also check that the system is not abused. Sealed envelopes are prepared by a statistician and may be used to allocate treatment from a central organisation or at individual centres by the coordinating physicians; the method of minimisation requires a central organisation. When sealed envelopes are distributed to centres it is difficult to maintain a detailed check of whether patients have been entered in the trial or excluded, unless randomisation can be carried out by a department such as the pharmacy, which is independent of the clinical trial. For this reason and others, centralisation of the logging of patient entry and randomisation is much preferred; the entire process can be accomplished efficiently by telephone and hence it used to be known as telephone registration or telephone randomisation. Today it is often implemented using fax, e-mail or the internet.

On entry to a clinical trial, patients are allotted a trial number, which serves as a unique identifier on all records (both written forms and letters, and computer databases). Trial numbers should have a simple format with a constant number of characters. The first character may be a letter used to identify the centre in a multicentre trial. For example, one letter combined with two digits allows 23 centres each entering up to 99 patients. (Note that the letters I, O and Z are excluded to avoid confusion with the numbers 1, 0, and 2.) The trial numbers are then recorded to the same fixed length, for example, B01 (not B1), D12.

The sealed-envelope technique

This technique (Gore, 1981b) was popular in clinical trials with a small number of stratifying factors and a small number of strata; its use has greatly declined over the past decade with the preference for centralised, computerised randomisation. However, for historical reasons (it is encountered in meta-analysis) and because the sealed-envelope technique is mirrored in the computerised randomisation used today, it is presented here. It is usually convenient to number the individual strata sequentially and then prepare a separate batch of envelopes for each. The envelopes are given a serial number within each stratum and ordered sequentially, starting from 1. It is usual to label the envelope with the title of the trial (perhaps abbreviated), the number of the stratum and an abbreviated description of the stratum characteristics, as well as the serial number. Each envelope contains a card labelled with the same information as the corresponding envelope, together with the identity of the treatment allocated. In addition, the cards may have space to enter the patient's name and trial number as well as the date of randomisation; they may be colour coded and used as an index of patients entered in the trial. Envelopes are kept and opened in strictly increasing order of the serial numbers in each stratum; only one envelope is used per patient and is opened only after the decision to randomise treatment has been made. The envelopes are usually destroyed after opening. The treatments designated on the cards are determined using random permuted blocks to ensure that the numbers of patients allocated to each treatment are balanced within each stratum at predetermined, but not necessarily constant, and undisclosed intervals.

The sealed-envelope technique is illustrated in Fig. 8.1 for an open clinical trial of amitriptyline compared with mianserin in patients with manic–depressive psychosis; patients are stratified by centre (hospitals A, B and C), gender and the number of previous episodes of affective disorder (less than three/three or more), giving three stratifying factors with three, two and two levels respectively. The total number of strata is then 12 ($3 \times 2 \times 2$). Thus 12 separate series of randomisation envelopes are prepared. If randomisation is centralised, the 12 series will be kept together at one location, whereas with local randomisation four separate series of envelopes will be distributed to each of the three centres. We assume that 20 patients have been entered in the trial with the characteristics, trial numbers and allocated treatments shown in Table 8.2. The next patient to enter (number 21) is a woman with three previous episodes of affective disorder under treatment at hospital A; being the 12th patient to enter from this centre, she receives trial number A12. Since she is the second female patient at hospital A with at least three affective episodes (a combination that we will assume characterises stratum 4), her treatment is allocated by opening envelope number 2 of the series for this stratum. Figure 8.1 shows that this patient is prescribed A (amitriptyline). Special care is required when using this method in double-blind trials to ensure that treatment is identified uniquely for each patient, so that there is no possibility of disclosure of the treatment given to a whole group of patients if the code is broken for one. When this type of randomisation is implemented on a computer, the output may be just a drug pack number, thus ensuring that the identity of allocated treatment is not disclosed to anyone.

The method of minimisation

An alternative to sealed envelopes (or stratified block randomisation), although one that is still infrequently used, is the method of minimisation (White & Freedman, 1978; Gore, 1981b); this aims to minimise some measure of imbalance between the numbers of patients assigned to the different treatments over each of the stratifying factors and requires centralisation of the randomisation procedure. A separate table is prepared for each stratum and used to indicate the numbers of patients within that stratum assigned to each treatment (usually by the trial number). When a patient is entered into the trial the tables for the corresponding strata are selected, the measure of imbalance is calculated with the new patient assigned to each treatment in turn, and the treatment that leads to the least overall imbalance is allocated.

The method is illustrated for the example above in Fig. 8.2, where the patient to be entered in the trial is again number 21, a woman with three previous episodes of affective disorder under treatment at hospital A. We assume here that our measure of imbalance is just the absolute difference between the total numbers of patients assigned to each treatment summed over the appropriate strata. The three tables for hospital A, women and at

115

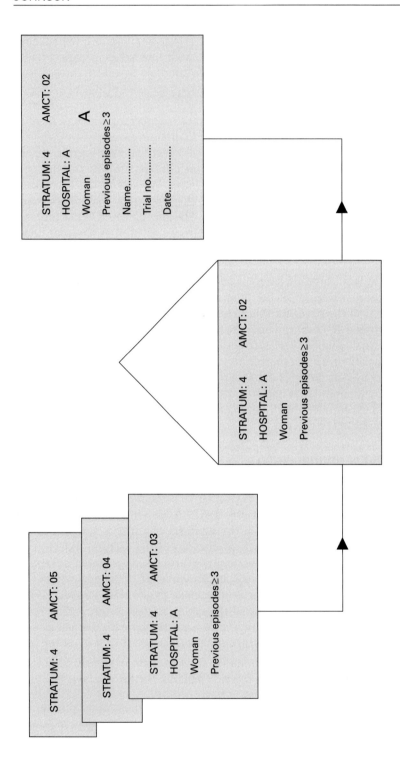

Fig. 8.1 Randomisation by the sealed-envelope technique. The second patient in stratum 4, a woman with three previous episodes of affective disorder under treatment at hospital A is allocated amitriptyline. Abbreviated clinical trial title AMCT.

Table 8.2 Treatment allocations for the first 20 patients entered in a hypothetical clinical trial comparing the efficacy of amitriptyline and mianserin in manic–depressive psychosis

Patient	Hospital	Gender	No. of previous episodes	Trial no.	Allocated treatment
1	A	F	1	A01	Mianserin
2	B	F	1	B01	Amitriptyline
3	A	F	2	A02	Amitriptyline
4	C	M	4	C01	Amitriptyline
5	C	F	2	C02	Mianserin
6	A	M	2	A03	Mianserin
7	A	F	2	A04	Amitriptyline
8	B	M	1	B02	Mianserin
9	A	F	2	A05	Amitriptyline
10	A	F	3	A06	Mianserin
11	C	F	6	C03	Mianserin
12	A	M	3	A07	Amitriptyline
13	C	F	2	C04	Amitriptyline
14	B	F	2	B03	Mianserin
15	B	F	4	B04	Amitriptyline
16	A	M	2	A08	Mianserin
17	A	F	1	A09	Amitriptyline
18	C	F	3	C05	Mianserin
19	A	M	2	A10	Mianserin
20	A	M	2	A11	Amitriptyline
21	A	F	3	?	?

The 21st patient is the 12th to enter the trial from hospital A, the second patient with the combination of characteristics – hospital A, female gender and at least three affective episodes. Her trial number is A12.

least three affective episodes are selected. Assignment of patient A12 to amitriptyline gives imbalances of $7 - 5 = 2$, $8 - 6 = 2$ and $4 - 3 = 1$ in these three tables and a total imbalance of $2 + 2 + 1 = 5$; assignment to mianserin leads to a total imbalance of $(6 - 6) + (7 - 7) + (4 - 3) = 0 + 0 + 1 = 1$. The smaller imbalance is achieved if the patient is assigned mianserin. If the total imbalance had been equal for the two treatments, the allocation could be made using a prepared list of random assignments.

There are many variants of this method, some of them superior to the one described above. It is possible to use alternative measures of imbalance, and to apply different weights to the imbalance for each stratifying factor. In addition, treatment assignment may incorporate biased randomisation

Hospital A			
A	M	A	M
A02	A01		
A04	A03		
A05	A06		
A07	A08		
A09	A10		
A11			

Imbalance with allocation to:
A (amitriptyline)   M (mianserin)
$7 - 5 = 2$ $6 - 6 = 0$

Women			
A	M	A	M
B01	A01		
A02	C02		
A04	A06		
A05	C03		
C04	B03		
B04	C05		
A09			

$8 - 6 = 2$ $7 - 7 = 0$

Previous episodes ≥ 3			
A	M	A	M
C01	A06		
A07	C03		
B04	C05		

$4 - 3 = 1$ $4 - 3 = 1$

Overall imbalance:

5   1

Fig. 8.2 Randomisation by the method of minimisation. Patient 21 (Table 8.2) is allocated mianserin since the overall imbalance of 1 is smaller than the overall imbalance of 5 with amitriptyline.

even when there is overall imbalance, so that the procedure is not entirely predictable, for example using a probability ratio of 0.8:0.2 in allocating treatment to restore balance, rather than the deterministic 1:0.

Design of trials

There are only a few basic designs used in clinical trials, although there are many variations. At one extreme lie the fixed sample size trials, in which the number of patients recruited is decided at the design stage, and at the other extreme lie the fully sequential trials, which proceed until some predetermined termination (or stopping) criterion or rule is fulfilled. With fixed sample size trials, in principle, there should be just one single analysis at the predefined end-point of the study, whereas in sequential trials analysis is repeated as the results of patient assessment become available. In practice, with fixed sample-size trials, especially those including prolonged follow-up or requiring patient recruitment to extend over more than 1 year, there are often repeat ('interim') analyses of response to treatment, which have not been anticipated at the design stage and that make no allowance for multiple 'looks' at the data (multiple comparisons). Such practices are undesirable since they inflate the false-positive (or type I error) rate (see Power and confidence, below). To resolve this problem a class of 'group sequential designs' (Pocock, 1978) was introduced, in which analyses are repeated at regular intervals throughout the trial; the maximum number of analyses is determined at the design stage. Here we restrict attention to just two types of fixed sample-size trial, namely parallel-group and cross-over designs. However, first we introduce some terminology that is common to all trial designs.

Patients

All patients considered for entry to a clinical trial are assessed at a screening examination, which may be extended over a baseline period of observation and evaluation, before randomisation. Patients who do not satisfy the entry criteria for the trial are obviously ineligible and are not usually pursued further; patients who satisfy all the entry criteria except those concerned with agreement to randomisation, and consequently are eligible to participate in the trial, may be subdivided into two groups: those who agree to participate (that is, give informed consent), who become trial entrants, and those who do not consent to take part, sometimes referred to as eligible, non-randomised, patients. Although these latter patients play no further part in the clinical trial itself and certainly cannot contribute to the assessment of efficacy, they are important in defining the population of patients to whom the results of the study may be applied, and should be reported in the CONSORT diagram (see Moher et al, 2001). Keeping a log of these patients as well as details of the baseline variables thus enables the identification of systematic differences between trial entrants and eligible non-randomised patients.

Parallel-group trials

In parallel-group trials patients are allocated at random to one of two, or perhaps more, treatment groups and should be followed-up and assessed in the manner dictated by the trial design. Usually this implies that patients will be followed-up for a set period or until a specific date; long-term trials may incorporate a mixture of the two. The follow-up evaluations include interim assessments after specified periods and final assessments, when patients are formally discharged from the clinical trial; sometimes there are no interim assessments. The information collected at interim assessments is standardised but may vary from one assessment to another; for example, in studies of antidepressant drugs, ratings of the severity of depression may be obtained weekly, whereas biochemistry tests may be performed only every 4 weeks. One basic format is shown in Fig. 8.3. The main analysis of such trials either compares summary measures of response in the different treatment groups, or models and compares the repeated measures (profiles) in the different groups.

An example is provided by Corney (1987), who investigated the effectiveness of a social work intervention in patients with depression in general practice; 80 women who agreed to take part in the clinical trial were allocated randomly to routine treatment by their general practitioners or referral to attached social workers. The women were assessed on entry to the study using the Clinical Interview Schedule (Lewis *et al*, 1988) and

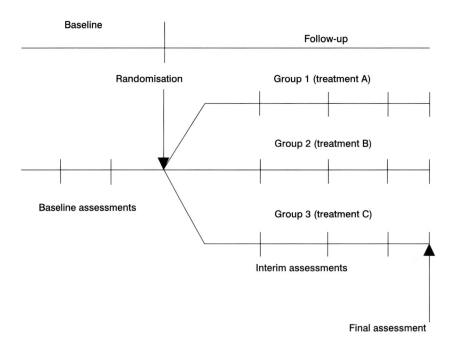

Fig. 8.3 Parallel-group clinical trials. The standard fixed-size three-treatment parallel-group design. Patients are screened, assessed over a baseline period and randomised to one of three treatment groups. The follow-up period may be of set duration as illustrated here or, especially in trials with extended follow-up, may vary from patient to patient.

the Social Maladjustment Schedule (Clare & Cairns, 1978), and reassessed after 6 months and 1 year. A simplified schematic representation (Hampton, 1981) of the results at 6 months is presented in Fig. 8.4.

An example of a different type is a clinical trial of continuation therapy in unipolar depressive illness in which 136 patients were randomly allocated to prophylactic treatment with lithium, amitriptyline or placebo on recovery from a depressive episode, and followed for 3 years or until relapse (Glen *et*

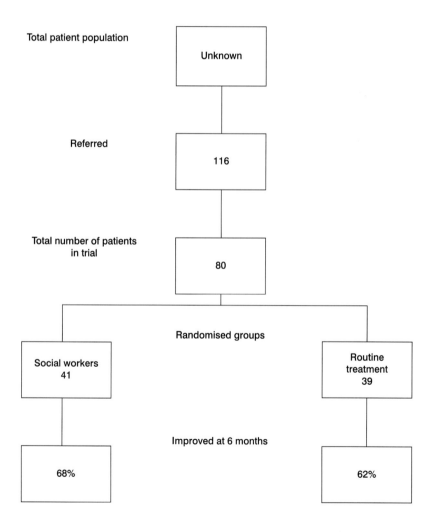

Fig. 8.4 A randomised parallel-group trial of social worker intervention in women with depression in general practice. Patients were assessed at 6 months (and again at 1 year) (for full details see Corney, 1987).

121

al, 1984) (Fig. 8.5). This study demonstrates both actuarial techniques (time to event data) that are particularly relevant for the analysis of clinical trials requiring prolonged observation of each patient and the pragmatic approach of comparing treatment policies by analysis based on 'intention to treat' (see Peto *et al*, 1976, 1977 and Clinical trials in practice, below). The diagram proposed by Hampton (Figs 8.4 and 8.5) is a forerunner of the CONSORT diagram used today and trialists are now required to estimate the size of the trial-eligible population reported in the top box, rather than designating it as unknown. Estimation of the number recorded here may be difficult but may be aided by keeping a log of all patients screened for entry in a trial.

Cross-over trials

In a cross-over trial patients receive more than one treatment and, whereas response in a parallel-group trial is assessed from differences *between* patients in different treatment groups, here the response is assessed from treatment differences within the same patients. Since the treatments are given sequentially within a short time span, they cannot be curative and are best chosen for the treatment of conditions associated with an underlying chronic disease. The basic two-period, two-treatment design is shown in Fig. 8.6. Patients are screened and assessed for entry in a similar manner to the parallel-group study and trial entrants are randomised to group 1, who receive treatment A during period 1 followed by treatment B during period 2, or to group 2, who receive treatment B during period 1 and treatment A during period 2. There is usually a 'washout period' between the two treatments, the main purpose of which is to eliminate the effect of treatment given in period 1 before starting treatment in period 2. The 'washout period' may also be used to repeat some baseline observations so that response to treatment can be expressed in terms of changes from a baseline, rather than in absolute values. The treatment periods are of the same duration and have the same pattern of interim followed by final assessments. The duration of the treatment periods need not be disclosed to patients or assessors, who would then be masked to the actual cross-over period. In principle the design may be extended to include more than two treatment periods, more than two treatments and more than two treatment sequences; such extensions are rare because of the severe logistic problems of actually following up the patients and the difficulties in analysis that result from patient default.

As an illustration, Fig. 8.7 shows the plan of an extended cross-over trial of reality orientation and reminiscence therapy in 15 elderly people with confusion (Baines *et al*, 1987). The five people in group C constitute a parallel control group. The cross-over is formed from the five people in group A, who received 4 weeks of reality orientation followed by 4 weeks without therapy and then 4 weeks of reminiscence therapy, and the five people in group B, who received a similar programme of therapy but with reminiscence therapy first. Five response measures were used and were assessed at 4-weekly

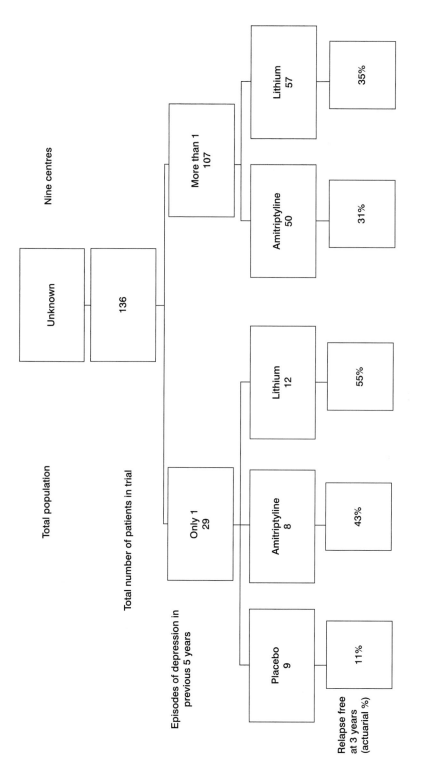

Fig. 8.5 Medical Research Council randomised double-blind parallel-group trial of continuation therapy in unipolar depressive illness. A pragmatic trial analysed by 'intention to treat' with patients followed for 3 years or until relapse (Glen *et al*, 1984).

intervals up to 16 weeks. It should have been appreciated at the design stage that the sample size was inadequate.

Cluster randomised trials

As Bradford Hill emphasised (see quotation on page 107), the randomised clinical trial can be applied to any (form of) treatment – patient education, referral and management strategies, as well as the 'more usual' drugs and psychotherapy. However, with the first three of these, in particular, it is not usually possible to randomise patients, individually, to alternative treatments since the different programmes are set up on an institutional basis and implemented in different general practices or hospitals. Randomising an individual patient could require their attendance at a practice or hospital, which is different from the one they usually attend and perhaps remote from their dwelling; this is not practical.

An example is a trial of the effectiveness of teaching general practitioners skills in brief cognitive–behavioural therapy, compared with usual practice, to treat patients with depression (King *et al*, 2002), in which 84 general practices were randomised to the two 'treatments' and 272 patients within these practices, who scored above threshold on the Hospital Anxiety and Depression Scale (Zigmond & Snaith, 1983), participated. A complication of such trials is that the responses of individuals within a practice (cluster) are correlated and, consequently, are less diverse than the responses of individuals in different practices (clusters). This correlation leads to some loss of efficiency compared with a trial in which patients are randomised

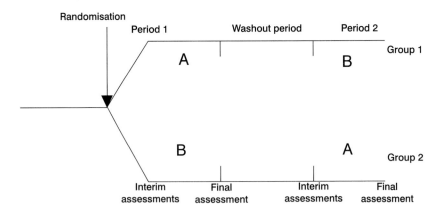

Fig. 8.6 The standard two-period, two-treatment cross-over trial: patients are screened, assessed over a baseline period and randomised to one of two treatment sequences, either treatment A, washout and treatment B (group 1) or treatment B, washout and treatment A (group 2).

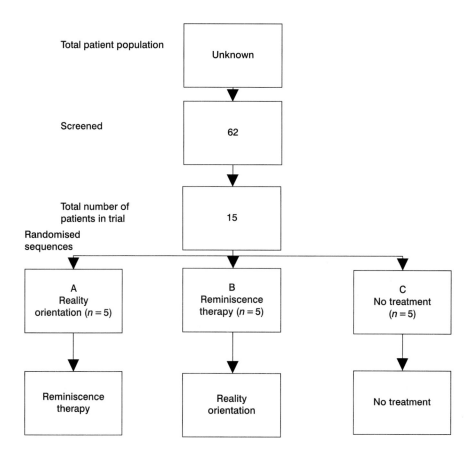

Fig. 8.7 Extended cross-over trial of reality orientation and reminiscence therapy in elderly people with confusion. The first two sequences form the cross-over; the third sequence is a 'no-treatment' control. The treatment periods lasted 4 weeks and were separated by 4 weeks. Assessment of six measures of outcome were made at 4-weekly intervals from the start of the trial (Baines *et al*, 1987). In conventional cross-over trials, only the two randomised treatment sequences are included. The 'no treatment' controls are an elaboration not necessary for the comparison of two forms of therapy.

individually, and this needs to be taken into account in both determination of sample size and analysis. Estimation of sample size requires both the number of practices (clusters) and the number of patients who will participate from each, together with a value for the intracluster correlation, even low values of which can exert a substantial effect. The simplest analysis is based on summary statistics calculated for each cluster; the alternative is to use a two-stage multilevel model for the individual patient data (see Donner & Klar, 2000).

There are two other areas of concern. First, *contamination* that results from sharing of information between the randomised clusters. For example, in trials of patient health education programmes, information provided to the institutions randomised to one treatment group might be circulated to the others. (Of course, individually randomised trials can also be affected by this 'treatment dilution bias'). Second, there might be failure to include *all* eligible patients within a cluster, either because they do not consent or because they are not identified (see Torgerson, 2001). In the trial of King *et al* (2002), for example, some patients who would have scored above threshold on the screening scale may not have been assessed.

Patient preference design

Another recent innovation is the patient preference design, which seeks to resolve the problem of obtaining outcome data for patients who do not consent to randomisation. Provided that they satisfy the other entry criteria, patients are offered any of the treatments under investigation and receive the treatment of their preference; those who do not have a preference are randomised in the usual way; all patients are followed up and assessed as required by the protocol. The analysis then seeks to integrate the data from the non-randomised patients with that from the randomised comparison. An example is a trial in primary care of drug treatment and counselling in patients with major depression (Chilvers *et al*, 2001); 103 patients expressed no preference and were randomised either to six sessions of counselling or to antidepressant drugs; 220 patients had a preferred treatment, 140 opting for counselling and 80 for drugs; outcome was assessed at 8 weeks and 1 year after entry using the Beck Depression Inventory (Beck *et al*, 1961) and the Short Form 36-item questionnaire (SF-36; Ware *et al*, 1993). Analysis compared the four groups at entry, the two randomised groups at 1 year, and in the absence of an interaction between treatment and preference, combined the randomised and patient preference groups to analyse outcomes.

Choice of design

The selection of a specific design for any clinical trial must be decided in consultation with a medical statistician. This discussion focuses not merely on the choice between a fixed-sized or sequential parallel-group design, or cross-over trial, but extends to assessment of response, frequency of data collection, sample size, recruitment period and any of the other functions listed in Box 8.2. Design must be dictated not merely by the diseases and treatments under evaluation but also by the exigencies of clinical practice. None the less there are fundamental differences between the basic designs mentioned above and some guidance about their use may be helpful.

Fully sequential designs (Armitage, 1975) are restricted to the very simple situation where there are just two treatments under comparison by a single measure of response or outcome, and where assessment is fairly rapid, at least by comparison with the period of patient entry. They are designed to provide rapid comparative assessment of outcome, especially when there are important differences in efficacy between treatments. Apart from requiring the specification of a stopping rule, they have two major disadvantages in that it is difficult both to incorporate information on prognostic factors and to assess efficacy on responses other than that selected at the design stage. Their major advantage over a comparable fixed-size, parallel-group trial lies in the exposure of fewer patients to an inferior treatment. Sequential trials have been used very rarely in psychiatry (see Joyce & Welldon (1965) for an interesting yet contentious example and Feely et al (1982) for an example comparing clobazam (a benzodiazepine) with placebo in the suppression of seizures associated with menstruation).

In cross-over trials (Jones & Kenward, 1989; Senn, 2002) at least two treatments are administered sequentially to each patient, and such designs are therefore useless in conditions or diseases such as anxiety and depression, which may be relieved for long and unpredictable periods by treatment. They may be useful in studying relief of side-effects, such as parkinsonism associated with the administration of neuroleptic medication for schizophrenia, or the relief of any acute condition associated with underlying chronic disease. However, they may give rise to ethical problems with the exchange of one treatment for another in patients who benefit from the treatment first administered, and they are complicated by patients who default during the first period of treatment (and are not available to receive the second). Because of problems associated with the prolonged observation of patients, cross-over trials should incorporate treatment periods that are reasonably short and rarely exceed 6 weeks. Their appeal stems from the beguiling assumption that since the differences between treatments are evaluated within patients, they require far fewer participants than a comparable parallel-group study. This may indeed be true but only with quite restrictive assumptions about the absence of differential carry-over effects (Hills & Armitage, 1979; Millar, 1983). The extension of cross-over trials to three or more treatments allows estimation of, and adjustment for, differential carry-over effects from one period of treatment to another, but only at a price of an even more extended trial and the administration of multiple treatments.

By far the most popular of all trial designs is the individually randomised, fixed-sample, parallel-group study that can be adapted, usually quite easily, to the study of any treatment, however complex, in any disease. Most issues of all general psychiatric journals that have appeared over the past 20 years contain at least one example. The design should be the first choice for any clinical trial in psychiatry and should be abandoned in favour of other designs only after careful appraisal. The main practical disadvantage of the design lies in the requirement for comparatively large numbers of patients, which may result in a recruitment period extending over several years. Such problems can be resolved by proper estimation of recruitment rates at the design stage and collaboration between many centres in a multicentre trial.

Clinical trials in practice

No clinical trial is perfect either in design or in execution, for no matter how carefully planned and conducted, the actual behaviour of patients as well as the data collected will be somewhat different from those originally envisaged. Just a few of the problems that should be anticipated are shown in Fig. 8.8. Patients who default during the baseline period before randomisation do not constitute a source of bias in the comparison of treatments, although they do pose a problem for recruitment to the trial if their numbers are substantial. Trial entrants who complete the schedule as detailed in the protocol are sometimes referred to as 'compliers', 'trial compliers' or 'completers', whereas those who do not are 'non-compliers' or 'non-completers'. This second group may be subdivided further into those patients who are followed up and assessed as required by the study design, but whose treatment is changed because of side-effects, those patients who simply do not take treatment as scheduled, and patients who do not complete the scheduled assessments, who are referred to as 'losses to follow-up'. Collectively these patients are 'deviations from protocol' or 'deviations from treatment'; the terms 'withdrawals from treatment' and 'withdrawals from protocol' are also used frequently, but should be avoided since they give the misleading impression that such patients are simply taken out of the trial at the time of deviation and are not followed up further. Occasionally patients who do not satisfy the entry criteria are randomised into a clinical trial; this may arise quite simply by mistake (they are entered in error) or because it later becomes clear that the patients have a different disease or condition from that specified by the protocol.

It is apparent that the problems described above and illustrated in Fig. 8.8 are just those encountered in the routine management of patients under normal clinical care. The designer of any clinical trial will then be faced with a major quandary in deciding whether to eliminate the non-compliers by intensive patient management or simply to assess the treatments as used in practice. Either approach requires elimination as far as possible of the losses to follow-up, for which only death (or perhaps migration) are reasonable excuses.

Explanatory and pragmatic trials

The two extremes are represented by explanatory trials and pragmatic trials. The objective of an explanatory trial is to answer a scientific question about the pharmacological activity of the drug or about the therapeutic value of a specific modality of treatment. Such studies require quite rigid scientific control, with the treatment groups differing only in the specific factor of interest. It can be appreciated that although explanatory studies are necessary for the development of pharmacological treatments, the search for active subcomponents of therapy and for the testing of scientific

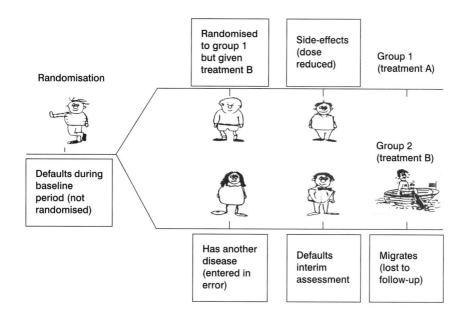

Fig. 8.8 Clinical trials in practice. Some of the problems that arise frequently in practice are illustrated in the context of a two-treatment parallel-group design. Given incorrect treatment, defaults interim assessment and lost to follow-up are deviations from protocol; dose reduction owing to side-effects is a deviation from protocol in a fixed-dose clinical trial but not in a variable-dose study.

theories, they provide limited information about the benefits and problems of treatment in routine clinical use.

Pragmatic trials are designed to answer questions of practical importance in the treatment of patients; they compare the policy of giving one treatment with the policy of giving another by analysing the trial data on the basis of the 'intention to treat', that is, all randomised patients are followed up and assessed as required by the protocol *irrespective* of changes in, or non-adherence to, the prescribed treatment. There appears to be little point in using placebo controls in such trials, since a placebo by itself is not a form of treatment prescribed in routine clinical practice. However, with psychiatric illnesses it is frequently difficult to obtain objective response criteria when the treatment is known, particularly when patients are followed up through interim assessments, so some form of placebo control may be necessary to enable an objective assessment of outcome. At the same time, the difficulties with using placebos should not be underestimated, given that most active treatments are associated with well-recognised side-effects.

A major problem with many clinical trials in psychiatry is that they are conceived and designed as explanatory studies aimed at answering a question of scientific importance (perhaps mainly of academic interest) but in a clinical environment where rigid control cannot be maintained. Protocol deviations, as exemplified by Fig. 8.8, mean that at the end of the study the investigator is faced with a difficult choice: either to abandon those patients who do not conform to the protocol and attempt an explanatory analysis of those who do (a procedure fraught with selection bias) or to abandon the explanatory analysis (and the question of scientific importance) by using all the available data in a pragmatic analysis, which attempts to answer a question of clinical relevance. The design as an explanatory study may vitiate and frustrate this process.

The problem can be resolved only partially. The investigators must summarise *all* known protocol deviations in their report and present an initial analysis of all trial entrants as randomised. Subsequent analyses on subgroups of patients may be conducted and reported, but there must be clear statements about which patients and which data were excluded, so that critical readers can form opinions about the validity of the investigators' claims and their robustness.

Missing data

Apart from deviations from protocol that arise from known changes in treatments and dosages, as well as non-adherence, it should be anticipated that patients may default follow-up assessment, resulting in missing data on treatment and clinical status. Such missing data must be anticipated at the stage of trial design, eliminated as far as possible by efficient follow-up procedures and catered for in the analysis by some method of imputation. More than a small amount of missing data suggests that the trial design, or the instruments chosen for assessment, or the primary outcomes themselves, are inappropriate.

There is a tendency in psychiatric studies to attempt quite frequent follow-up, often with batteries of psychometric tests and other assessments. However, the best tests available will be useless if patients cannot be persuaded to turn up for assessments or decline to undertake them. One solution lies in simplicity: increase the sample size, reduce the number of interim assessments and use a simple measure of response.

Choice of treatments

It is important to heed Bradford Hill's description quoted at the beginning of this chapter (page 107) and emphasise that clinical trials are 'applicable with ... any treatment'. Some may consider the clinical trial solely as a research vehicle for the licensing of new pharmaceutical products. This could not be further from the truth. Any treatment, whether drug, electroconvulsive therapy (ECT), counselling, psychotherapy, diet, intensity of follow-up, referral practice or complementary therapy is amenable to comparative evaluation by a clinical trial. Some argue vigorously that it is important to test scientific theories by looking contemporaneously at different presentations of the same drug, or at (side-chain) modifications of a proven agent, or at different forms of psychotherapy in explanatory trials. So be it, but in phase III studies it is generally worthwhile maximising the difference between the forms of treatment under study and thus answering a question of direct clinical relevance. For example, it is feasible to conduct a pragmatic trial comparing a policy of drug treatment (the exact choice left to each psychiatrist), a policy of ECT (again the specific form left to each psychiatrist) and a policy of psychotherapy (determined by the psychiatrist).

Primary and secondary outcomes

In any clinical trial there are usually several different types of outcome (efficacy, side-effects, quality of life, costs, etc.) and a multitude of ways of assessing them (e.g. many observer and self-completed rating scales for depression). Primary outcomes determine the basic design features of a trial, including its sample size and interval for follow-up, and should be chosen on the basis of objectivity, simplicity (interpretability), practicality and ease of collection. Secondary outcomes are clearly not as important but nevertheless are required to aid interpretation of primary effects, for example, process and active components (mechanism of action). In trials conducted today there are often at least three primary outcomes: efficacy (the comparative extent to which a policy of treatment works in practice), side-effects (the 'downside' of treatment) and costs (to gauge the 'cost-effectiveness' of treatment against a background of competition for scarce resources). Measurement of costs and the derivation of indices of 'cost-effectiveness' within clinical trials have generated much debate as well as much recent research in both economics and biostatistics – see for example the series of occasional 'Economics notes' in the *BMJ* and the two papers: Thompson & Barber, 2000; Thompson, 2002. Secondary outcomes should be chosen to support the primary ones and should be limited severely both in number and in scope.

A sample size (usually statistical power at 90%) calculation (see below) is required for *each* primary outcome (often without any adjustment for multiplicity), with the actual trial size determined by the least sensitive. If these calculations result in a much greater sample size for one of the primary end-points than for the others, then the possibility of using a more sensitive alternative should at least be explored. Once sample size has been determined for the primary outcomes, the sensitivity of each secondary outcome (power to detect specified differences) should also be explored. Any secondary outcome that (after adjustment) does not achieve at least 80% power to detect the relevant specified difference should be replaced or eliminated. The number of secondary outcomes should be restricted (perhaps to five at most), should not introduce an excessive burden on patient assessment, such as could impair assessment of primary outcomes, and should not require major changes to the overall design of the trial as determined by primary outcomes. Patient interviews and assessments must be structured to safeguard assessment of primary outcomes, with provision to sacrifice secondary outcomes if patients are overburdened. It is not unusual for a continuous rating scale to be used for both primary and secondary outcomes: the total scale itself may be primary, with its sub-scales secondary; or one sub-scale may be primary, with the total scale and other sub-scales secondary; or a cut-off point on the total scale may be used as the primary outcome, with the actual score on the continuous scale chosen as the secondary. In this situation it may not be sensible to repeat power calculations on the secondary outcomes; sample size should be determined by the primary measure.

Power and confidence

Many clinical trials and certainly most of those conducted in psychiatry give little if any consideration to the determination of the sample size at the design stage (Freiman *et al*, 1978; Johnson, 1998). Medical journals continue to publish useless studies with too few patients in each treatment group, without any indication of the implication of such sample sizes for the precision of the estimated differences between treatments. Thus one of the most important aspects of clinical trial design, namely the choice of sample size, is not based on some rational calculation but rather is left irresponsibly to be determined by the numbers of patients available at some clinic or hospital, or who can be studied within some convenient set period. One approach to the rational determination of sample size is via the concept of statistical power, which, although not a panacea for subjectivity, should prevent total wastage of valuable patient resources in unethical studies.

As an introduction to this concept we consider, as before, a parallel-group study with two treatment groups, one receiving amitriptyline and the other mianserin, in patients with a history of affective illness and a current episode of depression. We will assume that response to treatment is measured by a dichotomous variable categorised as 'response' or 'no response' on the basis of a clinical rating 8 weeks after randomisation and treatment. It is also assumed from the results of previous studies that about 30% of patients will be judged to respond on this measure. We wish to design a clinical trial that will detect at least a 15% difference in response between the treatments. By this we mean that if the difference in response rates is really as large as 15%, then a (two-tailed) statistical test of the difference in response rates actually observed in the trial will be significant at the 5% level of probability (that is, $P < 0.05$). In practice, as a result of sampling and response variation, we can never be absolutely certain that the observed difference in response rates will be significant at $P = 0.05$, even if there really is a 15% difference in efficacy. If we imagine that there is no difference in efficacy but the trial indicates a statistically significant difference, we will have obtained a false-positive result and committed a type I error, α (alpha); on the other hand, if there really is a difference in efficacy of at least 15% and the difference in the trial is statistically not significant (at $P = 0.05$), then we will have obtained a false-negative result and committed a type II error, β (beta). The best we can hope to achieve in designing the trial is to choose the sample size in such a way that we impose reasonable limits on these two types of error.

The type I error rate, α, is equal to the level of probability chosen for declaring the difference between response rates significant; in this example α is equal to 0.05 or 5%. So there is one chance in 20 of obtaining a false-positive result. If this is considered unacceptable, then we could lower the type I error rate by reducing the P value for significance to 0.01 or 1%. The type II error rate, β, is more difficult to calculate, being dependent upon the type I error, α, the sample size and the difference in efficacy to be detected. In practice, instead of working directly with β, statisticians think in terms of $1 - \beta$, or $100(1 - \beta)$, which is called the power or sensitivity of the trial. In our example, it is the probability that the outcome of the trial will be statistically significant at $P = 0.05$, given that there is at least a 15% difference in response rates. For most statistical tests, tables are available that show the power of the test to detect specified differences for a given β and sample size, as well as tables that show the required sample size to achieve selected power for specified differences and given α (Machin *et al*, 1997). Table 8.3 is an extract chosen to illustrate the example we are considering. In designing a clinical trial, we should select the power $1 - \beta$ to be at least 0.80 (and preferably 0.90), so that there is a chance of one in five or less (or one in ten or less) of missing an important difference between treatments. (The survey by Freiman *et al* (1978) demonstrates that the power of published studies to detect substantial differences is often very low; see also Johnson (1998).) It can be seen from Table 8.3 that with $\alpha = 0.05$, $\beta = 0.20$, power $= 1 - \beta = 1 - 0.20 = 0.80$, we require about 160 patients per treatment group. If we increase the power to 90%, giving a chance of one in ten of a false-negative result, then 220 patients per treatment group are required; if, in addition, α is reduced to 0.01 (i.e. 1%), then 240 patients per treatment group are required for a power of 80% and 305 patients per treatment group for a power of 90% (not shown in Table 8.3). If we are interested in detecting smaller differences in response rates, say of the order of 10%, then we require correspondingly larger sample sizes (with $\alpha = 0.05$ and power 80% we need 360 patients and with power 90% we require 480 patients in each treatment group). Compare these with the actual sizes of published trials!

When calculating the sample sizes necessary to achieve given type I and type II error rates, for specific response rates and differences between them at the design stage, we should also investigate the power of a given clinical trial to detect specific differences under alternative, imagined outcomes. Such calculations may be important in interpreting non-significant results. In Table 8.4 we show some hypothetical results from a clinical trial. Note

133

that the response rate in the amitriptyline group is in line with the expected response rate of 30%, whereas that in the mianserin group is 50%, a difference between treatments of 20%. From Table 8.3 we can see that with 40 patients per group the trial has a power of just over 40% to detect a 20% difference in response rates given that such a difference exists. So a non-significant χ^2 test is no surprise! With half this number of patients and similar response rates the situation is rather worse; now there is only about 25% power of detecting a 20% difference. Indeed, there is 50% power (an even chance!) of detecting a difference of 30% in response rates given that such a difference exists. With double the numbers of patients, that is 80 per treatment group, we have over 70% chance of detecting a real difference of 20%.

How should we interpret the results in Table 8.4(a), (b) and (c)? The temptation, indeed the usual practice, is to interpret a non-significant test as synonymous with no treatment difference. This is utterly fallacious! Instead of merely reporting the results of tests of statistical significance, we need to report the precision of our estimate of the difference in response rates for the two treatments. This can be done by giving a 95% confidence limit for the difference (Gardner & Altman, 1986). We note from Table 8.4 that the differences between response rates are always 50%–30% or 20%; the 95% confidence limits for this difference are −9% and 50% for Table 8.4(b), −1% and 41% for Table 8.4(a) and 5% and 35% for Table 8.4(c). The lesson is obvious. As the sample size increases, the precision of the estimate of the difference between treatments increases – the width of the 95% confidence interval decreases from 59%, through 42% to 30%. With small numbers

Table 8.3 Numbers of patients required in each of two groups to detect changes in response rates of 10%, 15% and 20% when the smaller response rate is 30% at a significance level $\alpha = 0.05$ (two-tailed)

Power	Difference in response rates		
(%)	10%	15%	20%
20	55	25	15
30	95	40	25
40	130	60	35
50	175	80	50
60	220	100	60
70	280	125	75
80	360	160	95
90	480	220	125

Example: to have 80% power of detecting a change in response rates from 30% to 45% requires 160 patients in each group.

our estimates of the difference between treatments are very imprecise and certainly insufficient to guide clinical practice.

Although the example above is centred on a dichotomous response variable, similar calculations can be performed for a continuous variable. The only complication is that we need to have an estimate of the variation in response. Let us assume that in the clinical trial in our example above, the Hamilton Rating Scale for Depression (HRSD; Hamilton, 1960) is used to assess affective status. We can assume that randomisation will balance the distribution of baseline HRSD scores in the two treatment groups and so use the scores after 8 weeks as our measure of response. The mean scores in the two groups at 8 weeks will then be compared with a t-test. Assume that we require 80% power to detect a difference of six points on the HRSD between treatment groups at $P = 0.05$ (smaller differences will be hard to detect and may not be clinically impressive). To carry out our sample size calculation we need an estimate of the standard deviation of the distribution of HRSD scores at 8 weeks. This information should be available from previous studies but we will assume estimates of 4, 6 and 8 units. Dividing the required difference of 6 units by the standard deviation provides a standardised difference or an effect size; here the effect sizes are 1.5, 1.0 and 0.75, respectively. Tables of the numbers of patients needed to achieve given power for set values of α and different values of the effect size are available (Machin et al, 1997). These indicate

Table 8.4 Hypothetical results from a clinical trial of the comparative efficacy of amitriptyline and mianserin

		Amitriptyline	Mianserin	Total
(a)	Response	12	20	32
	No response	28	20	48
	Total	40	40	80
	$\chi^2 = 3.3$, d.f. = 1, $P > 0.05$			
(b)	Reponse	6	10	16
	No response	14	10	24
	Total	20	20	40
	$\chi^2 = 1.7$, d.f. = 1, $P > 0.05$			
(c)	Response	24	40	64
	No response	56	40	96
	Total	80	80	160
	$\chi^2 = 6.7$, d.f. = 1, $P < 0.01$			

Response rates in amitriptyline and mianserin groups are 30% and 50% respectively.

χ^2 not corrected for continuity.

that we need group sizes of about 8, 17 and 30 for the three situations to achieve 80% power and 10, 22 and 40 for 90% power. In fact these sample sizes should be regarded with some caution since in practice HRSD scores at 8 weeks may not be normally distributed, thus invalidating direct application of the *t*-test to the raw scores. A square-root or logarithmic transformation may be necessary. In addition HRSD scores may also be obtained at interim assessments, say at weeks 1, 2, 4 and 6, in which case the analysis will become a repeated-measures analysis of variance with treatment differences assessed from the test for interaction effects, with a consequent increase in power; alternatively a global summary measure (such as the area under the score profile) could be used and may be preferable (Matthews *et al*, 1990).

With multiple-response variables the probability of a false-positive result (type I error) will be increased. So some adjustment for multiple comparisons may be necessary to retain an overall type I error rate α of about 5%. This will inflate the necessary sample size. One approach, known as the Bonferroni method (Godfrey, 1985), is to divide the overall type I error rate α by the number of response variables and use the resultant P value as the level of probability for declaring statistical significance. For example, with five response variables and $\alpha = 0.05$ (overall type I error rate), each response variable would be assessed using $P = 0.05/5 = 0.01$. There is some disagreement about when and how to adjust for multiple comparisons. In practice, primary outcomes, assuming there are not more than two or three, are often tested individually at $P = 0.05$ and adjustments for multiplicity are reserved for secondary outcomes (see Primary and secondary outcomes, above).

Apart from allowance for multiple comparisons, the sample size derived from a power calculation at the design stage should be increased by about 10% (not more) to account for loss to follow-up. If it is anticipated that loss to follow-up will amount to more than 10%, then the whole strategy for follow-up assessments should be re-examined with the specific intention of reducing it.

Equivalence trials

Most clinical trials seek to establish differences between two or more treatments or between different doses or intensities of the same treatment. Sometimes such differences may not be expected, for example when comparing two different drugs within the same class, such as two selective serotonin reuptake inhibitors. It must also be remembered that a non-significant difference between treatments in a clinical trial does not establish that the treatments are equivalent. Instead of designing trials to establish (very) small differences, trials are designed to demonstrate that the treatments are equivalent within defined limits (equivalence trials) or that one treatment is not moderately worse than another (non-inferiority trials). The latter is particularly useful when one treatment is much more expensive than another but slightly more efficacious. The principles underlying this type of trial are discussed by Jones *et al* (1996). The design of trials of this type requires specification of the average expected success (or failure) rate, the maximum allowable clinical difference for equivalence, sometimes called the limits for equivalence (for example, within 10%), a confidence level that is usually 5% (two-sided) for an equivalence study and 5% (one-sided) for non-inferiority trials, and finally a probability for demonstrating equivalence – this is analogous to power in significance testing and is set to at least 90%. Results are reported as a difference (or some other comparative summary statistic) in response rates between treatments with a 95% confidence interval. The treatments are accepted as equivalent if the limits of this confidence interval lie within the specified limits of equivalence or as non-inferior if the lower limit of the confidence interval falls short of the maximum allowable difference. Statistical significance testing plays no part in the analysis of these trials. Trials of this type require substantial sample sizes, usually in excess of 250 patients per group, a target that can be reduced substantially by widening the limits of equivalence from 10% to 15%, or even 20%. Such practices make no sense! In psychiatry, differences between treatments of 15% are substantial and treatments should not be accepted as equivalent within this limit; trials should adopt the 10% criterion.

Analysis

I have commented already on some of the important issues in the analysis of data collected during clinical trials; here I reiterate these and comment briefly on a few more, but for a full discussion the reader is referred to the list of further reading cited at the end of this chapter.

The first point to re-emphasise is that to carry out a sensible and informative analysis it is necessary to have a sufficient quantity of high-quality data. No amount of skilful adjustment or manipulation will compensate for more than a small amount of missing information. In psychiatric studies in particular, there is a tendency to collect far more data than can be justified by the sample size. Investigators should elect at the design stage to ask of every single item of information that it is intended to seek, whether it is essential; the objective should be to eliminate at least 50% of it. During the trial itself, there must be determined efforts to obtain the information required; there is no excuse for more than a tiny number of missing values on baseline variables, whereas missing values on response variables, especially the primary outcome(s), indicate that an alternative method of assessment is required. The first analysis conducted and reported should include all randomised patients and should reflect (at least initially) all features of the design including pre-stratification. Adjustment of the response variables for differences between treatment groups on distributions of baseline variables (post-stratification) should be made if such adjustment is considered important. The baseline variables for which to adjust should not be chosen on the basis of statistical significance tests comparing randomised groups; such tests are uninformative (Altman, 1985); they should be agreed by consensus as part of trial design.

When further analyses are reported it must be clear to the reader exactly which patients have been excluded and why. Treatment differences should be summarised not just by the results of statistical significance tests but in terms of 95% confidence limits for the difference, or relative risk. The power of the clinical trial to detect specified differences between treatment groups should be stated.

In many clinical trials patients are categorised as responders or non-responders, followed by attempts at analysis of baseline variables to distinguish one group from the other. Few clinical trials are sufficiently large to warrant such abuse and the practice should be abandoned, except perhaps within the context of a meta-analysis (National Heart, Lung and Blood Institute & National Cancer Institute, 1987).

The statistical analysis strategy

Since there are many ways of (a) analysing and summarising even a single outcome variable, (b) subdividing the total sample into different groups, (c) selecting baseline variables on which to adjust the outcome and (d) imputing missing values, the process of analysis is prone to subjective judgement and open to criticism that key decisions may be made in favour of, or against, one of the treatments. To circumvent such allegations, it is now becoming established practice to develop and document a complete analysis strategy prior to examination of the trial data; the strategy document should be approved by the trial management committee and the trial steering committee. Although the trial protocol will give a broad overview of the methods to be employed, it does not present sufficient detail to drive the complete analysis.

The statistical analysis strategy sets out on a variable-by-variable basis exactly how the data will be manipulated, analysed and summarised, at least for the primary (and usually secondary) outcomes. Once written, the main analysis of the trial data is reduced to following prescribed steps. The principal contents are shown in Box 8.3.

Although it is important that the conclusions drawn from a clinical trial are not subject to bias resulting from subjective, data-dependent decisions, it is also important that research data are used to their full potential, including the generation of ideas for future research studies. Data collected in clinical trials are frequently a resource for research projects, including theses, in both clinical medicine and biostatistics. The statistical analysis strategy is not intended to curtail these but it should require that the potentially subjective basis of such (exploratory) analyses is acknowledged.

Box 8.3 Prescribed steps for the main analysis of the trial data

- Basic principles underlying the analysis strategy
- Summary of the basic trial design, including randomisation
- Baseline data collected
- Follow-up data collected
- Descriptive analyses – representativeness of trial sample, baseline comparability of randomised groups, quality of therapy, adherence to therapy, inadvertent unmasking, losses to follow-up, available data, reliability of data
- Specification of groups for analysis – definition of intention to treat and per protocol samples
- For each primary (and secondary) outcome – definition, handling of missing values, imputation, methods of analysis and summarisation, covariates for adjustment
- Interaction tests between baseline characteristics and treatments (if intended)
- Examination and handling of differences between centres (if intended).

Meta-analysis

We have seen from the earlier discussion that many, perhaps most, of the clinical trials conducted in psychiatry are too small to provide reasonable power of detecting clinically important differences between treatments; they provide only rather imprecise estimates of comparative efficacy and cost-effectiveness. The solution to this problem is to conduct larger trials that have been specifically designed to provide meaningful results. However, the conclusions from a single trial, even a large one, usually require replication, preferably by further studies conducted in different centres and in other countries. Two trials with the same protocol, recruiting similar patients in a single hospital, will not yield identical estimates of comparative efficacy; however, they may be expected to yield estimates that are broadly comparable in magnitude. Several independent trials of the same treatments (or the same class of treatments), conducted in different centres and perhaps with different entry criteria, would be expected to exhibit more variation in outcome.

An important problem is how to summarise the information obtained from similar studies and when to synthesise it to form a broad overall conclusion. Before 1980, the solution was to write a mainly descriptive but critical (narrative) review article that set out and commented on the main characteristics of (sometimes arbitrarily) chosen studies, including their merits and demerits, and then attempted to integrate their results in a way that provided a convincing conclusion of the effectiveness (or ineffectiveness) of one of the studied treatments. The integration was sometimes an act of balancing significant and non-significant P values, which, as we have seen already from Table 8.4, does not provide a useful approach.

Since the mid-1970s, the need to formalise the process of review, to make it more objective and therefore accessible to scientific scrutiny has become widely appreciated. The result has been the emergence of a new discipline, which under the sobriquet of 'meta-analysis' has made an enormous impact, especially in medicine. There is now an extensive research literature linked to several hundred meta-analyses (or overviews as they are sometimes called). Here it is not possible to explore the subject in depth; interested readers will find methodological aspects in the books by Hedges & Olkin (1985), Wolf (1986), Egger *et al* (2001), Sutton *et al* (2000) and Whitehead (2002) and broad discussion centred on specific meta-analyses in the proceedings of a workshop (National Heart, Lung and Blood Institute & National Cancer Institute, 1987). An excellent example is provided by an overview of 25 randomised trials of antiplatelet treatment in over 29 000 patients with a history of transient ischaemic attacks, occlusive strokes, unstable angina or myocardial infarction (Antiplatelet Trialists's Collaboration, 1988).

Meta-analysis is a technique for combining the results from a collection of randomised clinical trials to provide an objective overview of their conclusions, usually in the form of one or more global measures of comparative efficacy or cost-effectiveness. Since these global measures are estimated from comparatively large numbers of patients, they will be much more precise than the estimate available from any single trial and consequently more likely to yield clinically useful results. Indeed, when comparing the incidence of rare events such as mortality in some trials, the thousands of patients included in a meta-analysis may provide the only method of demonstrating a small advantage for one treatment; and a small advantage translates into many lives worldwide. In addition, meta-analysis sometimes allows specific subgroup analyses, for example to examine dose effects or the response of patients characterised by specific disease presentation; such analyses are not feasible within a single trial because of small sample sizes. Of course, subgroup analyses should be defined in the meta-analysis research protocol and not appear as an interesting afterthought.

It must be strongly emphasised that meta-analysis is not a 'back-of-an envelope' exercise but a time-consuming and labour-intensive research investigation conducted according to a proper protocol for which there are established guidelines (Gerbarg & Horwitz, 1988; Boissel *et al*, 1989); it is also an area of controversy (Thompson & Pocock, 1991). Once the objectives of a meta-analysis of treatment efficacy have been established, there follows: (a) an intensive literature search to find all eligible published randomised clinical trials (those with historical or concurrent, non-randomised controls do not qualify because of selection and allocation bias); (b) contact with authors and other relevant investigators to seek information about eligible trials that have never been published (in an attempt to guard against the bias of publishing 'positive' ($P < 0.05$) results); (c) contact with all trialists to seek additional information, especially about randomised patients excluded from analysis, as well as details not appearing in published papers (if possible, obtain copies of the original data and do not assume automatically that published analyses are correct); (d) selection of the measures of treatment response (these should be obtainable for all trials); (e) selection of comparative summary statistics with which to quantify the results of each trial (for example effect sizes and odds ratios together with 95% CI); (f) selection of a statistical model for the variation of treatment effects among trials (fixed or random), as well as a strategy for examining heterogeneity and deciding whether an overview is feasible; (g) selection of a method of actually combining the separate effects to produce the overview (preferably through an underlying statistical model of the treatment effects themselves, rather than combining P values or test statistics); (h) clear presentation of the overview results as demonstrated by the study of antiplatelet treatment referred to above.

Some examples in psychiatry include a meta-analysis of 19 double-blind placebo-controlled trials of antidepressants and benzodiazepines v. placebo in (an unspecified number of) patients with panic disorders (Wilkinson *et al*, 1991); another of five randomised trials (in 99 patients) of lithium v. placebo augmentation in the acute treatment of depression (Austin *et al*, 1991); and more recently, a meta-analysis of 14 clinical trials (in 324 patients) of transcranial magnetic stimulation for the treatment of depression (Martin *et al*, 2003). Adams *et al* (2001) conducted a 'meta-review' by synthesising the findings from Cochrane reviews of depot antipsychotic drugs for people with schizophrenia; they found that depot antipsychotics are safe and effective, but also indicated that large trials are needed to examine longer-term outcomes. Finally, Stimpson *et al* (2002) performed a systematic review of clinical trials investigating pharmacological and psychological interventions for treatment-refractory depression and found that there is little evidence to guide the management of this illness. The conclusions from these last two reviews, that large pragmatic trials are still needed, exemplify another objective of meta-analysis, namely to establish whether or not yet more trials are required. Indeed, a systematic overview should be both the starting point and the finishing point for any clinical trial, the former to justify that it needs to be done, the latter to examine the effects of its results upon the evidence base.

One further remark is pertinent to forestall any misconceptions about meta-analysis. An individual clinical trial must satisfy relevant design criteria. In particular, as already remarked several times, a trial must have reasonable power to detect or eliminate a clinically important difference between randomised treatments; trials that cannot achieve this are unethical and constitute a waste of resources for both patients and doctors. No trial should be undertaken solely on the premise that although it cannot contribute much to clinical knowledge by itself, it may none the less be incorporated along with others in a meta-analysis.

141

Conclusion

The psychiatrist who wishes to conduct a clinical trial should seek advice from at least three experts: first, from a psychiatrist who has performed a clinical trial and can anticipate many of the clinical problems; second, from a doctor with experience of clinical trials in another medical discipline who can view the trial within the wider context of medicine; and finally, from a medical statistician (with some knowledge of psychiatry) who can tackle the problems of design and sample size. (Finding one may not be easy but they are around – see for example the Directory of Academic Statisticians (at http://www.swan.ac.uk/statistics/das/). To those who wish to proceed, it is hoped that these notes and the references at the end of the chapter will prove useful.

References

Adams, C. E., Fenton, M. K. P., Quraishi, S., *et al* (2001). Systematic meta-review of depot antipsychotic drugs for people with schizophrenia. *British Journal of Psychiatry,* **179**, 290–299.

Altman, D. G. (1985) Comparability of randomized groups. *Statistician,* **34**, 125–136.

Antiplatelet Trialists' Collaboration (1988) Secondary prevention of vascular disease by prolonged antiplatelet treatment. *BMJ,* **296**, 320–331.

Armitage, P. (1975) *Sequential Medical Trials* (2nd edn). Oxford: Blackwell.

Austin, M. P., Souza, F. G. & Goodwin, G. M. (1991) Lithium augmentation in antidepressant-resistant patients: a quantitative analysis. *British Journal of Psychiatry,* **159**, 510–514.

Baines, S., Saxby, P. & Ehlert, K. (1987) Reality orientation and reminiscence therapy: a controlled cross-over study of elderly confused people. *British Journal of Psychiatry,* **151**, 222–231.

Beck, A., Ward, C., Mendelson, M., *et al* (1961) An inventory for measuring depression. *Archives of General Psychiatry,* **4**, 561–571.

Blackwell, B. & Shepherd, M. (1967) Early evaluation of psychotic drugs in man: a trial that failed. *Lancet,* ii, 810–822.

Boissel, J. P., Blanchard, J., Panak, E., *et al* (1989) Considerations for the meta-analysis of randomised clinical trials. *Controlled Clinical Trials,* **10**, 254–281.

Butler, G., Cullington, A., Hibbert, G., *et al* (1987) Anxiety management for persistent generalised anxiety. *British Journal of Psychiatry,* **151**, 535–542.

Buyse, M. E., Staquet, M. J. & Sylvester, R. J. (eds) (1984) *Cancer Clinical Trials: Methods and Practice.* Oxford: Oxford University Press.

Chilvers, C., Dewey, M., Fielding, K. *et al* (2001). Antidepressant drugs and generic counseling for treatment of major depression in primary care: randomized trial with patient preference arms. *BMJ,* **322**, 772–775.

Clare, A. W. & Cairns, V. E. (1978) Design, development and use of a standardised interview to assess social maladjustment and dysfunction in community studies. *Psychological Medicine,* **8**, 589–604.

Cook, C. C., Scannell, T. D. & Lipsedge, M. S. (1988) Another trial that failed. *Lancet,* i, 524–525.

Corney, R. H. (1987) Marital problems and treatment outcome in depressed women: a clinical trial of social work intervention. *British Journal of Psychiatry,* **151**, 652–659.

Donner, A. & Klar, N. (2000) *Design and Analysis of Cluster Randomization Trials in Health Research.* London: Arnold.

Egger, M., Smith, G. D., Altman, D. G. (eds) (2001) *Systematic Reviews in Health Care: Meta-analysis in Context*. London: BMJ Books.

Everitt, B. S. & Wessely, S. (2004) *Clinical Trials in Psychiatry*. Oxford University Press.

Feely, M., Calvert, R. & Gibson, J. (1982) Clobazam in catamenial epilepsy: a model for evaluating anti-convulsants. *Lancet*, ii, 71–73.

Freiman, J. A., Chalmers, T. C., Smith, H., *et al* (1978) The importance of beta, the type II error and sample size in the design and interpretation of the randomized control trial. Survey of 71 'negative' trials. *New England Journal of Medicine*, **299**, 690–694.

Gardner, M. J. & Altman, D. G. (1986) Confidence intervals rather than P-values: estimation rather than hypothesis testing. *BMJ*, **292**, 746–750.

Gerbarg, Z. B. & Horwitz, R. I. (1988) Resolving conflicting clinical trials: guidelines for meta-analysis. *Journal of Clinical Epidemiology*, **41**, 503–509.

Girling, D. J., Parmar, M. K. B., Stenning, S. P., *et al* (2003) *Clinical Trials in Cancer: Principles and Practice*. Oxford: Oxford University Press.

Glen, A. I., Johnson, A. L. & Shepherd, M. (1984) Continuation therapy with lithium and amitriptyline in unipolar depressive illness: a randomized, double-blind, controlled trial. *Psychological Medicine*, **14**, 37–50.

Godfrey, K. (1985) Comparing the means of several groups. *New England Journal of Medicine*, **313**, 1450–1456.

Gore, S. M. (1981a) Assessing clinical trials – record sheets. *BMJ*, **283**, 296–298.

Gore, S. M. (1981b) Assessing clinical trials – restricted randomization. *BMJ*, **282**, 2114–2117.

Green, S. B. (1991) How many subjects does it take to do a regression analysis? *Multivariate Behavioural Research*, **26**, 499–510.

Guiloff, R. J. (ed.) (2001) *Clinical Trials in Neurology*. London: Springer-Verlag.

Hamilton, M. (1959) The assessment of anxiety states by rating. *British Journal of Medical Psychology*, **32**, 50–55.

Hamilton, M. (1960) A rating scale for depression. *Journal of Neurology, Neurosurgery and Psychiatry*, 23, 56–92.

Hamilton, M. (1967) Development of a rating scale for primary depressive illness. *British Journal of Social and Clinical Psychology*, **6**, 278–296.

Hampton, J. R. (1981) Presentation and analysis of the results of clinical trials in cardiovascular disease. *BMJ*, **282**, 1371–1373.

Hedges, L. V. & Olkin, I. (1985) *Statistical Methods for Meta-analysis*. London: Academic Press.

Hill, A. B. (1955) *Principles of Medical Statistics* (6th edn). London: Lancet.

Hills, M. & Armitage, P. (1979) The two-period crossover clinical trial. *British Journal of Clinical Pharmacology*, **8**, 7–20.

Johnson, D. A., Ludlow, J. M., Street, K., *et al* (1987) Double-blind comparison of half-dose and standard-dose flupenthixol decanoate in the maintenance treatment of stabilised out-patients with schizophrenia. *British Journal of Psychiatry*, **151**, 634–638.

Johnson, T. (1998) Clinical trials in psychiatry: background and statistical perspective. *Statistical Methods in Medical Research*, **7**, 209–234.

Jones, B. & Kenward, M. G. (1989) *Design and Analysis of Cross-over Trials. Monographs on Statistics and Applied Probability*, 34. London: Chapman and Hall.

Jones, B., Jarvis, P., Lewis, J. A., *et al* (1996) Trials to assess equivalence: the importance of rigorous methods. *BMJ*, **313**, 36–39.

Joyce, C. R. & Welldon, R. M. (1965) The objective efficacy of prayer: a double-blind clinical trial. *Journal of Chronic Diseases*, **18**, 367–377.

King, M., Davidson, O., Taylor, F., *et al* (2002). Effectiveness of teaching general practitioners skills in brief cognitive behaviour therapy to treat patients with depression: randomised controlled trial. *BMJ*, **324**, 947–950.

Lewis, G., Pelosi, A. J., Glover, E., *et al* (1988) The development of a computerized assessment for minor psychiatric disorder. *Psychological Medicine*, **18**, 737–745.

143

Machin, D., Campbell, M. J., Fayers, P., *et al* (1997) *Sample Size Tables for Clinical Studies* (2nd edn). Oxford: Blackwell Science.

Machin, D., Day, S. & Green, S. (2004) *Textbook of Clinical Trials*. Chichester: Wiley.

Martin, J. L. R., Barbanoj, M. J., Schlaepfer, T. E., *et al* (2003) Repetitive transcranial magnetic stimulation for the treatment of depression. *British Journal of Psychiatry* **182**, 480–491.

Matthews, J. N., Altman, D. G., Campbell, M. J., *et al* (1990) Analysis of serial measurements in medical research. *BMJ*, **300**, 230–235.

Meinert, C. L. (1986) *Clinical Trials: Design, Conduct and Analysis*. Oxford: Oxford University Press.

Millar, K. (1983) Clinical trial design: the neglected problem of asymmetrical transfer in crossover trials. *Psychological Medicine*, **13**, 867–873.

Moher, D., Schulz, K. F., Altman, D. G., for the CONSORT Group (2001) The CONSORT Statement: revised recommendations for improving the quality of reports of parallel-group randomised trials. *Lancet*, **357**, 1191–1194.

National Heart, Lung and Blood Institute & National Cancer Institute (1987) Proceedings of Methodologic Issues in Overviews of Randomized Clinical Trials Workshop. *Statistics in Medicine*, **6**, 217–409.

Overall, J. E. & Gorham, D. R. (1962) The brief psychiatric rating scale. *Psychological Reports*, **10**, 799–812.

Peto, R., Pike, M. C., Armitage, P., *et al* (1976) Design and analysis of randomized clinical trials requiring prolonged observation of each patient. I. Introduction and design. *British Journal of Cancer*, **34**, 585–618.

Peto, R., Pike, M. C., Armitage, P., *et al* (1977) Design and analysis of randomized clinical trials requiring prolonged observation of each patient. II. Analysis and examples. *British Journal of Cancer*, **35**, 1–39.

Pocock, S. J. (1978) The size of cancer clinical trials and stopping rules. *British Journal of Cancer*, **38**, 757–766.

Senn, S. (2002) *Cross-over Trials in Clinical Research* (2nd edn). Chichester: Wiley.

Stimpson, N., Agrawal, N. & Lewis, G. (2002). Randomised controlled trials investigating pharmacological and psychological interventions for treatment-refractory depression. Systematic review. *British Journal of Psychiatry* **181**, 284–294.

Sutton A. J., Abrams, K. R., Jones, D. R., *et al* (2000) *Methods for Meta-Analysis in Medical Research*. Chichester: Wiley.

Tabachnick, B. G. & Fidell, L. S. (2001) *Using Multivariate Statistics* (4th edn). Boston: Allyn and Bacon.

Thompson, S. (ed) (2002) Statistical methods in cost-effectiveness analysis. *Statistical Methods in Medical Research*, **11**, 453–551.

Thompson, S. G. & Barber, J. A. (2000) How should cost data in pragmatic randomised trials be analysed? *BMJ*, **320**, 1197–1200.

Thompson, S. G. & Pocock, S. J. (1991) Can meta-analysis be trusted? *Lancet*, **338**, 1127–1130.

Torgerson, D. J. (2001) Contamination in trials: is cluster randomization the answer? *BMJ*, **322**, 355–357.

Vallejo, J., Gasto, C., Catalan, R., *et al* (1987) Double-blind study of imipramine versus phenelzine in melancholia and dysthymic disorders. *British Journal of Psychiatry*, **151**, 639–642.

Ware, J. E., Snow, K., Kosinksi, M., *et al* (1993) *SF–36 Health Survey Manual and Interpretation Guide*. Boston, MA: Health Institute.

White, S. J. & Freedman, L. S. (1978) Allocation of patients to treatment groups in a controlled clinical study. *British Journal of Cancer*, **37**, 434–447.

Whitehead, A. (2002). *Meta-Analysis of Controlled Clinical Trials*. Chichester: Wiley.

Wilkinson, G., Balestrieri, M., Ruggeri, M., *et al* (1991) Meta-analysis of double-blind placebo-controlled trials of antidepressants and benzodiazepines for patients with panic disorders. *Psychological Medicine*, **21**, 991–998.

Wing, J. K., Cooper, J. E. & Sartorius, N. (1974) *The Description and Classification of Psychiatric Symptoms: An Instruction Manual for the PSE and Catego Systems*. Cambridge: Cambridge University Press.

Wolf, F. M. (1986) *Meta-Analysis: Quantitative Methods for Research Synthesis*. London: Sage Publications.

Wright, P. & Haybittle, J. (1979) Design of forms for clinical trials. *BMJ*, ii, 529–530; 590–592; 650–651.

Zigmond, A. S. & Snaith, R. P. (1983) The hospital anxiety and depression scale. *Acta Psychiatrica Scandinavica*, **67**, 361–370.

Further reading

Altman, D. G., Machin, D., Bryant, T. N., *et al* (eds) (2000) *Statistics with Confidence* (2nd edn). London: BMJ Books.

Altman, D. G., Schulz, K. F., Moher, D., *et al* (2001) The revised CONSORT statement for reporting randomized trials: explanation and elaboration. *Annals of Internal Medicine*, **134**, 663–694.

Chalmers, T. C., Smith, H., Blackburn, B., *et al* (1981) A method of assessing the quality of a randomised clinical trial. *Controlled Clinical Trials*, **2**, 31–49.

Chaput de Tonge, D. M. (1977) Aide-memoire for preparing clinical trial protocols. *BMJ*, i, 1323–1324.

Day, S. (1999) *Dictionary for Clinical Trials*. Chichester: Wiley.

Duley, L. & Farrell, B. (eds) (2002). *Clinical Trials*. London: BMJ Books.

Everitt, B. S. & Pickles, A. (1999) *Statistical Aspects of the Design and Analysis of Clinical Trials*. London: Imperial College Press.

Friedman, L. M., Furberg, C. D. & Demets, D. L. (1998) *Fundamentals of Clinical Trials* (3rd edn). New York: Springer.

Good, C. S. (ed.) (1976) *The Principles and Practice of Clinical Trials*. Edinburgh: Churchill Livingstone.

Good, P. I. (2002) *A Manager's Guide to the Design and Conduct of Clinical Trials*. Hoboken, New Jersey: Wiley.

Gore, S. M. & Altman, D. G. (1982) *Statistics in Practice*. London: British Medical Association.

International Conference on Harmonisation. *ICH Harmonised Tripartite Guideline E9: Statistical Principles for Clinical Trials*. http://www.ich.org/

Karlberg, J. & Tsang, K. (1998) *Introduction to Clinical Trials: Clinical Trials Research Methodology; Statistical Methods in Clinical Trials; The ICH GCP Guidelines*. Hong Kong: The Clinical Trials Centre, University of Hong Kong.

Matthews, J. N. (2000) *An Introduction to Randomised Controlled Clinical Trials*. London: Arnold.

McFadden, E. (1998) *Management of Data in Clinical Trials*. New York: Wiley.

Medical Research Council (1998) *MRC Guidelines for Good Clinical Practice in Clinical Trials*. London: MRC.

Mosteller, F., Gilbert, J. P. & McPeek, B. (1980) Reporting standards and research strategies for controlled trials. *Controlled Clinical Trials*, **1**, 37–58.

Piantadosi, S. (2005) *Clinical Trials: A Methodologic Perspective* (2nd edn). New York: Wiley.

Pocock, S. J. (1983) *Clinical Trials: A Practical Approach*. Chichester: Wiley.

Raven, A. (1993) *Clinical Trials: An Introduction* (2nd edn). Oxford: Radcliffe Medical Press.

Redmond, C. & Colton, T (eds) (2001) *Biostatistics in Clinical Trials*. Chichester: Wiley.

Senn, S. (1997) *Statistical Issues in Drug Development*. Chichester: Wiley.

The *BMJ* has published several series of papers. Each series has a variable number of papers published in different issues of the *BMJ*. Series include: *Understanding Controlled Trials*; *Methods in Health Services Research*; *Meta-analysis*; *Systematic Reviews in Health Care*; *Measuring Quality of Life*; *Getting Research Findings into Practice*; *Economic Notes*; and *Statistics Notes*. The series can be found at http://bmj.bmjjournals.com/series

CHAPTER 9

Using computers in research

Chris Freeman, Patricia Casey, Ula Nur and Peter Tyrer

This chapter is intended primarily for the new researcher who is not totally familiar with the handling of data. Computer enthusiasts and experienced researchers generally tell you that computers are easy to use and will save you a great deal of research time. This may be true when you are familiar with a particular statistics package, but it certainly is not so at the start. You will almost certainly find yourself wondering why you every bothered to try to use a computer at all and, unless you have a lot of data, you will probably find that on your first attempt it will take you longer to learn the system, prepare the data in the correct way and analyse the results than if you had done the whole thing by hand. For large amounts of data, whether they are studies with many participants or studies with a lot of data for each participant, computers are the only real answer. If, however, you have only 30 or 40 participants and 15–20 variables, you may find it much simpler to do things by hand, using a pocket calculator and paper and pencil, although this is no longer wise. Many calculators can perform simple descriptive statistics and carry out χ^2 and t-tests and the equivalent non-parametric tests. With few data the main reasons for using a computer would be either to learn the system for future use or to carry out certain statistical manipulations that would be difficult or impossible without the aid of a computer.

Even if you decide not to use a computer, it is a good idea to collect and code your data as if they were going to be used in this way. Whatever system you use, you will have to convert all your data into numbers and preparing a proper coding sheet, as described below, allows you to do this in a systematic way.

Using a computer – easy steps

The first steps are outlined in Fig. 9.1. First you will have to prepare your data in a particular way and this is dealt with more fully below. Each item of information you collect will need to be converted into a number and 'coded'.

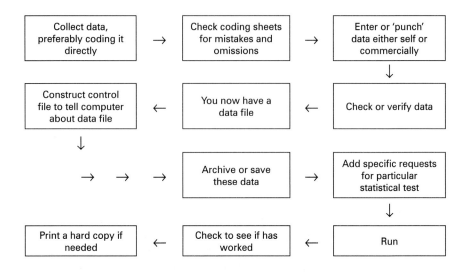

Fig. 9.1 The steps in using a computer to analyse data

Wherever possible, you should arrange for the coding to be part of the questionnaire that you are using, rather than have separate coding sheets. Each time you transpose the data, say from your original questionnaire to a coding sheet and then from the coding sheet to a computer, the chances of introducing errors increase. Even when you are using self-rating questionnaires that are given to patients, you can arrange for the coding to be down the right-hand margin (to be folded if you do not wish the patient to see the scoring system). Once your data have been coded, you will need to check for accuracy to ensure that there are no items of missing data or obvious mistakes, such as people being coded as age 12 when your study protocol states that the minimum age for entry to the study was 18 years. Next you have to enter the data on to a computer. If you have large amounts of data, it is best to organise for this to be done professionally. Entering large amounts of data is very tedious and it really is not cost-effective for you to be doing this. There are commercial organisations that will prepare and enter your data and they will almost certainly do it more accurately than you would have done. For a small extra charge you can ask for your data to be 'verified'. This usually means that the data are entered twice by two separate computer operators and then each item is cross-checked by the computer. The term 'punching' is often used for this process. This comes from the time when punch tape or punch cards with small holes were used as a means of entering data.

Once your data have been entered you will have what is called a data file. On a printout this will look just like horizontal columns of figures. The computer can do nothing with these data until it is given instructions about what the figures represent. Programs such as Excel, Access and the Statistical Package for the Social Sciences (SPSS) will already have asked for data definition, but there are still benefits from having a simple text file provided that it is properly coded.

Recording data

One of the most infuriating aspects of research is to forget to record data at an interview and then find out later, long after the event has passed, that the data are missing. It is therefore desirable to establish a fairly simple sequence of forms together with checklists to ensure that all the relevant data have been collected. It is particularly important to check patients' self-ratings immediately after they have been recorded to ensure that all the appropriate questions have been answered and that there have been no confusing responses (e.g. two or more items ticked when only one was requested). This will allow the relevant amendments to be made at the time. Remember, once the patient has left the interview room the opportunity has been lost and if you attempt to fill in the missing data you will be guessing at best or will be biased at worst.

Initially most data are recorded on record forms and ideally are simultaneously coded so that they can be transferred directly to a computer (e.g. by keeping a copy that converts the response into a number). Most trainees will not have this degree of help and it is often useful to cut out a template of the form with the numbered scores next to the individual responses to aid the scoring system.

Checking the accuracy of your data

No matter how careful you have been, there will be mistakes in your data. Some mistakes you will never be able to discover. For example, if someone has been coded as aged 47 rather than 45, you will not be able to see this mistake unless you check each item by hand, which will take you as long as, if not longer than, entering the data all over again. There are some simple things that you can do to check the accuracy of your data. You could leave some columns in your coding sheets blank so that if numbers are present in these columns when coding is complete then something has been miscoded. A common mistake is for each item of data to be one column out because a key has been pressed twice. You could also make some simple visual checks. For example, if column 43 is where information about in-patient or out-patient status is coded, and you know that in-patients were coded 1 and out-patients coded 2 and no other codes were used, then you can run your eye down that particular column and make sure it contains only 1s and 2s. Another way of checking your data is to run the data through a program that gives simple descriptive statistics such as maximum and minimum values and ranges. This will allow you to check that you have no obvious mistakes, such as patients with scores on the Hamilton Rating Scale for Depression (HRSD; Hamilton, 1967) of 87 when the maximum score is 40 or patients aged 99 when the oldest patient in your study was 65. Other items are relatively simple to check; for example, if your study has 60 patients, 30 in an experimental group and 30 in a control group, check that the computer has the correct numbers recorded in each group.

There is a tendency for the inexperienced trainee to collect too many rather than too few data from each patient. This needs to be addressed at the planning/writing stage, but when recording the results it will come up again. The danger is that the trainee, having collected many data with a great deal of effort, often feels it necessary to code and store every single item on a computer file in the hope that something of interest may turn up when the data are analysed. Although there are a few exceptions when important new information is derived from data that was not originally considered important (perhaps the discovery of penicillin might be one example), in general the collection of too many data impedes subsequent analysis and creates a great deal of extra work.

Separating manual and computer records

After checking the coding sheets for errors or omissions, the data necessary for computer analysis need to be coded. Although ideally the hand-recorded data should be automatically recorded on a form that can be directly fed into the computer, this can be a mixed blessing, as quite frequently data can be further simplified before entering into a computer.

Problems in coding

There are many elementary errors that can make coding of data much more complicated and difficult than it would otherwise be. These can be discussed under seven headings.

Data recorded in wrong order

Many data in research are collected to fit in with the needs of a clinical interview or with other practical considerations and may not look satisfactory when recorded directly on a record form. This does not matter; as long as each variable is correctly identified, it makes absolutely no difference in which order they appear on the computer file. People often have problems in adapting to changes in order; computers do not.

Too many data

This problem has already been mentioned. There is a general statistical rule of thumb when analysing data that a ratio of at least 5 to 1, and preferably 10 to 1, between the number of patients and number of variables being analysed is ideal. Thus if the data are collected on 200 patients, about 20 key variables need analysis. This does not mean that the total number of variables studied should be limited to 20 or less, since other variables may be used later to examine other aspects of the study such as outcome. However, it does mean that the major analysis should be limited to that number. For example, in Fig. 9.2 the investigator may be interested in whether the living circumstances (column 12) influence the outcome of depressive illness treated by different methods. The data in column 12 can therefore be used to split the total population of patients with depression into four groups that can then be analysed separately.

However, there is a limit to this sort of exercise, which at the level of publication is known as 'salami slicing', which is again determined by the number of patients. If the number is small, then separating the total into four or more groups is likely to lead to such small numbers in each analysis group that the analysis is hardly worth carrying out.

An irritating minor problem is to allocate too few columns for data when preparing the coding key. If you think that a patient might score over 100 for an item (so that three columns of data are necessary), then allow for this in advance. If you are mistaken you have lost nothing; if you have to create an extra column later, the rest of the data will need to be recoded.

Another consideration is the tendency to create type 1 errors (false-positives) purely because so many different analyses are being carried out. The investigator needs to bear in mind continually that statistics is concerned with probabilities and if apparently random data are analysed, 1 in 20 of the comparisons is likely to be significant at $P<0.05$ and 1 in 100 significant at $P<0.01$. This complicates interpretation of the results and it is preferable to avoid this confusion by reducing the number of variables before analysis.

Often extra data that are not envisaged at first are added later. Quite apart from spoiling the variable/case ratio, this adds to the problem of interpretation. Often investigators can only be cajoled into helping in an investigation if they can do a 'small project' of their own choosing. Such 'add-on' studies should be avoided wherever possible.

Coding errors

By leaving blank columns in the data file (Fig. 9.3) some errors can be detected. Another simple way of reducing errors is to leave the coding of data until the time of analysis. For example, column 16 in Fig. 4.2 (marital status) could be coded by letters (single=S, married=M, separated/divorced=D, widowed=W) and these letters later converted into the appropriate numbers before analysis. On the data file (Fig. 9.3) the columns of letters stand out in the same way as blank columns and errors are detected easily.

Before analysis it is also wise to check the distribution of the data to ensure that the scores are within the correct ranges. For example, if the total score

Study no.	☐	☐	☐	☐	Cols 1–4
Card no:				☐	Col 5
Interviewer:				☐	Col 6
Date of birth (27.2.56)					
Code as weeks and year	☐	☐	☐	☐	Cols 8–11

Living circumstances
       Lives alone=1
       Lives with family of origin=2
       Lives with partner=3
       Lives with children=4

Not known (missing data)=9	☐	Col 12

Educational attainment
Code in number of years of continuous education

Not known=99	☐	☐	Cols 13–14

Who referred for help
       General practitioner=1
       Other specialist=2
       Self-referral=3
       Other=4

Not known=9	☐	Col 15

Marital status
       Single=1
       Married=2
       Separated/divorced=3
       Widowed=4

Not known=9	☐	Col 16

Length of time from GP referral
to being seen by specialist
Code as number of weeks
       Not applicable=88

Not known=99	☐	☐	Cols 17–18

Number of previous episodes of depression
       None=1
       One to three=2
       Four to six=3
       Seven or more=4

Not known=9	☐	Col 20

Initial HRSD score

0–17 items	☐	☐	Cols 21–22
18–21 items	☐	☐	Cols 23–24
Total score	☐	☐	Cols 25–26

Treatment group
       Antidepressant therapy=1
       Cognitive therapy=2

Social work therapy=3	☐	Col 31

HRSD score after 4 weeks

0–17 items	☐	☐	Cols 32–33
18–21 items	☐	☐	Cols 34–36
Total score	☐	☐	Cols 36–37

Fig. 9.2 Example of coding sheet used to obtain background information for a study of depressive illness in general practice

on the HRSD (columns 25–26) shows a maximum of 89 and a minimum of 0, the higher score must be an error, as it exceeds the maximum score on the scale. Identification of scores that differ from the others (outliers) is valuable because a certain proportion of these are likely to be errors.

Missing data

Missing data are a major source of problems. The data may be missing because they were not collected in the first place or have been lost. Apart from reducing the likelihood of this by having checklists at the beginning or end of the record forms, it is necessary for someone to monitor missing data and repeatedly remind investigators of the need to obtain these. This usually makes the monitor extremely unpopular, but the bliss of avoiding 'data nagging' is such that missing data are kept to a bare minimum.

Sometimes missing data are unavoidable (e.g. patients who drop out from a clinical trial). In such cases, space needs to be set aside in the computer file for these data so that they can be coded accordingly. If this space is not made available, the computer will 'read' the file as though the data that follow those that are missing are the numbers it is looking for. Thus, in Fig. 9.3 the data from the last row are all missing and have been recorded appropriately. If the file ended at column 19, the computer would look for the first seven digits of the next line to place as 'data' and would therefore misrecord all subsequent items of information.

Missing values should be coded clearly; a different code should be given to items left missing (i.e. where the participant refused to answer, skipped the question by mistake, items were not asked or were irrelevant for the specific participant). Unfortunately missing data cannot be avoided in medical, epidemiological and other fields of research, even if great effort is put into planning the study and data collection. These difficulties have led researchers to think about developing methods to handle missing data when faced with this problem (Dempster *et al*, 1977; Little & Rubin, 1987).

Input ignorance

If, as is commonly the case, the researcher decides not to put data into the computer file directly but employs a commercial organisation or a research assistant to input the data, it is important to realise that the data clerk is bound to be ignorant of many aspects of the data. It is therefore wise to be absolutely certain of the data file before it is handed over for data input.

It can be almost guaranteed that a handwritten record form given to a data clerk for conversion to a computer file will be entered incorrectly in the first instance. This is because the investigator assumes knowledge of the data that the data clerk does not have. This can include:

- assumption of knowledge that appears to be self-evident (e.g. the case number in Fig. 9.3 when repeated measurements are used)

- assuming that a code has already been allocated for missing data but not actually put down on the record form
- non-allocation of space for missing data
- ambiguity of information, such as recording '1 or possibly 2' for data, in which case the data clerk has no means of knowing which is preferred
- simple misreading of long lists of numbers which have no intrinsic meaning.

In view of this, and the universal availability of personal computers and data organisers, it is much better to make an immediate record of the data roughly in the form in which it is to be entered, preferably as a simple numerical file (e.g. Fig. 9.3) together with a coding key. It does not matter if this file is saved in a word processing program; the additional information necessary for word processing can be removed from this before analysis when it is saved as a simple text file.

Unnecessary calculation

Frequently the investigator is tempted to perform calculations on data before computer entry. Thus, for example, the mean score of a set of variables that is already being coded is calculated as an additional variable. When the score is a single figure (e.g. the HRSD score) it is very simple to add up the total,

001713	08563131299	3240428	1203
			462
001724	62949912106	4199641	
001736	29941212107	9999999	
001811	12495991403	3190019	1101
			538
001821	64399216401	4921199	
001832	11121349612	6413911	
001912	14634141302	1280129	1101
			123
001923	21299461666	1 2129969	
001933	11234671432	9999999	

Fig. 9.3 Example of a data file based on the coding shown in Fig. 9.2. All data are missing from the last row and are coded accordingly. Column 19 has been left blank. The number 1 entered in this column is a mistake. Four blank columns separate the follow-up data.

but when the individual scores are larger or when complicated algorithms are used to derive a research diagnosis, there is no point in calculating this separately. It is much more convenient to enter the data on to the file and subsequently to write a short program to do the necessary calculations (without any errors) as the first stage in analysis.

Post-hoc analyses

There is another error that is easy to commit after all data have been collected. The investigator is so proud of his work that he wishes to see the maximum benefit extracted from it. If the main analyses show no new findings of significance then, there is a temptation to dredge through the data to find some meaning. Do not do this unless you have a clear hypothesis beforehand.

What software will I need?

To use your computer for research the minimum requirements are:
- a word processing package
- a program for producing a spreadsheet
- a statistical package
- a graphics package.

The first thing to check is what local agreements there are either within the Health Service or within your local university department to make software available at a cheap rate. Many universities buy site licences for software, which means that a package whose full price might be £500 can be obtained for less than £100 per annum. Please note that many licences have to be renewed on an annual basis. Remember that software is copyright protected and it is illegal simply to copy your friend's. Pirated software is also the main route by which computer viruses are spread.

Do not become a software junkie. Most modern software packages are extremely powerful and flexible and take time to learn properly. Stick to two or three well-tried packages and do not clutter up your hard disk with things that you will probably never use.

Word processing

This should be the first software package that you buy because it will allow you to write letters, alter page layouts, check your spelling, keep address lists, etc. The power of word processing packages has increased markedly in the past few years and most now allow you to construct tables, import pictures or graphs and do some of the tasks one would expect from a desktop publishing package. The market leader at present is undoubtedly Microsoft Word. It is usually wise to use updated versions of Microsoft Windows when they become available, as these are usually genuinely improved versions and have better protection against viruses.

A reference management system

Although this is not on the above list, we would recommend that this is the second piece of software you buy. This software allows you to store and retrieve references in a standard format which looks on the screen a bit like a file card. The management system can sort references alphabetically or numerically but most importantly can transform the reference style to comply with a huge range of different journal formats. You will save hours of time and effort if you begin to collect and type in your references on a reference management system. Reference Manager (http://www.refman. com), now in version 11, is the most frequently used. It allows the searching of internet databases and can organise references into any journal format, which is a boon when resubmitting papers to different journals.

Spreadsheets and databases

Many of the functions of these two pieces of software overlap and you may decide that you can do without one or the other. A spreadsheet is just as it sounds, it really is a huge flat table which can be up to thousands of columns wide and thousands of lines long. It is a means of entering and storing numerical and simple alphabetical data. Spreadsheets allow you to carry out simple statistics and transformations on the data and often quite complex calculations between various columns. Many were designed for use in financial planning rather than biomedical research. The better ones allow importing and exporting of data from many sources, including text files and many statistical packages. The best examples are Excel and Lotus 123, which are available for both PC and Macintosh systems. You may find that if you buy one of the statistical packages described here you will not need a spreadsheet because these come built into the statistics package.

Databases are best considered as series of files stacked in a filing cabinet drawer, each individual having a separate sheet. They allow the collection and recording of much more comprehensive data. Sophisticated packages, such as Filemaker-Pro, can be arranged so that your computer screen looks identical to your hardcopy questionnaire, with data entered in much the same way. The database can reorder your patients numerically or alphabetically, select certain subgroups from the population and produce tables of age, gender or summary data of any of the variables you have entered. Again, checking the ability of the database to import and export data from other sources is important. Other examples are d-BaseIV, FoxBase and 4th Dimension.

Statistical packages

SPSS

SPSS is Statistical Package for the Social Sciences and is available for all major operating systems. It is an excellent package for handling many data and can deal with thousands of variables on thousands of cases. Many beginners enjoy using this package because it is very easy to use. The package has a good data editor, which allows the user to enter data and attributes easily (i.e. missing values, value labels, etc). Although all the statistical analysis and graphics can be carried out using pull-down menus, this package also allows the user to write programs using the command syntax. SPSS carries out a wide variety of statistical manipulations and is good at summarising and presenting data graphically. SPSS introduced multilevel modelling, a procedure for data with hierarchical or nested structure, in its versions SPSS 11, 12.

STATA

STATA is a powerful statistical package, which can also be used as a programming language. STATA has a number of versions for different operating systems, for example Windows, LINUX, Macintosh and UNIX. Although this statistical package was mainly command driven, pull-down menus for most of its applications and routines were introduced in its latest versions, STATA 8 and 9 (http://www.stata.com). The software comes with a comprehensive manual on procedures and commands, which documents easy-to-follow examples on how to use and interpret most of the statistical techniques supported by the package. One can also review the implemented commands and options using a very efficient help system. The graphics were the major limitation of STATA. However, the graphics were greatly improved for STATA 8. The new graphics provide a more attractive design and much more programming flexibility.

SAS

This once stood for Statistical Analysis Software and was introduced in the 1970s to analyse agricultural data. It is a highly efficient system but is not usually recommended for individual researchers starting out on a research programme.

BMDP

BMDP stands for Biomedical Data Processing, a package from the University of California. It has recently been purchased by SPSS, Inc. and is now relatively little used.

Other packages

Recently a number of very powerful statistical packages have appeared. These include S-PLUS, which uses the S language for statistical applications. It is not recommended for beginners.

Writing and submitting your paper

Much of the focus in this chapter has been on the benefits of using computers for data coding and analysis. However, there are other benefits for researchers. All university libraries and their associated hospitals have computer links. Online access to most of the journals held by the library is available to university departments on request. The library must be contacted in order to open an account for your department. In some circumstances it may also be possible for a university employee to open such an account for use at home. Thus you will be able to read papers online, take copies and download to your reference manager, all from your own desk.

It is worth bearing in mind that many international journals are now computerised. Most now only accept papers online, although others continue to combine this with postal methods. Unfortunately, the user-friendliness of online submission varies greatly, with some being simple (consisting of a basic e-mail system) but others being frustratingly difficult to navigate. Some journals require prior registration to use this facility. However, a telephone call to the journal manager, who will talk you through the procedure, can save hours of time. Close scrutiny of the journal's instructions to authors also helps.

Conclusions

This has been only a very brief introduction to the use of computers and the only way to learn is to sit down at a keyboard and practise. As well as producing statistical analyses, computers can help you in other ways. There are some very sophisticated graphics packages now available which will allow you to display your data in many different ways. Once you have entered your data on to a mainframe computer you can store them safely and keep them for many years. Most mainframe systems have an archiving storage facility to allow you to do this. You can also move your data around the country. There is a network called JANet (Joint Academic Network) that links Edinburgh, Newcastle, Cambridge, Manchester, Bristol, Exeter, Southampton, Oxford and London universities. There are gateways from this network to Europe and to America, so you can take your data with you if you move or even if you emigrate. At present, the main sources for further information on using computers for statistical analysis are the statistical manuals themselves. I do not know of any book that sets down the principles in a simple way for the first-time user. It is unfortunate that many of these manuals assume a great deal of prior knowledge about computing and statistics. If you are going to use computers on a regular basis, it is best that you try to become familiar with one statistical package and ask for help if you need to use other packages. Many university departments run regular computing courses aimed at learning a specific package, and it is worth enquiring at your nearest department of computer science about such courses.

References

Dempster, A. P., Laird, N. M. & Rubin, D. B. (1977) Maximum likelihood from incomplete data via EM algorithm. *Journal of The Royal Statistical Society. Series B (Methodological)*, **39**, 1–38.

Hamilton, M. (1967) Development of a rating scale for primary depressive illness. *British Journal of Social and Clinical Psychiatry*, **6**, 278–296.

Little, R. J. A. & Rubin, D. B. (1987) *Statistical Analysis with Missing Data*. New York: Wiley.

SPSS (2003) *SPSS Base 12.0 User's Guide*. Chicago, IL: SPSS.

Stata Corporation (2003) *Stata Release 8.0*. College Station, TX: Stata.

CHAPTER 10

Principles of psychological assessment

Simon Gilbody, Stephen Morley and Philip Snaith

The aims of this chapter are threefold: to provide the reader with an introduction to basic issues that surround measurement of psychological and behavioural variables; to provide a series of guidelines that potential researchers may use when setting up projects (throughout this chapter the reader will find checklists that summarise major points); and to provide a useful bibliography for those who wish to explore the issues of psychological assessment in more depth.

Background

Research in psychiatry covers a very wide range of problems and raises a variety of measurement problems, which include: case identification; assessing the severity of a disorder; assessing personality, mood, intellectual performance and behavioural activity; and assessing outcomes of treatment. Measures may be required to categorise people on salient dimensions or to index change during therapeutic trials. To meet these demands a series of techniques is used, ranging across observer rating scales for interviews, behavioural observation studies, self-rating scales for personality and mood measurement, and self-monitoring methods (usually 'diaries'). Measures may have group-referenced norms, which enable a person to be located with respect to a defined target population, or, at the other extreme, personal questionnaire techniques that provide sensitive measurement tailored to one person may be used. Given this range of measurement problems and methods, is it possible to provide a framework by which the researcher can evaluate their requirements, select an appropriate measure and interpret the results that arise from their investigation?

The concepts of validity and reliability, developed by psychometricians, provide such an evaluative framework and have great utility; this chapter provides an overview of these concepts and shows that they are closely intertwined and can be placed within the notion of 'generalisability' which has so far not penetrated psychiatric research. In addition, the appropriation of standardised psychological instruments as measures of outcome –

especially in clinical trials – has required that the notion of sensitivity to change be added to validity and reliability when examining the utility of an instrument. Each of the issues of validity, reliability and sensitivity to change will be explored in this chapter, with illustrative examples drawn from the literature.

Validity

On beginning research one is often asked to state whether a selected measure is reliable and valid. Generally this question is misleading because it implies that there are single indices of reliability and validity, and that the measure is reliable and valid for all occasions on which it is used. It also implies that a test has inherent validity. This is strictly not true; what is validated is an interpretation of data obtained by the test under specified conditions, and a test that has validity under one set of measurement conditions may not be valid when applied to another problem in another context, although the situation may be superficially similar. Validity is explored from a number of perspectives which are outlined below.

Content validity

Content validity is concerned with whether the instrument adequately probes the specific domain that one requires; that is, does it measure what it purports to measure? For example, a test of mathematical reasoning would have no content validity as a measure of verbal ability (although it may have considerable predictive validity and construct validity – see below). Content validity is a serious problem in psychiatry, especially as when making a diagnosis one must consider the selection of appropriate symptoms, the required level of severity of the symptoms and the time frame in which these symptoms are to be measured (Williams *et al*, 1980). A scale will have content validity if it does not contain elements that could be attributable to other processes or variables that are not the focus of the disorder to be studied. In order to establish content validity, investigators must have clearly articulated 'maps' of what they want to measure.

Example: measuring depression in physical illness

The importance of content validity is illustrated by the measuement of depression in physical illness. The problem here is that the traditional psychiatric concept of depression includes the presence of 'biological symptoms' such as loss of appetite and sleep disturbance. These symptoms are often present in physical illness although the person may not be depressed. It is therefore necessary to map a revised concept of depression in this group of people and to develop a measuring instrument according to the revised map that does not rely on symptoms that can arise primarily through ill health and are not attributable to depression. Zigmond & Snaith (1983) developed such an instrument: the Hospital Anxiety and

Depression (HAD) scale. Table 10.1 compares the sub-scales of the HAD with those of the widely used Beck Depression Inventory (BDI; Beck *et al*, 1961).

Arguments about the content validity of instruments are therefore concerned with the specification of theories about what one is trying to measure. There are no empirical methods of justifying content validity – one cannot refer to correlations between the test and other measures as an index of content validity. Content validity is obtained only by developing a conceptual map of what one wants to measure and considering what other factors would contaminate the measure. It is therefore important when planning a research project to define carefully the variable one wishes to

Table 10.1 Comparison of the sub-scales of the Beck Depression Inventory (BDI) and the Hospital Anxiety and Depression (HAD) scale

BDI	HAD
Items shared by the BDI and HAD	
Pessimism	Current enjoyment
Current dissatisfaction	Current laughter
Sad feeling	Feeling cheerful
Feel unattractive	Loss of interest in appearance
Discouraged about the future	Anticipated enjoyment
Effort to work	Slowed down
BDI items not in the HAD	
Past failure	
Punishment	
Self-blame	
Crying	
Loss of interest in others	
Guilt	
Disappointment in self	
Self-harm	
Irritable	
Decision difficulties	
*Sleep	
*Appetite	
*Weight loss	
*Concern with health	
*Libido	

*These might be a result of physical illness rather than depression.

measure, the populations to be assessed and the conditions under which the measurement is to take place. Potential measuring instruments can then be inspected for their content and the way in which the content was derived. One then chooses the 'best-fit' measure. In some cases it may be necessary to tailor the instrument to one's own needs or develop a new measure. A checklist for content validity is given in Box 10.1.

Criterion validity

Criterion validity determines whether a measure discriminates between people who are known to be dissimilar on a feature external to the measure itself. Many measures are developed as a cost-effective way of classifying people without the need for extensive interviews by clinicians. The criterion validity of these tests is therefore very important and their development will include calibration against a reliable external criterion – or 'gold standard'. The General Health Questionnaire (GHQ; Goldberg, 1978) is a common instrument whose criterion validity has been established for several different forms.

Concurrent validity

There are two main types of criterion validity. The first, concurrent validity, is established when the measure and criterion are measured at the same time. For example, a sample of patients from general practice complete the GHQ and are given a structured interview for psychiatric diagnosis (e.g. the Present State Examination (PSE); Wing *et al*, 1974). The classification of the patients by the PSE is the criterion against which the GHQ is to be validated. When developing an instrument, various cut-off scores will be explored to determine which provides the maximum discrimination between the known groups.

Predictive validity

The second aspect of criterion validity is predictive validity, whereby the criterion is measured later. In psychiatry, measures with predictive validity are typically used to determine a person's likely response to treatment (e.g. the Newcastle Scale for response to electroconvulsive therapy; Kerr *et*

Box 10.1 Checklist for content validity

- Specify carefully what you want to measure
- Inspect measures already available
  - How well do their contents match what you want to measure?
  - How were the contents of these instruments derived?
  - Does this match your requirements?

al, 1974) or the course of illness (e.g. the Kendrick Battery for dementia; Kendrick, 1985). Usually the content of the test is related to the outcome, but this is not necessarily so. None the less, the content of tests with predictive validity is often determined by the causal models espoused by researchers.

Specificity and sensitivity

Criterion validity is often presented in terms of the specificity and sensitivity of the test (Streiner & Norman, 2003). These terms are explained in Fig. 10.1, which shows the distribution of cases by allocating them according to whether they exceed the cut-off score of the test and meet the validating criterion (gold standard). There are four possible states:

- true positive, those defined as positive by both test and criterion
- true negative, those defined as negative by both test and criterion
- false positive, those incorrectly defined as positive by the test
- false negative, those incorrectly defined as negative by the test.

The sensitivity of the test is defined as the proportion of positive cases that are correctly identified. The specificity of the test is the proportion of negative cases that are correctly identified. The sensitivity and specificity change with the cut-off score, and there is some degree of 'trade-off' between these two dimensions of criterion validity. By choosing a high cut-off score, one can be reasonably sure that most of those without a disorder will score below the cut-off (high specificity), but many cases will also score below this level and will be missed (low sensitivity). Conversely, by lowering the score threshold, more cases will be picked up (high sensitivity) but this will be at the expense of incorrectly identifying a substantial proportion of people without the disorder as being unwell

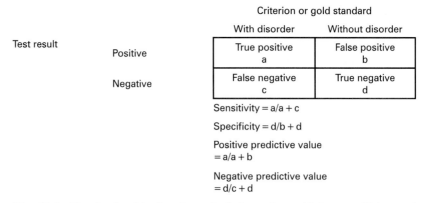

Fig. 10.1 The 2×2 table for the calculation of sensitivity, specificity and predictive values

(lower specificity). The trade-offs between sensitivity and specificity can be neatly represented by using the receiver operator characteristic (ROC) curve (Zweig & Campbell, 1993). A series of 2×2 tables for different cut-off points are constructed and the sensitivity and specificity are calculated separately for each point. An ROC curve is then constructed for a test by plotting the false-positive rate (1 − specificity) against the true positive rate (sensitivity) for each of these cut-offs. An ideal test is one that would have both high specificity and sensitivity, and the curve would follow the path of the upper left-hand corner. A hypothetical example of a ROC curve of a test with good sensitivity and specificity is given in Fig. 10.2. A way of quantifying the performance of a test instrument is calculated from the area under the ROC curve. A line of equivalence is seen with an uninformative test (sensitivity + specificity = 1) and the area under the curve is 0.5. A perfect test has an area under the curve of 1.0 but this is never achieved in practice.

The trade-offs between sensitivity and specificity are context specific and in setting a cut-off one has to consider whether it more important to identify all cases, or to ensure that all those without a disease are not wrongly identified as being 'cases'. Screening tests are used throughout medicine and the ROC analysis has been widely used to inform these trade-offs – although this technique is only now becoming more widespread in psychiatry.

Example: screening for depression in the general hosptial

The use of ROC curves in psychological assessment is illustrated by a study of depression in a general hospital. Harter *et al* (2001) used the GHQ and HAD instruments to screen for depression and anxiety in a general hospital population of 206 patients with musculo-skeletal disease. They administered the Composite International Diagnostic Interview (M-CIDI; Wittchen, 1994) to consecutive patients in order to obtain standardised psychiatric diagnoses. Sensitivities and specificities for each of the cut-off points on the GHQ and HAD were then obtained to produce ROC curves for depression and anxiety in patients with musculo-skeletal disease (Fig. 10.3). The curves showed that HAD performs better than the GHQ in this population, with the ROC curve lying more in the upper left quadrant. This performance is quantified by an area under the curve for the HAD of 0.79 (95%CI 0.73–0.85) *v.* 0.68 for the GHQ (95%CI 0.61–0.75). Formal statistical tests of differences in areas under the curve show this not to have reached statistical significance (test for equality of areas $P=0.11$)

Cross-validation

It is always important to cross-validate a test, that is, to establish whether the test maintains criterion validity when applied to another sample. In most cases the cross-validation takes place in a sample very similar to the original sample, but some published tests have their criterion validity

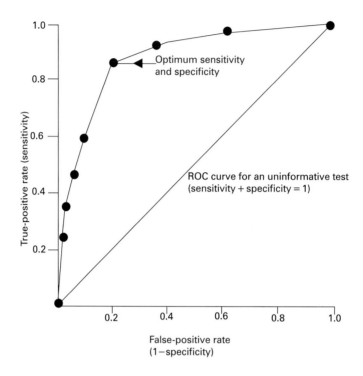

Fig. 10.2 A hypothetical receiver operator characteristic (ROC) curve for a screening test.

established over a number of populations and the details are published in their manuals.

One important caveat to the notion of cross-validation needs to be borne in mind when interpreting results: the impact of prevalence on the predictive power of a test. Sensitivities and specificities are fundamental characteristics of a test and do not vary according to the prevalence of a disorder within a population. Hence, a screening test with good sensitivity and specificity will have a similar sensitivity in psychiatric out-patients (with a high prevalence of psychiatric diagnoses) and in the general population (where the prevalence of psychiatric problems rarely rises above 8–10% (Meltzer *et al*, 1995). However, the predictive value of a positive test (the proportion of people with a positive test who turn out to have the disorder) does change (see Fig. 10.1). The positive and negative predictive values are perhaps the most informative for clinicians using tests in routine practice (Sackett *et al*, 1991). A checklist for criterion validity is given in Box 10.2.

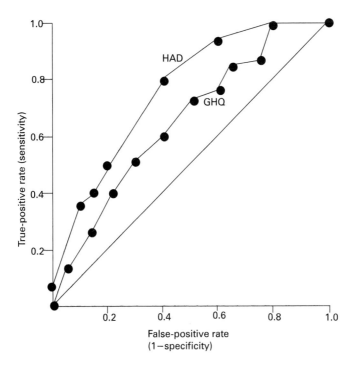

Fig. 10.3 Receiver operator characteristic (ROC) curve for the ability of the General Health Questionnaire (GHQ) and the Hospital Anxiety and Depression (HAD) scale to detect depression in patients with musculo-skeletal disease (Harter *et al*, 2001).

Construct validity

Many things that we wish to measure in psychiatry have no single criterion that can be entirely determined. In this case the construct validity of the measure can be exhaustively specified. Unlike criterion validity, construct validity is not measurable in a single operation or study and evidence for it must be obtained through a series of inter-related studies.

'Construct validity is evaluated by investigating what qualities a test measures, i.e., by demonstrating that certain explanatory constructs account to some degree for the performance on the test.' (American Psychological Association, 1954)

The construct validity of the test is therefore intimately connected with the theory that underpins the test. For example, Eysenck's well-known

167

Box 10.2   Checklist for criterion validity

- Define the criterion you are interested in very carefully
- Does this match the established criterion of the tests?
- Under what conditions was criterion validity established? Do they correspond to your conditions?
- Over what range of conditions has the criterion validity been established? Is there evidence that it is robust?

---

construct of neuroticism (Eysenck, 1970) contains many predictions about what variables should be associated with each other. No one variable uniquely validates Eysenck's construct but the pattern of interrelations observed over the years provides convincing evidence that such a construct exists and is useful. Intelligence is another well-known construct for which there is persuasive evidence.

In order to establish construct validity the theoretical relationships between variables must be specified unambiguously; this will include exploration of potentially confounding variables (alternative explanations). Next, the empirical relationships between the variables must be explored and data obtained. Lastly, the collected evidence must be weighed and assimilated, and decisions about the validity of the construct made.

The central feature of construct validity is the explication of the theoretical construct. Cook & Campbell (1979) give four tests that can be applied to determine whether a construct has validity.

- Do independent variables change dependent variables in the direction and manner predicted by the theory?
- Do the independent variables fail to alter measures of related but different constructs?
- Do the proposed dependent variables tap items that they are meant to measure?
- Is it true that the dependent measures are not dominated by irrelevant factors?

Convergent and divergent validity

In classic psychometric technique, construct validity can be determined by establishing convergent and divergent validity (Campbell & Fiske, 1959). Convergent validity is established when measures that are predicted to be associated (because they measure the same thing) are found to be related. Divergent validity is established when the measures successfully discriminate between other measures of unrelated constructs. For example, one would expect that different measures of abnormal illness behaviour (Pilowsky, 1969) would be related (correlated) but that they would not be related to measures of neuroticism, a construct that is supposedly independent. If the measures of abnormal illness behaviour are correlated with neuroticism, then one might have doubts as to the validity of the construct of abnormal illness behaviour because neuroticism is well established as a construct and it could be argued that it is in some senses more fundamental than abnormal illness behaviour. A case example of using neuroticism and abnormal illness behaviour, as measured by the Illness Behaviour Questionnaire (IBQ), is given by Zonderman *et al* (1985).

Example: construct validity of the IBQ

Pilowsky (1969) proposed that people who have inappropriate or mal-adaptive ways of responding to their health could be said to exhibit abnormal illness behaviour. This category was said to include the more traditional concepts such as hysteria, hypochondriasis and conversion reaction. As a consequence of his proposal Pilowsky developed the IBQ to measure abnormal illness behaviour. Zonderman *et al* (1985) attempted to replicate Pilowsky's original research on the IBQ (Pilowsky & Spence, 1975) and to confirm the structure of the sub-scales of the questionnaire. They also explored the construct validity of the IBQ by correlating it with various personality measures. If the IBQ has good construct validity it should not be strongly correlated with personality measures. However, Zonderman *et al* (1985) found that all sub-scales of the IBQ were correlated with three separate measures of neuroticism. In contrast, there were few correlations with aspects of personality such as extroversion and 'openness'. This suggested that the IBQ overlaps considerably with the construct of neuroticism. Zonderman *et al* (1985) noted that this might be interpreted as offering support for the construct validity of the IBQ because neuroticism is known to be related to complaints about bodily symptoms. Against this positive finding must be set the fact that the sub-scales of the IBQ do not have any demonstrable discriminant validity, that is, they all seem to measure the same thing. Consequently, Zonderman *et al* (1985) argued that previous studies that claimed to have demonstrated that the IBQ can separate patients with chronic pain (presumed to be without an organic cause) from other patients are open to reinterpretation. It is possible that the higher scores on the IBQ might represent truthful responses by a person seeking help for bodily complaints which worry them. At present interpretation of IBQ scores is far from clear.

A checklist for assessing construct validity is given in Box 10.3 and alternative explanations for negative evidence in Box 10.4.

Face validity

'Face validity' is the least technical type of validity. A test or measure has face validity if it is judged to measure what it is supposed to measure. There is no way of determining the face validity of a test using statistical methods. It is determined by whether the researcher and his or her colleagues agree

---

Box 10.3 Checklist for construct validity

- Is there a theoretical rationale that underpins the measure you are interested in?
- Is it well articulated so that predictions about the relationships between measures are made?
- Is there evidence of a consistent pattern of findings involving different researchers, methods, populations and other theoretical structures over time?

---

that the measure looks as if it is measuring what it is supposed to measure. High face validity can be both an advantage and a disadvantage. It is probable that patients will be more cooperative if they can see that the test is actually measuring something of relevance to them. On the other hand, tests with high face validity may make the purpose of the test so obvious that it is easy for the patient to dissimulate.

Reliability

The traditional concept of reliability is concerned with the repeatability of measurement and by implication its vulnerability to error. A common assumption is that a measure is intrinsically reliable or unreliable under all conditions, but it is possible for a test to be highly reliable under one condition and very unreliable under another. Indeed, for certain purposes it is desirable for measures to have this mixed combination of reliabilities. A reliability coefficient is a statement about how far the measure is reproducible under a given set of conditions. The basic procedure for establishing reliability is to obtain two sets of measurements and compare them, usually by means of the correlation coefficient. The different reliability coefficients reflect changes in the conditions under which the measures were used. There are several reliability coefficients in common use.

Box 10.4 Evaluating negative evidence – alternative explanations

- The measure lacks validity as a measure of the construct
- The theoretical framework is incorrect
- The procedure used to test the relationship was faulty
- There is low construct validity because the other variables were measured unreliably.

Test–retest reliability

Test–retest reliability is established by administering the measure to a group of people on two occasions separated by a designated period of time. A perfectly reliable test would have a correlation coefficient of 1.0, indicating that the participants scored exactly the same on both occasions. This never happens as there are several influences that will change the participant's performance on the second occasion. For example, the person's intrinsic state may have changed, or they may be fatigued or bored so that careless errors are made. In addition, more difficult test items might be more likely to be solved correctly on the second occasion (a special problem in tests of intellectual ability). If the interval is sufficiently long, the person will have matured. A major class of error is known as 'reactivity'. This refers to the process whereby the act of measurement induces a change in the object of measurement. For example, measuring people's attitudes to sexual behaviour may prompt them to reconsider their attitudes and change them. A little reflection will produce numerous other confounding sources of change that the test–retest correlation may tap.

A low test–retest reliability may not mean that the measure is 'poor' but that it is susceptible to one of several influences. Clearly the relevance of test–retest reliability will be determined by the construct being measured. For example, if one is concerned with fluctuations in mood during the day it would be inappropriate to select an instrument with high test–retest reliability. This would indicate that it is relatively stable and possibly insensitive to short-term mood changes. One solution would be to select a measure with good 'alternate forms' reliability or high internal consistency, and low test–retest reliability.

Alternate forms reliability

In alternate forms reliability the same people are given different but equivalent forms of a test on two occasions. The forms of the measure are carefully developed to ensure equivalence as far as possible. This procedure is especially useful if one suspects that there may be a significant learning effect as a result of the first administration which would seriously bias a second testing on exactly the same measure. Many tests of intellectual ability have alternate forms, as do several personality questionnaires, for example the Eysenck Personality Inventory (Eysenck & Edwards, 1964). As the tests must be administered on two separate occasions, the alternate forms reliability coefficient is subject to the same sources of error as test–retest reliability. On the whole this form of reliability is rarely examined in measuring instruments used in psychiatry.

Internal consistency measures of reliability

This type of reliability focuses on the reproducibility of measurement across different items within a test, that is, reproducibility of content. To establish the internal consistency of a measure, the test is administered once to a pool of participants and the interrelationship between items on the test is assessed. There are several methods of establishing internal consistency, including the split-half coefficient, the Kuder–Richardson (K–R 20) method and Cronbach's α. All of these reliability coefficients are obtained by intercorrelating participants' scores on items within a test. If the test is reliable, that is, has internal consistency, then scores on the items should be positively correlated with each other and the internal consistency coefficients will be high. Simple, non-technical guides to these various methods can be found in introductory psychometric texts (Anastasi, 1968; Cronbach, 1970; Carmines & Zeller, 1979). Internal consistency overcomes the problems of errors introduced by re-administering a test. However, the assumption of internal reliability procedures is that items in the test measure more or less the same thing. Since the items tap different constructs one would expect the internal consistency of the test to be reduced. This of course relates to the notions of construct and content validity, which have already been discussed.

Interrater reliability

Many measures in psychiatry cannot be repeated in time and the object of measurement is not a construct that can be sampled in different forms, as is required for a measure of internal consistency. The paramount example of this is a diagnostic interview, where a person's mental state will need to be examined at a particular time. Similar problems arise when the overt behaviour of a person has to be assessed, as, for example, with the Clifton Assessment Procedures for the Elderly (CAPE; Gilleard & Pattie, 1979). When this problem arises, reliability can be assessed by comparing the ratings of two independent observers to determine the extent to which they agree in their observations. There are a number of statistics that are used to compute reliability (Fig. 10.4). The most common metric that is quoted in quantifying reliability is Cohen's kappa (Cohen, 1968).

Agreement on the total score, achieved by summing all the items on a rating scale, is often computed in the form of a correlation coefficient. This will give an estimate of the global reliability of the measure, but it is possible to investigate the reliability of the scale in much more detail by calculating the reliability for each item using one of the measures in Fig. 10.4. This will enable the investigator to determine which aspects of behaviour are poorly defined or difficult to discriminate. This may form a basis for revising the rating scale or improving the training of raters. Generally speaking, a reliability measure based on kappa is recommended because it takes into account the fact that raters can agree by chance. Kappa can also be calculated for scales that categorise respondents according to more than two levels of severity (Cohen, 1968). Hall (1974) and Streiner & Norman (2003) provide good worked examples for determining

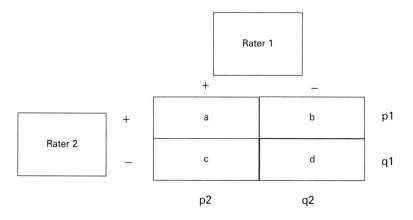

Fig. 10.4 Calculation of a reliability coefficient for a two-point categorical scale

kappa. Most statistical computer programs allow the calculation of kappa statistics, together with their confidence intervals.

Which reliability coefficient?

Just because studies of the reliability of an instrument have been published, it does not mean that it can be automatically used as a research instrument. First, one must assess the type of reliability that has been established and the conditions under which it was examined. This must be compared with the requirements of the planned research. Consider an instrument developed to measure anxiety that is known to have high test–retest reliability. You wish to measure change in a group of patients after they have been given a drug. If there is no change in their score, how should this be interpreted? The two major alternative explanations are that the drug is ineffective or that the instrument is insensitive to change. Knowing that there is a high test–retest correlation would mean that the latter explanation could not be eliminated. In this case it would seem that the scale is designed to measure the enduring trait of anxiety rather than a transient condition or state of anxiety. In practice it would be necessary to select a measure with low test–retest reliability but with high internal consistency. In this example we can see the link between reliability and validity. The selection of a test that is sensitive to change will be facilitated if it has already been established that the test is sensitive to various experimental manipulations that are known to alter anxiety, that is, the test's construct validity has been investigated and established.

Second, it cannot be assumed that because reliability has been ascertained in a previous study it 'carries over' to other studies. This is particularly true of studies that involve direct observation of behaviour (including interviewer rating scales). In these studies the measuring instrument is the observer, not the scale itself, and it is necessary to ensure that the observers are suitably trained in the definitions of criterion behaviour used by the scale. Even when it has been demonstrated that two observers can reach high levels of agreement during training, it must not be assumed that this reliability will be maintained over the period of study. It is always necessary to conduct reliability probes during the study by sampling the ratings of two or more observers. The picture is further complicated in direct observational studies, as it is possible for the observers to remain highly reliable, as assessed by interrater agreement, but yet to drift from the original criteria. Under certain conditions it is possible for observers to be highly reliable but inaccurate. This phenomenon of 'observer drift' has been studied by behavioural psychologists and it is known to be influenced by the expectations that the observers have about the patients. Therefore in research involving direct observation, considerable care must be taken to ensure that reliability and accuracy are maintained throughout the study (Hartman, 1982, 1984).

A checklist for assessing reliability is given in Box 10.5.

Recent advances

The selection of psychological assessment instruments draws heavily on the science of measurement and psychometrics, and the theoretical foundations were largely laid in the 1950s and 1960s (e.g. Stevens, 1951; Nunnally, 1967). Many of these notions of validity and reliability are as relevant today as they were at the time of their first conception and the examples given have hopefully illustrated how they might be applied in psychological assessment.

No science is static and the science of psychological assessment has evolved and grown. The following section highlights some more recent advances and empirical observations for the interested reader. Five topics will briefly be considered: (a) the concept of generalisability; (b) the measurement of

---

Box 10.5 Checklist for reliability

- What types of reliability have been established for the measure?
- Under what conditions were these types of reliabilities established? For example, what groups of people were tested and when and where were they tested?
- How closely do your conditions correspond to the original ones?
- Do you need to establish reliability for measures in your study? This will almost certainly be necessary for studies involving direct observations of patients.

outcome; (c) the application of systematic reviews and meta-analysis of psychometric instruments; and (d) the abuse of psychometric instruments by investigators.

The concept of generalisability

The astute reader will be aware that the two concepts of validity and reliability are interwoven. They both relate to the wider question of how far one can make a general statement about the data collected. In other words, given that one has collected data in a certain form, how far is one entitled to generalise from these data to other conditions? For example, one would have little confidence in observations collected by a single observer, but consistent data collected by several observers would give confidence that the phenomenon existed in some sense. On the other hand, a measure with predictive validity would enable a general statement to be made about behaviour across time. In both of these examples we are generalising from one set of observations to another and we have some measure of confidence in these generalisations as provided by reliability and validity coefficients.

One advantage of the concept of generalisability is that it forces one to think about the type of generalised statements that one would like to be able to make at the end of a study. The purpose of most research is to provide additional information about a problem that will extend beyond the particular study. Table 10.2 outlines the different domains of generalisability described by Cronbach *et al* (1972) and indicates the sort of questions that one needs to ask about a study.

The facets correspond to traditional notions of reliability and validity. For example, the time facet corresponds to test–retest reliability. Cornbach, who introduced the generalisability theory, demonstrated how it is possible to consider more than one facet at a time by using statistical methods of analysis of variance. For an introductory discussion of the concept of generalisability, see Streiner & Norman (2003).

Using psychological instruments to measure outcome

The preceding discussion has highlighted the use of psychological instruments as 'one-off' assessment tools which are used to decide whether a disorder or attribute is present or absent and to quantify magnitude or severity. The ROC analysis exemplifies the application of scientific rigour to this process. However, in many cases psychological instruments are not used on a one-off basis but are used to measure change over time within individuals or groups of individuals. This measurement of change over time is central to the notion of the measurement of *outcome*.

It was Avedis Donabedian who first coined and popularised the term '*outcome*' in his influential description of the three components of the quality of care: *structure, process and outcome* (Donabedian, 1966). Outcome

175

Table 10.2 The main facets of generalisability and the typical questions considered

Main facets	Typical questions
Observers/scorers	Can the results be extended across different observers (e.g. interviewers and test scorers, independent markers of an IQ test)?
Time	Are the data consistent on different occasions of measurement?
Settings	Are the observations in one setting consistent with observations in another setting? How far can we gneralise between the various settings?
Participants	How far can the observations be generalised from one person to another?
Item/behaviour	How do the items on a test, or different behaviours, relate to each other?

measures are now used for a number of purposes including: evaluation of healthcare policy; evaluation of the effectiveness of treatments; making individual decisions in routine clinical practice; economic evaluation and resource allocation; and clinical audit. Not surprisingly, no one instrument is suitable for each and every one of these purposes. In judging the ability of an instrument to be used as a measure of outcome, the attribute of 'sensitivity to change' has to be examined in addition to validity and reliability (Fitzpatrick *et al*, 1992). If an instrument is unable to detect underlying changes in health or psychological status, then it is not suitable for use as an outcome measure.

The notions of sensitivity to change and responsiveness are at variance with traditional notions of reliability and validly. For example, an instrument may be reliable and valid in that it consistently differentiates between those with a disorder and those without, but it may not be sufficiently sensitive to detect subtle but clinically important changes in the individual over a period of time (Guyatt *et al*, 1992). The usual technique that is used for the measurement of health status (where notions of sensitivity to change have been most comprehensively examined) is to select only those items that most sensitively measure changes in an attribute of interest, in order to construct a measure of outcome. Similarly, attributes of validity and reliability are necessarily examined within groups of patients and groups of observers, and methods of validation are tested using statistical analyses that take into account the inherent variance of instrument scores within groups of patients or populations. However, in applying well-validated and reliable instruments to the individual patient, it is often difficult to know whether changes that are observed over time reflect the natural measurement variance of an instrument within the individual or genuine change in the underlying state of health. This is a problem that is rarely appreciated by those who adopt psychometrically robust instruments for individual patient care and audit (Dunn, 1996).

The key message is to not assume that a psychological instrument that is valid and reliable can be automatically adopted as a measure of outcome in a clinical trial or in individual patient care and audit. For a more complete examination of this issue in the field of psychiatry, see Gilbody *et al* (2003), and for an examination of the methods that are used to examine responsiveness see Streiner & Norman (2003).

Systematic reviews and meta-analysis of psychological assessment instruments

One of the major advances in health services research over the past decade has been the development of systematic review and meta-analysis and their application to a whole variety of questions (Mulrow & Cook, 1998; see also Chapter 4). These methods have largely been used to investigate the effectiveness of interventions through the synthesis of groups of trials. This approach has proved fruitful in psychiatry, since many of the trials that are conducted are of limited sample size and the results vary between trials, often as a result of genuine sampling variance. The same is true for studies that investigate reliability and validity, and it is possible that the application of systematic reviews to studies of diagnostic and screening instruments might prove equally useful. Statistical pooling can be used to increase the precision and generalisability of estimates of sensitivity and specificity (Deeks, 2000).

The techniques for synthesising validation and reliability studies for diagnostic tests are already well advanced in other branches of medicine but have not generally been applied in psychiatry. One notable example is a review commissioned by the US Agency for Health Research and Quality, which examined the sensitivity and specificity of common screening questionnaires for depression (Pignone *et al*, 2002; Williams *et al*, 2002). This review demonstrated that studies can be combined using meta-analysis to construct a summary ROC (sROC) curve, which gives the best well-powered estimates of sensitivity and specificity for a variety of cut-off points. These techniques are likely to be more widely applied in the future and it will be no more reasonable to use the results of a single validation study to select an instrument than it is to use the results of a single trial to select a treatment when systematic reviews are available.

The abuse of psychological instruments by researchers

Biases creep into all areas of evaluative research and part of the process of becoming a critical reader is to become aware of these biases in order to spot them when they do occur. One such bias has emerged in recent years with respect to psychological rating scales – the use of unpublished and 'cannibalised' scales by trialists, with the aim of showing treatments in their best light.

There has long been scepticism about the selective publication of results from trials – so-called publication bias (Gilbody & Song, 2000). A subtle variation on this theme seems to be the publication of the results of studies that used unpublished rating scales and non-standardised versions of existing rating scales. Marshall *et al* (2000) compared the results of 300 trials that used unpublished or non-standardised versions of scales (i.e. those scales where only certain items from a standardised scale had been used to measure outcome) with matched trials that used a standardised version of a psychological rating scale. They found that trials that used unpublished or non-standardised scales were twice as likely to show a positive result as trials using only published rating scales. They concluded that when using modified versions of published scales researchers would selectively report only those items from a rating scale that had shown a between-group difference, in order to demonstrate a statistically significant result for their trial. Using unpublished scales, where validity and reliability are not in the public domain, and using non-standardised versions of published scales should therefore be avoided. Moreover, the results of trials using these scales are potentially biased and should be treated with a degree of scepticism.

Conclusions

The selection of an appropriate set of measures for research requires very careful consideration. Just because a test or rating scale has been published does not mean that it is appropriate for all uses. Readers should be aware of considering only the face validity of measures – that if a measure looks good, it is good. The selection of an appropriate measure requires very careful specification of the research hypothesis and possible alternative rival hypotheses. This is usually achieved only after reflection and discussion with experienced colleagues. Once the central issues have been decided it becomes clearer what measurement is required. At this stage a literature search may reveal that certain instruments have been repeatedly used. Some of these studies should be carefully investigated to document the known details of reliability and validity of the instrument. It is also useful to contact others who have used the instruments to obtain their opinion. Finally, when a measure is selected, plans must be drawn up to determine what aspects of reliability or validity will need to be monitored in the planned study. On occasions the researchers will be left with no option other than to develop their own measure or to modify a previously published instrument. In that case extensive provision for the study of the reliability and validity of the instrument must be made.

References

American Psychological Association (1954) Technical recommendations for psychological tests and diagnostic techniques. *Psychological Bulletin*, (suppl. 51), 1–38.

Anastasi, A. (1968) *Psychological Testing* (3rd edn). London: Macmillan.

Beck, A. T., Ward, C. H., Mendelson, M., *et al* (1961) An inventory for measuring depression. *Archives of General Psychiatry*, **4**, 561–571.

Campbell, D. T. & Fiske D. W. (1959) Convergent and discriminant validation by the multi-trait multi-method matrix. *Psychological Bulletin*, **56**, 81–105.

Carmines, E. G. & Zeller, R. A. (1979) *Reliability and Validity Assessment*. Beverly Hills, CA: Sage Publications.

Cohen, J. (1968) Weighted kappa: Nominal scale agreement with provision for scaled disagreement or partial credit. *Psychological Bulletin*, **70**, 213–220.

Cook, T. D. & Campbell, D. T. (1979) *Quasi-experimentation. Design and Analysis Issues for Field Settings*. Chicago, IL: Rand McNally.

Cronbach, L. (1970) *Essentials of Psychological Testing* (3rd edn). New York: Harper and Row.

Cronbach, L. J., Gleser, G. C., Nanda, H., *et al* (1972) *The Dependability of Behavioral Measurements: Theory of Generalizability for Sores and Profiles*. New York: Wiley.

Deeks, J. (2000) Evaluations of diagnostic and screening tests. In *Systematic Reviews in Health Care* (eds M. Egger, G. Davey Smith & D. G. Altman), pp. 248–282. London: BMJ Books.

Donabedian, A. (1966) Evaluating the quality of medical care. *Milbank Memorial Fund Quarterly*, **44** (suppl.), 166–206.

Dunn, G. (1996) Statistical methods for measuring outcomes. In *Mental Health Outcome Measures* (eds G. Thornicroft & M. Tansella), pp. 3–15. Berlin: Springer-Verlag.

Eysenck, H. J. (1970) *Structure of Human Personality* (3rd edn). London: Hodder.

Eysenck, H. J. & Edwards, S. (1964) *The Eysenck Personality Questionnaire*. Windsor: NferNelson.

Fitzpatrick, R., Ziebland, S., Jenkinson, C., *et al* (1992) Importance of sensitivity to change as a criterion for selecting health status measures. *Quality in Health Care*, **1**, 89–93.

Gilbody, S. M. & Song, F. (2000) Publication bias and the integrity of psychiatry research. *Psychological Medicine*, **30**, 253–258.

Gilbody, S. M., House, A. O. & Sheldon, T. (2003) *Outcomes Measurement in Psychiatry: A Critical Review of Patient Based Outcomes Measurement in Research and Practice (CRD Report Number 24)*. York: University of York.

Gilleard, C. & Pattie, A. (1979) *Clifton Assessment Procedures for the Elderly*. Windsor: NferNelson.

Goldberg, D. (1978) *Manual of the General Health Questionnaire*. Slough: National Foundation for Educational Research.

Guyatt, G. H., Kirshner, B. & Jaeschke, R. (1992) Measuring health status: what are the necessary measurement properties? *Journal of Clinical Epidemiology*, **45**, 1341–1345.

Hall, J. N. (1974) Inter-rater reliability of ward rating scales. *British Journal of Psychiatry*, **125**, 248–255.

Harter, M., Reuter, K., Gross-Hardt, K., *et al* (2001) Screening for anxiety, depressive and somatoform disorders in rehabilitation – validity of HADS and GHQ-12 in patients with musculoskeletal disease. *Disability and Rehabilitation*, **23**, 737–744.

Hartman, D. P. (1982) *Using Observers to Study Behavior. New Directions for Methodology in Social and Behavioral Science, no. 14*. San Francisco: Jossey-Bass.

Hartman, D. P. (1984) Assessment strategies. In *Single Case Experimental Designs. Strategies for Studying Behavior Change* (2nd edn) (eds D. H. Barlow & M. Hersen), pp. 107–139. New York: Pergamon.

Kendrick, D. C. (1985) *Kendrick Cognitive Tests for the Elderly*. Windsor: NFER/Nelson.

179

Kerr, T. A., Roth, M. & Schapira, K. (1974) Prediction of outcome in anxiety states and depressive illnesses. *British Journal of Psychiatry*, **124**, 125–133.

Marshall, M., Lockwood, A., Bradley, C., *et al* (2000) Unpublished rating scales: a major source of bias in randomised controlled trials of treatments for schizophrenia. *British Journal of Psychiatry*, **176**, 249–252.

Meltzer, H. Y., Gill, B., Petticrew, M., *et al* (1995) *OPCS Surveys of Psychiatric Morbidity in Great Britain*. London: TSO (The Stationery Office).

Mulrow, C. D. & Cook, D. (eds) (1998) *Systematic Reviews: Synthesis of Best Evidence for Healthcare Decisions*. Philadelphia, PA: American College of Physicians.

Nunnally, J. (1967) *Psychometric Theory* (2nd edn). New York: McGraw-Hill.

Pignone, M. P., Gaynes, B. N., Rushton, J. L., *et al* (2002) Screening for depression in adults: a summary of the evidence for the U.S. Preventive Services Task Force. *Annals of Internal Medicine*, **136**, 765–776.

Pilowsky, I. (1969) Abnormal illness behaviour. *British Journal of Medical Psychology*, **42**, 347–351.

Pilowsky, I. & Spence, N. D. (1975) Patterns of illness behaviour in patients with intractable pain. *Journal of Psychosomatic Research*, **19**, 279–287.

Sackett, D. L., Haynes, R. B., Guyatt, G. H., *et al* (1991) *Clinical Epidemiology: A Basic Science for Clinical Medicine*. Boston, MA: Little Brown.

Stevens, S. (1951) Mathematics, measurement and psychophysics. In *Handbook of Experimental Psychology* (ed. S. Stevens), pp. 1–14. New York: Wiley.

Streiner, D. & Norman, G. (2003) *Health Measurement Scales: A Practical Guide to Their Development and Use* (3rd edn). Oxford: Oxford University Press.

Williams, J. W., Pignone, M., Ramirez, G., *et al* (2002) Identifying depression in primary care: a literature synthesis of case-finding instruments. *General Hospital Psychiatry*, **24**, 225–237.

Williams, P., Tarnopolsky, A. & Hand, D. (1980) Case definition and identification in psychiatric epidemiology: review and assessment. *Psychological Medicine*, **10**, 101–114.

Wing, J. K., Cooper, J. E. & Sartorius, N. (1974) *The Measurement and Classification of Psychiatric Symptoms*. London: Cambridge University Press.

Wittchen, H. U. (1994) Reliability and validity studies of the WHO Composite International Diagnostic Interview (CIDI): a critical review. *Journal of Psychiatric Research*, **28**, 57–84.

Zigmond, A. S. & Snaith, R. P. (1983) The Hospital Anxiety and Depression Scale. *Acta Psychiatrica Scandinavica*, **67**, 361–370.

Zonderman, A. B., Heft, M. W. & Costa, P. T. (1985) Does the illness behaviour questionnaire measure abnormal illness behavior? *Health Psychology*, **4**, 425–436.

Zweig, M. H. & Campbell, G. (1993) Receiver-Operating Characteristics (ROC) plots: a fundamental evaluation tool in clinical medicine. *Clinical Chemistry*, **39**, 561–577.

Further reading

There are a number of classic textbooks on psychometrics that will prove useful to the interested reader and which are detailed below. Perhaps the most useful and up-to-date textbook is that by Streiner and Norman (2003), which has recently been updated and includes clear elaborations on all concepts covered in this chapter.

Carmines, E. G. & Zeller, R. A. (1979) *Reliability and Validity Assessment*. Beverly Hills, CA: Sage Publications.

This small text provides an excellent introduction to traditional psychometric concepts, is invaluable and contains good examples of how the various formulae are applied.

Lemke, E. & Wiersma, W. (1976) *Principles of Psychological Assessment*. Chicago, IL: Rand McNally.

This is more extensive than Carmines & Zeller's text but it is beautifully laid out with excellent examples. Each chapter has appended test questions.

Nunally, J. C. (1978) *Psychometric Theory* (2nd edn). New York: McGraw-Hill.

This is one of the standard texts on psychometrics. It is comprehensive and contains advanced coverage of psychometric theory and practice.

Streiner, D. & Norman, G. (2003) *Health Measurement Scales: A Practical Guide to Their Development and Use* (3rd edn). Oxford: Oxford University Press.

Compendia of psychological, quality of life and health status measures

There has been substantial effort in recent years to summarise the key attributes of common and not so common rating scales. These books are a substantial resource for researchers and will make the selection of the right instrument much easier. Clear summaries of the scope, practicality, cost, copyright and psychometric qualities are given for hundreds of measures.

American Psychiatric Association (2000) *Handbook of Psychiatric Measures*. Washington: American Psychiatric Association Press.

A massive undertaking and phenomenal resource for psychiatric researchers. Also available on CD–ROM with printable versions for public domain measures. Ask your library to get it.

Bowling, A. (2004) *Measuring Health: A Review of Quality of Life Measurement Scales* (3rd edn). Buckingham: Open University Press.

Summarises the common psychological and, most importantly, quality of life measures for researchers and practitioners. Inexpensive and includes very useful introductory chapters on the key concepts.

McDowell, I. & Newell, C. (1996) *Measuring Health: A Guide to Rating Scales and Questionnaires*. Oxford: Oxford University Press.

A more comprehensive version of Bowling; again with excellent introductory chapters on psychometrics and the best guide to depression measures that is available.

CHAPTER 11

Rating scales in psychiatry

Peter Tyrer and Caroline Methuen

One of the most difficult tasks for aspiring research workers is choosing a rating scale. In an ideal world this should not be a difficult decision. Certain problems require special evaluation and, provided the problem has been recognised before, a suitable rating scale will exist for the purpose. If the rating scale is well established and is clearly the leader in the area, it will choose itself and there should be clear instructions on what training and expertise the researcher will need before the scale (or questionnaire) is applied. However, in practice choosing a rating scale is seldom this straightforward. This is mainly because there are too many rating scales and it is extremely difficult for the novice, and often even the expert, to choose the right scale easily. In previous editions of this book we have described a large number of rating scales, but this has only been a selection from a much larger pool; in the ensuing 10 years the abundance of new scales has made it impossible to cover the territory adequately. This chapter is therefore a general guide which should enable the researcher to identify the most appropriate scales for their area of interest, but a little more research will be required before the final choice of a scale is made. Hence we have given the main references for a large number of scales in the absence of space for an adequate review of each, on the premise that the wider the pool the better the eventual selection.

Choosing a rating scale

Figure 11.1 indicates the bumpy journey that the researcher will have to take before feeling confident that the right instrument has been chosen for the problem under investigation. The scales published in this chapter are by no means exhaustive so do not feel that it is unjustified for you to use a scale of your own choosing if you cannot find a measure for the subject under review in the pages below.

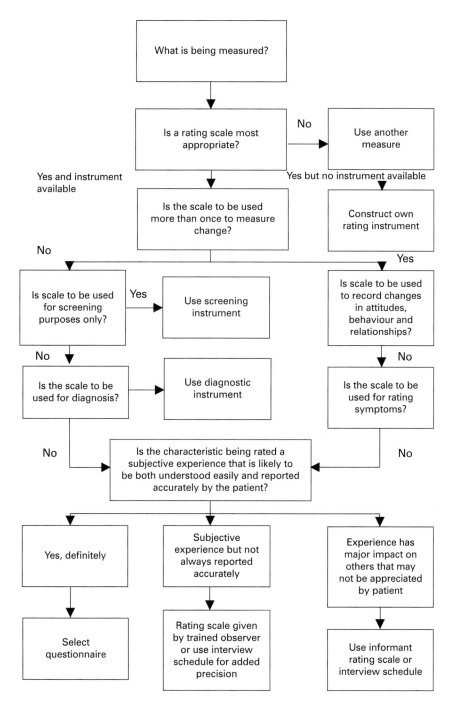

Fig. 11.1 Flow chart for selection of rating instruments in psychiatric research.

What is being measured?

Rating scales may not always be necessary in a study. As the use of rating scales involves administering an interview to an individual (patient or informant), the procedure is liable to natural attrition in any study, ranging from refusal to take part through to inability to follow-up. However, some other measures (e.g. admission to hospital) can be obtained from other sources and are more likely to yield complete data. There is also a strong and unnecessary tendency for junior researchers to collect as much data as possible without regard to its purpose. Investigators should elect at the design stage to ask whether every single item of information is essential, with the objective of eliminating at least half. The main advantage of simpler methods using few variables is that larger numbers of patients can often be accessed and so more robust findings are likely to emerge. It is therefore reasonable for the researcher to ask the question 'Can I get away without using a rating scale in this project?' It will save a tremendous amount of time and trouble if rating scales and questionnaires are avoided.

What is being measured and why?

There are three main reasons uses for rating scales in psychiatry. The first is as a screening instrument which identifies a population with the condition of interest but could include some people without the condition. A screening instrument should have high sensitivity even though this may be achieved at the expense of low specificity (see Chapter 10).

The second reason for using a rating scale is to identify a feature that is felt to be important. Quite often this is a psychiatric diagnosis, but it could be any characteristic. The point of using the rating scale is to more accurately measure this characteristic and thereby improve the quality of the research, and also to compare the findings with other studies. First, for example, if one wanted to assess whether a specific personality disorder was associated with childhood physical abuse, the researcher might consider it necessary to assess such abuse (e.g. using the Child Trauma Questionnaire) rather than simply asking the patient a yes/no question.

The third reason for using an instrument is to record change, either spontaneously or following some type of intervention. This raises several other important questions. Is the instrument easy to administer, does repeated assessment lead to practice effects and is the administration of the instrument prone to bias of any sort?

The answer to these questions should determine the nature of the rating instrument selected and whether it is to be self-administered (i.e. a questionnaire) or administered by another person such as a researcher.

Source of information

Reliability always tends to increase with more structured scales and with trained interviewers. There is an understandable tendency to select such instruments (especially when trained interviewers are available) in order to improve the quality of the study, but, long before this, it needs to be asked who is providing the information and why. Thus, for example, if an intervention designed to reduce depression is being tested, it is appropriate to use a structured interview schedule of established reliability (e.g. Schedule for Affective Disorders and Schizophrenia; Endicott & Spitzer, 1978) for assessment, but if the person concerned has relatively mild symptoms that could be hidden from a stranger, it would be more appropriate to assess the patient with a self-rating scale (e.g. Hamilton Rating Scale for Depression; Hamilton, 1960).

Almost all psychiatric symptoms have both a subjective element and an objective one that is shown to others. In some instances there may be a gross disparity between the two (e.g. in the features of psychopathy), but it is rare to have one feature only. For this reason many investigators use both self-rating questionnaires and more 'objective' rating scales, although in practice these often show good levels of agreement.

One of the main advantages of the questionnaire is that it reduces the potential for bias because a patient is more likely to describe their own feelings accurately than an investigator who is involved in a comparison of treatments and has some knowledge of what these are. Often bias is unwitting and one advantage of recording both self-rated and observer-rated symptoms is that similar results with both types of instrument suggest a minimum of bias.

Devising your own instrument

Although there is a natural tendency for researchers to develop their own instruments on the premise that there is no scale available to measure a particular feature, this position is increasingly untenable as instruments become available for all aspects of psychiatric illness and treatments. There is also considerable concern that new and untested scales yield much larger effect sizes than well-established scales (i.e. overstate the difference between treatments; Marshall *et al*, 2000).

Although there are still circumstances when a new rating scale might be necessary for a specific project, it is important for researchers to be aware that such a scale should be evaluated and the results of the evaluation should be published before the scale is used in the planned study. This will invariably involve much more work than using an established scale. Nobody should believe that using a specially derived scale for a project is going to be a short cut to success.

In deciding on a new rating scale the investigator will have to make a distinction between a simple dichotomous scale, an interval scale and a visual analogue scale (Fig. 11.2). There is often a wish to modify an existing scale and although under some circumstances this is justifiable, it must not be done without a great deal of thought, as comparisons with data using the original scale would thereby be rendered invalid.

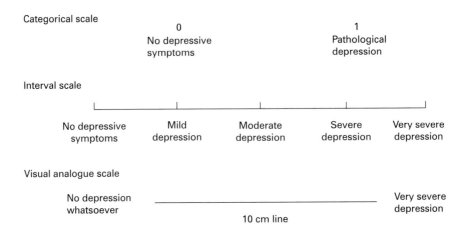

Categorical scale

0
No depressive
symptoms

1
Pathological
depression

Interval scale

No depressive
symptoms

Mild
depression

Moderate
depression

Severe
depression

Very severe
depression

Visual analogue scale

No depression
whatsoever

Very severe
depression

10 cm line

Fig. 11.2 Examples of types of rating scale: categorical scale, interval scale (implying dimensions, e.g. Likert scale) and visual analogue scale (the participant is asked to place a vertical mark across the line at the point that best describes current feelings; this is measured to give a 'depression score').

Finding a rating scale

The rest of this chapter lists the main scales for each area of psychiatry. This is a repetitive exercise but it is clear from talking to novice researchers that the listing of these scales is important. We decided that the main criterion for the inclusion a scale should be the extent of its use (as the wider the use of a scale the better will be comparability with other studies). We have therefore calculated the citation rate per year of each scale since the year of publication and only those scales that are widely cited in the literature (with a cut-off point of 4.0 per year for general scales and 2.0 per year for specific ones) have been included. Although we are well aware that some of the most commonly used scales are not quite as good as some others and have only achieved their status by a combination of primacy, luck and salesmanship, their frequency of use is still the best single criterion for the research worker in making a choice. Where the details of scales are not available in the published references the researcher is advised to search for these on the internet. This is now much easier with improved search engines such as Google, and any scale which is searched for using the author's name and title of the scale should be found easily. The most popular scales are frequently copyrighted and distributed by commercial publishers. For those that are less widely used but seem to be appropriate for a study it does no harm to get in touch with the originator(s). They will be flattered (unless of course the scale is so widely used it has led to many previous enquiries) and may offer extra help in starting the project. This may even be worthwhile

Table 11.1 Rating scales and questionnaires for depression

Author(s)	Type of assessment	Citation rate per year and comments
Hamilton (1960)	Hamilton Rating Scale for Depression (HRSD)	199.5 (the original and, to many, still the best)
Beck et al (1961)	Beck Depression Inventory (BDI)	186.2 (competing for the crown with enthusiasm – generally preferred in more recent studies)
Zigmond & Snaith (1983)	Hospital Anxiety and Depression Scale (HAD)	133.0 (currently the most frequently used self-rating scale, equally good for anxiety)
Montgomery & Åsberg (1979)	Montgomery–Åsberg Depression Rating Scale (MADRS)	83.2 (derived from the Comprehensive Psychopathological Rating Scale (CPRS) and may be of special value when multiple pathology is being assessed; very often used in short-term studies of interventions, particularly drugs)
Zung (1965)	Zung Self-Rating Depression Scale	78.9 (the original self-rating scale; still widely used)
Brink et al (1982)	Geriatric Depression Scale (GDS)	71.9 (clear preference for this scale in studies of older adults)
Beck et al (1974b)	Hopelessness Scale	38.9 (very frequently used in studies of suicide)
Cox et al (1987)	Edinburgh Postnatal Depression Scale (EPDS)	33.1 (the established scale for assessing depression in relationship to childbirth) Also see Cox & Holden (2003)
Seligman et al (1979)	Attributional Style Questionnaire	22.4
Alexopoulos et al (1988)	Cornell Scale for Depression in Dementia	22 (an example of a special area in which a general scale may not be accurate)
Carney et al (1965)	ECT Scale (Newcastle)	21.4 (was once very widely used but less so recently, as the distinction between depressive syndromes is less often required)
Kandel & Davies (1982)	Six-Item Depression Mood Inventory	15.4
Brown & Harris (1978)	Life Events and Difficulties Scale (LEDS)	11.2 (the definitive life events assessment scale – needs prior training – listed here as the work was primarily concerned with depression)
Zuckerman (1960)	Multiple Affect Adjective Checklist (MAACL)	8.5. (checklists used to be very common methods of assessing mood states but are now less often used)

continued

187

Table 11.1 *continued*

Author(s)	Type of assessment	Citation rate per year and comments
Robinson *et al* (1993)	Pathological Laughter and Crying Scale	8.2
Raskin *et al* (1969)	Raskin Three-Area Depression Rating Scale	7.9
McNair & Lorr (1964)	Profile of Mood States (POMS)	7.63 (a very widely used simple scale, but not used so much in recent years)
Snaith *et al* (1971)	Wakefield Self-Assessment Depression Inventory	6.97 (now replaced mainly by Hospital Anxiety and Depression Scale)
Steiner *et al* (1980)	Premenstrual Tension Syndrome Scale (PMTS)	6.8
Snaith *et al* (1976)	Leeds Scales for the Self-Assessment of Anxiety and Depression	6.71 (as for Wakefield Scale)
Lubin (1965)	Depression Adjective Check-List (DACL)	6.3
Sunderland *et al* (1988)	Dementia Mood Assessment Scale	5.6
Costello & Comfrey (1967)	Costello's Scales for Measuring Depression and Anxiety	5
Berrios *et al* (1992)	Guilt Scale	3.9

Table 11.2 Rating scales for mania

Author(s)	Type of assessment	Citation rate per year and comments
Young *et al* (1978)	Young Mania Rating Scale	21.5 (a short scale now well established in research studies of all kinds and the clear leader)
Bech *et al* (1986)	Bech–Rafaelsen Rating Scale for Mania	3.6 (particularly useful when severe depression (melancholia) also being measured, as Bech–Rafaelsen Rating Scale for Melancholia can also be used)
Altman *et al* (1994)	Clinician-Administered Rating Scale for Mania (CARS–M)	3.5 (good psychometric properties but not widely used)

with the more established scales, and can sometimes lead to a great deal of extra help in both using and analysing results.

Depression and mania

Depression (next to anxiety) is probably the most common psychiatric symptom and so there are many scales for its measurement. However, only five (Table 11.1) are used frequently in current research studies and the choice is not as difficult as might have been expected. In contrast, mania is less common and there are considerably fewer scales, of which the Young Mania Rating Scale is the most often chosen (Table 11.2). For studies in which both mania and depression are investigated the Bech–Rafaelsen scales for both mania and melancholia (Bech *et al*, 1986) may be most appropriate. As depression can occur in so many different clinical contexts there is scope for many other instruments for its measurement. The Edinburgh Postnatal Depression Scale (Cox *et al*, 1987) (Table 11.1) is probably the best example of a more specialised scale, but all of the specialised scales closely correlate with the general scales and have overlapping questions.

Cognitive function and impairment (including assessments specific to old age)

Although mood disturbance may be the most common psychiatric symptom, cognitive function, in its many forms, is probably most frequently assessed. It is now accepted that something more than clinical questioning is needed to assess cognitive functioning and this is demonstrated by the success of the Mini Mental State Examination (MMSE; Table 11.3) and its modified form (3MS; Teng & Chui, 1987) as part of clinical assessment (Aquilina & Warner, 2004). The ordinary assessment of mental state is being supplemented by a more formal measure that can be scored and helps to quantify any impairment. As the average age of the population increases, so will the use of these scales.

Eating disorders

The symptomatology and related clinical features of eating disorders show important differences from other syndromes in psychiatry and require assessment with appropriate specialised scales. Although self-rating scales are commonly used, there is a problem with their validity at some stages of illness, particularly in severe anorexia when patients often deny obvious symptomatology (Halmi, 1985). The two most frequently used scales are the Eating Attitudes Test (Garner & Garfinkel, 1979) and the Eating Attitudes Inventory (Garner *et al*, 1983), but bulimia is often assessed using different scales (Halmi *et al*, 1981; Henderson & Freeman, 1987) (Table 11.4). However, no one scale achieves clear primacy in this area.

Table 11.3 Scales for assessment of cognitive function and old age symptomatology

Author(s)	Name of scale	Citations per year and comments
Folstein *et al* (1975)	Mini Mental State Examination (MMSE)	528.9 (The ultimate success of a rating scale is to be incorporated into standard clinical practice. The MMSE has now achieved this status – at least for the time being.)
Hughes *et al* (1982)	Clinical Dementia Rating (CDR)	68.1
Hachinski *et al* (1975)	Ischemia Score	66.1
Blessed *et al* (1968)	Blessed Dementia Rating Scale (BDRS) Information – Memory – Concentration Test (IMCT)	62.7
Gottfries *et al* (1982*a,b*)	Gottfries–Brane–Steen Dementia Rating Scale (GBS)	61
Reisberg *et al* (1982)	Global Deterioration Scale (GDS)	55.7
Katz *et al* (1963)	Index of Activities of Daily Living	52.7 (included here as this assessment is so often linked to cognitive assessment but could also be included under social function)
Cummings *et al* (1994)	Neuropsychiatric Inventory (NPI)	50.4
Mohs *et al* (1983)	Alzheimer's Disease Assessment Scale (ADAS)	42.5
Lawton & Brody (1969); Lawton (1988*a,b*)	Instrumental Activities of Daily Living (IADL) Scale	41.3 (as for Katz *et al* 1963)
Pfeiffer (1975)	Short Portable Mental Status Questionnaire (SPMSQ)	41.2
Plutchik *et al* (1970)	Geriatric Rating Scale (GRS)	34
Teng & Chui (1987)	Modified Mini-Mental State (3MS) Examination	26.7
Neugarten *et al* (1961)	Life Satisfaction Index (LSI)	19.5
Roth *et al* (1988)	Cambridge Mental Disorders of the Elderly Examination (CAMDEX)	17.7 (increasingly being used in non-US studies)
Katzman *et al* (1983)	Orientation–Memory–Concentration Test (OMCT)	17
Broadbent *et al* (1982)	Cognitive Failures Questionnaire (CFQ)	16.8
Lawton *et al* (1982)	Multilevel Assessment Instrument (MAI)	16.5

continued

Table 11.3 *continued*

Author(s)	Name of scale	Citations per year and comments
Copeland *et al* (1976)	Geriatric Mental State Schedule (GMS)	15.8
Copeland *et al* (1986)	Geriatric Mental State Schedule and Diagnostic Schedule (AGECAT)	15.7
Teri *et al* (1992)	Revised memory and behaviour checklist	14.8
Hodkinson (1972)	Mental Test Score	14.3
Lawton (1975)	Philadelphia Geriatric Center Morale Scale	13.9
Wells (1979)	Checklist Differentiating Pseudo-Dementia from Dementia	13.7
Gelinas & Gauthier (1999)	Disability Assessment for Dementia (DAD)	12.6
Inouye *et al* (1990)	Confusion assessment method (CAM)	11.9
Greene *et al* (1982)	Relative's Stress Scale	10.1
Greene *et al* (1982)	Behaviour and Mood Disturbance Scale	10
Knopman *et al* (1994)	Clinicians Interview-Based Impression (CIBI)	10
Soloman *et al* (1998)	Seven minute neurocognitive screening battery	9.8
Pattie & Gilleard (1979)	Clifton Assessment Procedures for the Elderly (CAPE)	9.6
Reisberg (1988)	Functional Assessment Staging (FAST)	9.6
Trzepacz *et al* (1988)	Delirium Rating Scale (DRS)	9.3
Jorm & Jacomb (1989)	Informant Questionnaire on Cognitive Decline in the Elderly (IQCODE)	9.3
Shader *et al* (1974)	Sandoz Clinical Assessment–Geriatric (SCAG) Scale	8.2
Cohen-Mansfield *et al* (1989)	Cohen-Mansfield Agitation Inventory (CMAI)	8.1
Kopelman *et al* (1990)	Autobiographical Memory Interview (AMI)	7.4

continued

Table 11.3 *continued*

Author(s)	Name of scale	Citations per year and comments
Gurland *et al* (1976, 1977)	Comprehensive Assessment and Referral Evaluation (CARE)	6.7
Logsdon & Gibbons (1999)	Quality of Life in Alzheimer's Disease (QoL–AD)	6.6
Hall *et al* (1993)	Bilingual Dementia Screening Interview	5.6
Reisberg & Ferris (1988)	Brief Cognitive Rating Scale (BCRS)	4.7
Spiegel *et al* (1991)	Nurses' Observation Scale for Geriatric Patients (NOSGER)	4.6
Hope & Fairburn (1992)	Present Behavioural Examination (PBE)	4.6
Patel & Hope (1992)	Rating Scale for Aggressive Behaviour in the Elderly – The RAGE	4.5
Wilkinson & Graham-White (1980)	Edinburgh Psychogeriatric Dependency Rating Scale (PGDRS)	4.5
Jorm *et al* (1995)	Psychogeriatric Assessment Scales (PAS)	4.2
Allen *et al* (1996)	Manchester and Oxford Universities Scale for the Psychopathological Assessment of Dementia (MOUSEPAD)	4 (close to getting an award for the most inventive acronym for a scale)
Qureshi & Hodkinson (1974)	Abbreviated Mental Test (AMT)	4
Helmes *et al* (1987)	Multidimensional Observation Scale for Elderly Subjects (MOSES)	3.6
Adshead *et al* (1992)	Brief Assessment Schedule Depression Cards (BASDEC)	3.4 (simple assessment using cards in similar situations to those for Cornell Scale for Depression in Dementia)
Sclan & Saillon (1996)	BEHAVE–AD	3.1
Kendrick *et al* (1979)	Kendrick Battery for the Detection of Dementia in the Elderly	2.8
Meer & Baker (1966)	Stockton Geriatric Rating Scale (SGRS)	2.7
Kuriansky & Gurland (1976)	Performance Test of Activities of Daily Living (PADL)	2.6
Bucks *et al* (1996)	Bristol Activities of Daily Living Scale	2.6
Schwartz (1983)	Geriatric Evaluation by Relative's Rating Instrument (GERRI)	2.5
Hersch (1979)	Extended Scale for Dementia (ESD)	2.3

Table 11.4 Instruments for the measurement of symptoms and attitudes in eating disorders

Author(s)	Name of scale	Citations per year and comments
Garner *et al* (1983)	Body Dissatisfaction Subscale of the Eating Disorder Inventory (EDI)	56.7 (The EDI is the most commonly used measure with a range of sub-scales – better for anorexia than bulimia)
Stunkard & Messick (1985)	Eating Inventory	42.1
Garner & Garfinkel (1979)	Eating Attitudes Test (EAT)	40.8
Halmi *et al* (1981)	Binge Eating Questionnaire	22
Cooper *et al* (1987)	Body Shape Questionnaire	16.5
Van Strien *et al* (1986)	Dutch Eating Behaviour Questionnaire (DEBQ)	16.1
Cooper & Fairburn (1987)	Eating Disorders Examination (EDE)	15.9 (semi-structured interview covering both bulimia and anorexia)
Morgan & Russell (1975)	Morgan–Russell Assessment Schedule (MRAS)	15.9 (often used in long-term outcome studies)
Gormally *et al* (1982)	Binge Eating Scale	12.7
Henderson & Freeman (1987)	Bulimic Investigatory Test, Edinburgh (BITE)	12.2 (short (33-item) questionnaire suitable for surveys)
Hawkins & Clement (1980)	Binge Scale	11.8
Smith & Thelen (1984)	Bulimia Test (BULIT)	8.6
Slade & Russell (1973)	Anorexic Behaviour Scale (ABS)	7.0
Johnson (1985)	Diagnostic Survey for Eating Disorders (DSED)	5.5
Slade *et al* (1990)	Body Satisfaction Scale (BSS)	3.1
Fichter *et al* (1989)	Structured Interview for anorexia and Bulimia Nervosa (SIAB)	3
Ben-Tovim & Walker (1991)	Ben-Tovim Walker Body Attitudes Questionnaire (BAQ)	2.9
Slade & Dewey (1986)	Setting Conditions for Anorexia Nervosa (SCANS)	2.3

193

General functioning and symptomatology

Psychiatry as a discipline used to be criticised because it did not use the language of science and measurement and so could be interpreted in so many different ways. The discipline responded (some might say overreacted) to this criticism by introducing a much more rigid and reliable set of diagnoses, the *Diagnostic and Statistical Manual for Mental Disorders* (3rd edn) (DSM–III) (American Psychiatric Association, 1980). By introducing operational criteria for the definition of each diagnosis a much greater level of reliability was achieved, but it is well known that improvements in reliability are often achieved at the expense of validity. This was a central issue of the life work of Robert Kendell (1925–2002), who pointed out that the only valid diagnosis was the one that demonstrated a 'point of rarity' between it and other diagnoses, in the same way that many organic diagnoses do in medicine. In fact, almost every psychiatric diagnosis is best perceived as a continuum or dimension rather than a separate and discrete category. This is not a criticism of the diagnostic process, since the identification of a psychiatric diagnosis may still be extremely useful in clinical practice; what must not be assumed is that clinical utility is the same as clinical validity (Kendell & Jablensky, 2003). This basic understanding of psychiatric diagnoses as a continuum is one of the reasons why scales measuring general functioning and symptomatology are becoming more popular; they are recording the dimensions.

Researchers will also wish to measure global psychopathology when the population being studied is a heterogeneous one in which all aspects of symptomatology need to be detected. Epidemiological studies of whole populations and cohort studies that examine change and new pathology over time are the most common examples. Many of the scales are linked to diagnoses, particularly DSM ones, and this probably explains why the SCID group (Structured Clinical Interviews for DSM Diagnoses) are so popular (Table 11.5). However, research workers should note that DSM–V is going to be very different from its predecessors and it is wise not to be too attached to measurement scales that are related to a changing system.

Satisfaction and needs

There is now a realisation of the importance of the consumer in mental health services, and although the word 'user' is not entirely satisfactory, the balance of influence is gradually shifting towards those who receive treatment from those who do the treating. We therefore have a range of relatively new instruments to measure need and satisfaction with services that are now becoming *de rigeur* in many research arenas. The best known of these is probably the Camberwell Assessment of Need (CAN; Phelan

Table 11.5 Scales for general functioning and symptomatology

Author(s)	Name of scale	Citations per year and comments
Spitzer *et al* (1990*a,b, d*)	Structured Clinical Interview for DSM–III–R (SCID)	165.6 (simple and straightforward scales that lack some subtlety but are widely used because of their DSM links)
Spitzer *et al* (1990*c*)	Structured Clinical Interview for DSM–III–R personality disorders (SCID–II)	162.7
Robins *et al* (1981)	Diagnostic Interview Schedule (DIS)	135.1
Wing *et al* (1974)	Present State Examination and Catego Program (PSE)	112.4 (now being replaced by SCAN, which incorporates much of the old PSE)
Endicott *et al* (1976)	Global Assessment Scale (GAS), later to become Global Assessment of Functioning (GAF)	76.3 (a scale that is now an axis of pathology – Axis 5 in the DSM classification) (may be separated into symptomatology and functioning components)
Goldberg (1972)	General Health Questionnaire (GHQ)	59.0 (the doyen of quick screening for common mental disorders)
Scheier & Carver (1985)	Life Orientation Test (LOT)	53.6
Derogatis *et al* (1973)	Symptom Check-List (SCL-90)	50.8 (very popular quick assessment of psychopathology but coming to the end of its useful life)
Derogatis *et al* (1974)	Hopkins Symptom Checklist (HSCL)	45.2 (linked to SCL-90)
Robins *et al* (1988)	The Composite International Diagnostic Interview (CIDI)	44.0 (rapidly becoming the benchmark for national epidemiological studies (except in the UK, where CIS–R is still used)
Åsberg *et al* (1978)	Comprehensive Psychopathological Rating Scale (CPRS)	33 (has the advantage of being linked to sub-scales for depression, anxiety, and obsessional and schizophrenic pathology)
Wing *et al* (1990)	SCAN – Schedules for Clinical Assessment in Neuropsychiatry	30.9 (the successor to the PSE, shortly to come out in a revised form (SCAN–II))
McGuffin *et al* (1991)	Operational criteria for psychotic illnesses	28.5 (useful when information needs to be obtained from notes and other records – may be converted to several diagnostic systems)
Millon (1981)	Millon Clinical Multiaxial Inventory (MCMI)	27 (a very popular personality assessment even though it does not match with DSM or ICD)

continued

Table 11.5 *continued*

Author(s)	Name of scale	Citations per year and comments
Goldberg *et al* (1970)	Clinical Interview Schedule (CIS)	20.4 (see also CIS–R)
Aitken (1969)	Visual Analogue Scales	20.1 (these are often useful when making self-ratings or in contructing one's own scales)
Dupuy (1984)	Psychological General Well-Being (PGWB) Index	19
Lewis *et al* (1992)	Clinical Interview Schedule – Revised (CIS–R)	17.8 (a scale specially developed for epidemiological studies with lay interviewers – has now mainly replaced the CIS)
Raskin & Crook (1988)	Relative's Assessment of Global Symptomatology (RAGS)	7
Spitzer *et al* (1970)	Psychiatric Status Schedule (PSS)	6.7
Brodman *et al* (1949)	Cornell Medical Index	6.6
Spanier (1987)	Dyadic Adjustment Scale	5.4
Luborsky (1962)	Health Sickness Rating Scale (HSRS)	5.3 (the forerunner of the GAF)
Burnam *et al* (1983)	Spanish Diagnostic Interview Schedule	5.1
Helzer & Robins (1981)	Renard Diagnostic Interview	4.8
Endicott & Spitzer (1972)	Current and Past Psychopathology Scales (CAPPS)	4.7
Marmar *et al* (1986)	California Psychotherapy Alliances Scales (CALPAS–T/P)	3.8
Power *et al* (1988)	Significant Others Scale (SOS)	3.8
Parloff *et al* (1954)	Symptom Check-List (SCL)	3.6
Lorr *et al* (1962)	Lorr's Multidimensional Scale for Rating Psychiatric Patients	2.3
Spitzer *et al* (1967)	Mental Status Schedule (MSS)	2.3

Table 11.6 Scales for the assessment of need and satisfaction

Author(s)	Name of scale	Citations per year and comments
Phelan *et al* (1995)	Camberwell Assessment of Need (CAN); CANE (Elderly), CANDID (Intellectual Disability), CANFOR (Forensic Psychiatry), CANSAS (Short Appraisal Schedule)	16.1 (now the most widely used scale in the area; the sub-scales have yet to be widely used)
Beecher (1959)	Measurement of Subjective Responses (MSR)	15.1 (useful in assessing the placebo effect)
Larsen *et al* (1979)	Consumer Satisfaction Questionnaire (CSQ)	14.5 (is rapidly becoming the most commonly used scale for measuring general satisfaction)
Amador *et al* (1993)	Scale to Assess Unawareness of Mental Disorder	13.1
Harding *et al* (1980)	Self Report Questionnaire (SRQ)	11.7
Bech (1993)	Psychological General Well-Being Schedule (PGWBS)	11.4
Bunney & Hamburg (1963)	Bunney–Hamburg Mood Check-list	10.8
Brewin *et al* (1987)	MRC Needs for Care Assessment	7.9 (the predecessor to CAN and probably its catalyst)
Ruggeri & Dall'Agnola (1993)	Verona Service Satisfaction Scale (VSSS)	6.2 (specifically developed for measuring satisfaction with mental health services)
Birchwood *et al* (1994)	Insight Scale (for Psychosis)	6.1 (the measurement of insight is becoming increasingly important in research studies)
Markova & Berrios (1992)	Insight Scale	3.8
Shipley *et al* (2000)	Patient Satisfaction Questionnaire	2.3
Tantam (1988)	The Express Scale and Personality Questionnaire	2.3

et al, 1995) and its many successors (CANSAS, CANFOR, CANDID, etc.), the latest being CAN–M for mothers. However, there are many others that attempt to assess patients' experiences and feelings towards their condition and treatment in a variety of settings (Table 11.6).

Self-harm

Self-harm has come to replace the earlier term 'parasuicide' and the misleading one 'attempted suicide' as a description of the behaviour of those who do not usually carry out their acts of harm with the intention of killing themselves, but who might do so by accident and are at much greater risk of successful suicide in the future (Jenkins *et al*, 2002; Zahl & Hawton, 2004). The chances of repeat attempts and successful suicide are greater when suicidal intent is greater (Zahl & Hawton, 2004) and so measures of this and other elements of risk are useful) (Table 11.7). There is evidence that such scales are successful in predicting self-harm (Tyrer *et al*, 2003).

Sexual behaviour

Although sexual behaviour has rarely been measured systematically in many psychiatric studies when it is clearly relevant (e.g. in patients with schizophrenia on antipsychotic drugs), such measurement is now

Table 11.7 Scales for the assessment of self-harm

Author(s)	Name of scale	Citations per year
Beck *et al* (1974*a*)	Beck Hopelessness Scale	43.7[1]
Beck *et al* (1979)	Scale for Suicide Ideation (SSI)	12.7
Beck *et al* (1974*b*)	Suicidal Intent Scale (SIS)	12
Motto *et al* (1985)	Risk Estimator for Suicide	4.2
Pallis *et al* (1982)	Post-Attempt Risk Assessment Scale	2.6
Plutchik *et al* (1989)	Suicide Risk Scale (SRS)	2.5
Buglass & Horton (1974)	Risk of Repetition Scale	2.3
Tuckman & Youngman (1968)	Scale for Assessing Suicide Risk of Attempted Suicides	2.3
Kreitman & Foster (1991)	Parasuicide Risk Scale	2.3

1. By far the most quoted and used scale, although hopelessness not strictly a self-harm measure.

becoming both more accepted and acceptable in research studies. For this reason a greater number of scales is given in Table 11.8 than is strictly necessary as their citation rate has been fairly low.

Substance use, dependence and withdrawal

The assessment of substance misuse is prone to error, mainly because the reliability of the information is often so uncertain. Hence there is an increasing tendency to use modern techniques such as hair analysis to obtain independent evidence of drug use. Table 11.9 includes some scales that are becoming established assessments for research studies; AUDIT, MAST, CAGE and SDS are the most frequently used. Most scales in Table 11.9 are concerned with dependence.

Increasingly it is becoming necessary to record symptoms of withdrawal following the cessation of illicit or prescribed drugs. Because each group of substances has different withdrawal effects (in addition to many common ones) it is probably preferable to select a scale to suit the substance (Table 11.10) rather than use a general scale.

Personality assessment and persistent behaviours

Personality assessment is one of the more difficult subjects to tackle in research. Like IQ, we like to think of personality as stable, but empirical studies have shown it is much less stable than we would like to think. However, when assessing personality we are not just assessing present

Table 11.8 Scales for the assessment of sexual function and behaviour

Author(s)	Name of scale	Citations per year
Lopiccolo & Steger (1974)	Sexual Interaction Inventory	50
Wilhelm & Parker (1988)	Intimate Bond Measure (IBM)	4
Hoon *et al* (1976)	Sexual Arousal Inventory (SAI)	3.9
Nichols & Molinder (1984)	Multiphasic Sex Inventory (MSI)	2.8
Eysenck (1971)	Eysenck Inventory of Attitudes to Sex	1.9
Golombok & Rust (1985)	Golombok–Rust Inventory of Sexual Satisfaction (GRISS)	1.6
Derogatis (1978)	Derogatis Sexual Functioning Inventory (DSFI)	1.3
Frenken & Vennix (1981)	Sexual Experience Scales (SES)	1.2

Table 11.9   Scales for the assessment of substance use and dependence

Author(s)	Name of scale	Citations per year and comments
Saunders et al (1993)	Alcohol Use Disorders Identification Test (AUDIT)	45.3 (used for the identification of hazardous and harmful alcohol consumption)
Selzer (1971)	Michigan Alcoholism Screening Test (MAST)	42.1
Mayfield et al (1974)	CAGE Questionnaire	27.6
Gossop et al (1995)	The Severity of Dependence Scale (SDS)	13.8 (used in heroin, amphetamine and cocaine dependence)
McLennan et al (1980)	Addiction Severity Index	5
Skinner & Allen (1983)	Alcohol Dependence Scale (ADS)	2.8
Chick (1980)	Edinburgh Alcohol Dependence Scale	2.3
Halikas et al (1991)	Minnesota Cocaine Craving Scale	2.2
Smith et al (1996)	Paddington Alcohol Test (PAT)	2.1 (used to detect hazardous drinking in patients presenting as emergencies)
Horn et al (1974)	Alcohol Use Inventory	2.1
Litman et al (1983)	Coping Behaviour Inventory (CBI)	2
Litman et al (1984)	Effectiveness of Coping Behaviour Inventory (ECBI)	1.9
Washton et al (1988)	Cocaine Abuse Assessment Profile (CAAP)	1.1
Skinner & Goldberg (1986)	Drug Abuse Screening Test (DAST)	1.1

Table 11.10   Scales for the assessment of substance use withdrawal problems

Author(s)	Name of scale	Citations per year
Chaney et al (1978)	Situational Competency Test (SCT)	8.7
Gross et al (1973)	TSA and SSA	5.9
Raistrick et al (1983)	Short Alcohol Dependence Data (SADD)	4.4
Tyrer et al (1990)	Benzodiazepine Withdrawal Symptom Questionnaire	4.2
Handelsman et al (1987)	Objective Opiate Withdrawal Scale (OOWS)	3.5
Handelsman et al (1987)	Subjective Opiate Withdrawal Scale	3.5
Annis (1986)	Situational Confidence Questionnaire	2.7
Sutherland et al (1986)	Severity of Opiate Dependence Questionnaire (SODQ)/Opiate Subjective Dependence Questionnaire (OSDQ)	2.4

personality function but characteristic function over a long period. This cannot be done easily but there are many attempts to shorten the assessment process in order to fit in with the multiple assessments being performed over a short time period. Most assessments are carried out using the DSM recommendations for personality disorders, even though these are now recognised to be grossly unsatisfactory and redundant in research terms (Livesley, 2001). Persistent behavioural problems such as aggression are also included in Table 11.11. There is also a very important group of instruments that measure risk of violence and these are becoming more commonly used in research studies as their predictive quality improves. The Psychopathy Checklist–Revised (PCL–R; Hare, 1991) is the best known but there are also many others (Dolan & Doyle, 2000).

Anxiety and associated disorders

Anxiety is ubiquitous, easy to measure but difficult to interpret. There has been much argument over the differences between state and trait anxiety and their significance, the meaning of the association of anxiety and depression (the two are intimate) and the importance of anxiety to the course and development of phobic, obsessional, hypochondriacal, pain, post-traumatic and fatigue disorders. These subjects are therefore included in Tables 11.12 and 11.13.

Sleep

Despite being somewhat relegated to the sidelines of psychiatry in recent years, sleep problems remain very prominent symptoms of mental illness. It is always possible to assess sleep problems from individual items in scales for depression and anxiety but for general sleep satisfaction and performance it is preferable to use one of the scales in Table 11.14.

Schizophrenia and related psychotic disorders

Although there continues to be debate over the issues of insight, adherence to therapy and the relationship between schizotypy and schizophrenia, the core assessment of schizophrenic pathology involves assessment with relatively few instruments, of which the Schedule for Affective Disorders and Schizophrenia (SADS) and Scales for the Assessment of Positive and Negative Symptoms (SAPS and SANS) are the most popular, and are gradually replacing the Brief Psychiatric Rating Scale (BPRS; Overall & Gorham, 1962) from the lead position it has held for most of the past 40 years (Table 11.15). The major change has been in the recognition of positive and negative symptoms and the need to record them separately. The different therapeutic profile of drugs such as clozapine has helped in this differentiation, as has

Table 11.11 Scales for assessing personality and persistent behavioural problems

Authors	Name of scale	Citations per year and comments
Spitzer *et al* (1990*c*)	Structured Clinical Interview for DSM–III–R Personality Disorders (SCID–II)	162.7
Buss & Durkee (1957)	Buss–Durkee Hostility and Guild Inventory	23.6
Spielberger *et al* (1985)	State–Trait Anger Expression Inventory (STAXI)	23.2
Pfohl *et al* (1983)	Structured Interview for DSM–III Personality Disorders (SID–P)	17.9
Yudofsky (1986)	Overt Aggression Scale (OAS)	17.3 (may also be used in modified form as the Modified Overt Aggression Scale (MOAS) (Sorgi *et al*, 1991))
Hathaway & McKinley (1967)	Minnesota Multiphasic Personality Inventory (MMPI)	16.6
Gunderson *et al* (1981)	Diagnostic Interview for Borderline Patients	15.6
Loranger *et al* (1985)	Personality Disorder Examination (PDE)	14
Tyrer & Alexander (1979)	Personality Assessment Schedule (PAS)	13.8
Rosenbaum (1980)	Self Control Schedule	13.2
Barron (1953)	Barron Ego Strength	10.9
Hare (1980)	Psychopathy Checklist (PCL)	10.2 (the best predictor of aggressive behaviour in psychiatric patients (Monahan *et al*, 2001); was revised in 1990 (PCL–R) and again in 2004; special training is required which is unlikely to be possible within the budget of simple research projects)
Hyler & Reider (1987)	Personality Diagnostic Questionnaire – Revised (PDQ–R)	9.8
Morey *et al* (1985)	Modified Minnesota Multiphasic Personality Inventory (MMPI)	9.1

continued

Table 11.11 *continued*

Authors	Name of scale	Citations per year and comments
Schwartz & Gottman (1976)	Assertiveness Self-Statement Test (ASST)	6.3
Glass *et al* (1982)	Social Interaction Self-Statement Test (SISST)	6.2
Palmstierna & Wistedt (1987)	Staff Observation and Aggression Scale (SOAS)	5.8
Baron *et al* (1981)	Schedule for Interviewing Schizotypal Personalities (SSP)	5.2
Conte *et al* (1980)	Borderline Syndrome Index (BSI)	5
Robson (1989)	Robson's Self-Esteem Scale	4.3
Bell (1981)	Bell Object Relations Self-Report Scale	3.8
Mann *et al* (1981)	Standardized Assessment of Personality (SAP)	3.7
Hyler *et al* (1982)	Personality Diagnostic Questionnaire (PDQ)	3.5
Galissi *et al* (1981)	Checklist of Positive and Negative Thoughts	3.2
Lorr & Youniss (1983)	Interpersonal Style Inventory (ISI)	2.1

Table 11.12   Scales for hypochondriasis, health anxiety, pain and fatigue

Author(s)	Name of scale	Citations per year
Fukuda *et al* (1994)	Chronic Fatigue Syndrome – case-defining symptoms	87.4 (important for examining chronic fatigue and formalising description of cases)
Melzack (1987)	McGill Pain Questionnaire (MPQ)	29.6
Chalder *et al* (1993)	Fatigue Scale	22.6
Pilowsky & Spence (1975)	Illness Behaviour Questionnaire (IBQ)	7.4
Kellner (1987)	Symptom questionnaire	7.2 (now mainly of historical interest)
Barsky *et al* (1990)	Somatosensory Amplification Scale (SSAS)	7.1 (may be useful to detect health anxiety)
Salkovskis *et al* (2002)	Health Anxiety Inventory (HAI)	2.3 (specifically used for health anxiety, which is not quite the same as the old concept of hypochondriasis)

Table 11.13 Scales for assessment of anxiety and related symptoms

Authors	Name of scale	Citations per year and comments
Zigmond & Snaith (1983)	Hospital Anxiety and Depression Scale (HADS)	133.0 (the anxiety version (HADS–A) can also be combined with the depression component (HADS–D) to score mixed anxiety–depressive symptoms (cothymia) (Tyrer, 2001))
Spielberger *et al* (1983)	Spielberger State–Trait Anxiety Inventory (STAI)	121.4 (commonly used in repeated measures studies – in which both present state and trait anxiety are measured separately)
Goodman *et al* (1989*a,b*)	Yale–Brown Obsessive Compulsive Scale (Y–BOCS)	81.1 (the standard scale for measurement of obsessive–compulsive symptoms – clearly now pre-eminent)
Beck *et al* (1988)	Beck Anxiety Inventory (BAI)	49.8 (beginning to usurp the Hamilton scale)
Hamilton (1959)	Hamilton Anxiety Scale (HAS)	45.6 (an observer-rated scale that remains standard but has been criticised for its emphasis on somatic symptoms that may reflect physical illness)
Taylor (1953)	Taylor Manifest Anxiety Scale (TMAS)	44.4 (really a measure of trait anxiety)
Marks & Mathews (1979)	Brief Standard Self-Rating Scale for Phobic Patients	36.2 (the most common self-rating for common phobic symptoms)
Keane *et al* (1988)	Mississippi Scale for Combat-Related Post-traumatic Stress Disorder	35.8
Watson & Friend (1969)	Fear of Negative Evaluation Scale (FNE)	28.3
Watson & Friend (1969)	Social Avoidance and Distress Scale (SAD)	28.3
Chambless *et al* (1984)	Body Sensations Questionnaire and the Agoraphobic Cognitions Questionnaire	20
Chambless *et al* (1985)	Mobility Inventory for Agoraphobia	18.8
Wolpe & Lang (1964)	Fear Survey Schedule (FSS)	14.9
Zung (1971)	Zung's Anxiety Status Inventory (ASI)	13.6
Alderman *et al* (1983)	Crown-Crisp Experiential Index (CCEI)	13.1
Hodgson & Rachman (1977)	Maudsley Obsessional-Compulsive Inventory	13.1

continued

Table 11.13 *continued*

Authors	Name of scale	Citations per year and comments
Beck *et al* (1987)	Cognitions Checklist–Anxiety (CCL–A)	10.8 (relevant in monitoring cognitive–behavioural therapy)
Davidson *et al* (1997)	Davidson Trauma Scale (DTS)	10.6
Cooper (1970)	Leyton Obsessional Inventory	9.6
Sanavio (1988)	Padua Inventory	8.3
Steinberg *et al* (1990)	Structured Clinical Interview for DSM–III–R Dissociative Disorders (SCID–D)	7
Crown & Crisp (1966)	Middlesex Hospital Questionnaire (MHQ)	6.9
Endler *et al* (1962)	Stimulus Response Inventory	6.6
Foa *et al* (1998)	Obsessive–Compulsive Inventory (OCI)	6.0 (42-item inventory that has recently been introduced in shortened form (Foa *et al*, 2002) which may be superseding the original)
Snaith *et al* (1982)	Clinical Anxiety Scale	5.5 (an attempt to compensate for the over-somatic representation of the Hamilton scale)
Gelder & Marks (1966)	Gelder–Marks Phobia Questionnaire	5.1
Bandelow (1995)	Panic and Agoraphobia Scale	5.1
Davidson & Miner (1997)	Brief Social Phobia Scale	5.0
Tyrer *et al* (1984)	Brief Anxiety Scale	4.2 (linked to Comprehensive Psychopathological Rating Scale (CPRS))
Snaith *et al* (1978)	Irritability–Depression–Anxiety Scale (IDA)	3.7 (probably the only measure of irritability available)

Table 11.14 Scales for the assessment of sleep disorders

Author(s)	Name of scale	Citations per year
Carskadon (1986)	Multiple Sleep Latency Test (MSLT)	30.1
Guilleminault (1982)	Sleep Questionnaire and Assessment of Wakefulness (SQAW)	7.5
Ellis *et al* (1981)	St Mary's Hospital Sleep Questionnaire	3.6
Parrott & Hindmarch (1978)	Sleep Evaluation Questionnaire (SEQ)	3.1
Hoddes *et al* (1972*a,b*)	Stanford Sleepiness Scale (SSS)	3.1

the focus of psychological treatments on negative symptoms (Sensky *et al*, 2000). Standard scales for the measurement of adverse effects are also included here. The clear preference for the measurement of akathisia is the Barnes scale (1989) and for tardive dyskinesia the Tardive Dyskinesia Rating Scale (TDRS; Simpson, 1988), but there are several competitors for primacy when other abnormal movements are being measured.

Childhood disorders

There are an astonishingly large number of scales in child and adolescent psychiatry; this is as much an expression of wonderment as one of criticism, and there are now many more than the 22 we listed in the previous edition of this book. This is also discussed at some length in Chapter 12. It is a pity that for so many areas there are no clear preferences or obvious front-runners. For specific areas the scales may select themselves. The Parental Bonding Instrument (PBI; Parker *et al*, 1979) is one such example; it has almost become a *sine qua non* of the assessment of early relational attachment. For other subjects it has become common for scales developed in adult practice to be adapted for children. Well-known examples include the Kiddie–SADS (K–SADS; Puig-Antich & Chambers, 1978) and the Leyton Obsessional Inventory – Child Version (Berg *et al*, 1986; Table 11.16). There has been considerable recent interest in attention-deficit hyperactivity disorder in children and in the autistic spectrum of disorders, and some recently introduced instruments are likely to be widely used (e.g. Holmes *et al*, 2004; Hansson *et al*, 2005).

When choosing instruments in child psychiatry it is important to ensure that the age range over which the instrument has been validated is the same as the population for which the researcher requires the instrument. Please refer to Chapter 12 for further advice.

Table 11.15   Scales for the assessment of schizophrenia and related psychotic disorders (including adverse effects)

Author(s)	Name of scale	Citations per year and comments
Endicott & Spitzer (1978)	Schedule for Affective Disorders and Schizophrenia (SADS)	146.8
Overall & Gorham (1962)	Brief Psychiatric Rating Scale (BPRS)	123.3 (the oldest scale but still has many merits and is likely to be relevant however diagnostic practice changes)
Bernstein & Putnam (1986)	Dissociative Experiences Scale (DES)	44.4
Andreasen (1982*a,b*)	Scale for the Assessment of Negative Symptoms (SANS)	42.7 (steadily increasing in use as the importance of negative symptoms in treatment outcome grows)
Barnes (1989)	Barnes Akathisia Rating Scale (BARS)	34.1 (the standard scale for recording akathisia)
Andreasen (1984)	Scale for the Assessment of Positive Symptoms (SAPS)	22.5
Andreasen *et al* (1992)	Comprehensive Assessment of Symptoms and History CASH)	20.7
Simpson (1988)	Tardive Dyskinesia Rating Scale (TDRS)	12.9
Andreasen (1979)	Thought, Language and Communication Rating Scale (TLC)	11.2
Claridge & Broks (1984)	Schizotypy Questionnaire (STQ)	10.6
Birchwood *et al* (1990)	Social Functioning Schedule (SFS)	5.5 (included here as it was specially prepared for the measurement of social function in schizophrenic patients)
Kendler *et al* (1983)	Dimensions of Delusional Experience Scale	3.7

Table 11.16   Scales for the assessment of childhood disorders

Author(s)	Name of scale	Citations per year
Conners (1969)	Conners Rating Scales	33.1
Herjanic & Campbell (1977)	Diagnostic Interview for Children & Adolescents (DICA)	33.1
Parker *et al* (1979)	Parental Boding Instrument (PBI)	33
Puig-Antich & Chambers (1978)	Kiddie–SADS (K–SADS)	27.2
Kovacs (1985)	Children's Depression Inventory (CDI)	26.3
Reynolds & Richmond (1978)	Revised Children's Manifest Anxiety Scale	26.3
Wechsler (1949)	Wechsler Intelligence Scale for Children	23.3
Achenbach (1978); Achenbach & Edelbrock (1979)	Child Behaviour Check-List (CBCL)	21.7
Puig-Antich *et al* (1980)	Kiddie–SADS–E (K–SADS–E)	19.9
Ward *et al* (1993)	Wender Utah Rating Scale (WURS)	18.7
Achenbach & McConaughy (1987a,b)	Empirically-Based Assessment of Child and Adolescent Psychopathology	14
Hodges *et al* (1982)	Child Assessment Schedule (CAS)	12.4
Harris (1963)	Goodenough–Harris Figure Drawing Test	12.3
Castaneda *et al* (1956)	Children's Manifest Anxiety Scale (CMAS)	10.1
Birleson (1981)	Depression Self-Rating Scale (DSRS)	9.4
Costello *et al* (1984)	Diagnostic Interview Schedule for Children (DISC)	7.7
Richman & Graham (1971)	Behavioural Screening Questionnaire (BSQ)	7.2
Berg *et al* (1986)	Leyton Obsessional Inventory – Child Version	6.2
Poznanski *et al* (1979)	Children's Depression Rating Scale (CDRS)	6
Carey (1970)	Carey Infant Temperament Scale	5.7
Ambrosini *et al* (1989)	Kiddie–SADS–III–R (K–SADS–III–R)	5.1
Lefkowitz & Tesing (1980)	Peer Nomination Inventory for Depression	5
Elliott *et al* (1983)	British Ability Scales – Revised (BAS–R)	4.9
Ullman *et al* (1984)	ADD–H Comprehensive Teacher Rating Scales (ACTeRS)	4.3
Reynolds *et al* (1985)	Child Depression Scale (CDS)	4

continued

Table 11.16 *continued*

Author(s)	Name of scale	Citations per year
Wing & Gould (1978)	Handicap, Behaviour and Skills (HBS)	3.9
Rutter (1967)	Rutter B(2) Scale	3.7
Quay & Peterson (1975)	Behavior Problem Checklist (BPC)	3.3
Zatz & Chassin (1983)	Children's Cognitive Assessment Questionnaire (CCAQ)	2.9
Matson *et al* (1991)	Diagnostic Assessment for the Severely Handicapped (DASH)	2.1

Social and behavioural measurement

The recording of social function is becoming a much more prominent part of measurement generally as it is now realised that functioning is probably more important than symptoms in determining the extent of pathology (Tyrer & Casey, 1993). Whether patients are admitted to hospital, either voluntarily or compulsorily, is determined much more by their general roles in society and their general functioning than by any independent measure of 'illness' *per se*. This is now recognised in multi-axial classification systems, in which social function and disability are given an axis for their domain, and in the growth of scales for recording social function in every medical condition. The scale that is cited more than any other is SF–36, the shortened form of an original medical outcomes scale which is so constructed as to record function in any disorder (Ware & Sherbourne, 1992). It is therefore used in many conditions, which explains its wide usage. It basically comprises one multi-item scale assessing eight health concepts: limitations in physical activities because of health problems; limitations in social activities because of physical or emotional problems; limitations in usual role activities because of physical health problems; bodily pain; general mental health (psychological distress and well-being); limitations in usual activities because of emotional problems; vitality (energy and fatigue); and general health perceptions. Sleep may also be included here. SF–36 is not always ideal for many psychiatric studies but is now such a benchmark measure that it should always be considered if general functioning is being measured.

Table 11.17 gives a comprehensive list of scales that encompass the range of subjects covered by social function and behaviour. Some of these are highly specific, if not idiosyncratic, but because of the frequent need for a specific instrument all are included.

Table 11.17 Scales for the assessment of social functioning

Author(s)	Name of scale	Citations per year
Ware & Sherbourne (1992)	Short Form 36 (SF–36) of Medical Outcomes Scale (MOS)	365.5
Holmes & Rahe (1967)	Social Readjustment Rating Scale	107.5
Kanner *et al* (1981)	Hassles Scale	49.9
Kanner *et al* (1981)	Uplifts Scale	49.9
Crowne & Marlowe (1960)	Marlowe–Crowne Social Desirability Scale (M–CSDS)	47.8
Sarason *et al* (1983)	Social Support Questionnaire (SSQ)	35.1
Russell *et al* (1978)	University of California, Los Angeles Loneliness Scale	30.5
Horowitz *et al* (1988)	Inventory of Personal Problems	25.8
Weissman & Bothwell (1976)	Social Adjustment Scale Self-Report (SAS–SR)	25.2
Jarman (1983)	Jarman Index	20.1
Paykel *et al* (1971)	Interview for Recent Life Events	12.5
Vaughan & Leff (1976)	Camberwell Family Interview (CFI)	11.6
Katz & Lyerly (1963)	Katz Adjustment Scale–Relatives Form (KAS–R)	10.6
Honigfeld & Klett (1965)	Nurses' Observation Scale for Inpatient Evaluation (NOSIE)	9.5
Aman *et al* (1985)	Aberrant Behavior Checklist	8.6
Derogatis (1976)	Psychosocial Adjustment to Illness Scale (PAIS)	8.4
Morosini & Magliano (2000)	Social and Functioning Assessment Scale (SOFAS)	7.9
Henderson *et al* (1980)	Interview Schedule for Social Interaction (ISSI)	7.9
Wykes & Sturt (1986)	Social Behaviour Schedule (SBS)	7.8
Gurland *et al* (1972)	Structured and Scaled Interview to Assess Maladjustment (SSIAM)	6.1
Kellner & Sheffield (1973)	Symptom Rating Test (SRT)	6.1
Doll (1965)	Vineland Social Maturity Scale	5.7
Tennant & Andrews (1976)	Life Events Inventory	5.6
Clare & Cains (1978)	Social Maladjustment Schedule (SMS)	4.9
Holmes *et al* (1982)	Disability Assessment Schedule (DAS)	4.5
Platt *et al* (1980)	Social Behaviour Assessment Schedule (SBAS)	4.3
Connor *et al* (2000)	Social Phobia Inventory (SPIN)	4
Margolin *et al* (1983)	Areas of Change Questionnaire (ACQ)	3.8
McFarlane *et al* (1981)	Social Relationship Scale (SRS)	3.5

continued

Table 11.17 *continued*

Author(s)	Name of scale	Citations per year
Jenkins *et al* (1981)	Social Stress and Support Interview (SSSI)	2.9
Tyrer (1990); Tyrer *et al* (2005)	Social Functioning Questionnaire (SFQ)	2.8
Paykel *et al* (1971)	Social Adjustment Scale (SAS)	2.8
Levenstein *et al* (1993)	Perceived Stress Questionnaire (PSQ)	2.8
Hurry & Sturt (1981)	MRC Social Role Performance Schedule (SRP)	2
Olson *et al* (1978)	Family Adaptability and Cohesion Evaluation Scale (FACES)	1.9
Affleck & McGuire (1984)	Morningside Rehabilitation Status Scales (MRSS)	1.9
Baker & Hall (1983)	Rehabilitation Evaluation Hall and Baker (REHAB)	1.8
Linn *et al* (1969)	Social Dysfunction Rating Scale (SDRS)	1.7
Strauss & Harder (1981)	Case Record Rating Scale (CRRS)	1.7
Remington & Tyrer (1979)	Social Functioning Schedule (SFS)	1.7
Schooler *et al* (1979)	Social Adjustment Scale 11 (SAS 11)	1.6
Crandall *et al* (1992)	Undergraduate Stress Questionnaire (USQ)	1.6
Moos (1974)	Ward Atmosphere Scale (WAS)	1.6
Ditommaso & Spinner (1993)	Social and Emotional Loneliness Scale for Adults (SELSA)	1.4
Brugha *et al* (1987)	Interview Measure of Social Relationships (IMSR)	1.4
Cohen & Sokolowsky (1979)	Network Analysis	1.3

Neuropsychological assessment

This is another rapidly expanding area and in most instances there will be a clear indication that will help in the choice of instrument. The measurement of intelligence was one of the first ratings in psychology and it has a worthy tradition in the WAIS, for which special training is required. However, many of the other scales can be used by research trainees but it is wise to seek advice for most of these first as they are not 'off the shelf' instruments (Table 11.18).

Table 11.18 Scales for neuropsychological assessment and intellectual disability

Authors	Name of scale	Citations per year and comments
Wechsler (1958)	Wechsler Adult Intelligence Scale (WAIS)	299.9 (the established successor to the early IQ tests; the latest version of this is WAIS–III; Fjordbak & Fjordback, 2005)
Teasdale & Jennett (1974)	Glasgow Coma Scale	98.7
Benton *et al* (1983)	Digit Sequence Learning	50.8
Nelson (1982)	National Adult Reading Test (NART)	46 (a good measure of verbal intelligence that is quick to measure)
Wechsler (1945)	Wechsler Memory Scale (WMS)	38.8
Goodglass & Kaplan (1972)	Boston Diagnostic Aphasia Examination (BDAE)	35.5
Nelson (1976)	Modified Card Sorting Test (MCST)	33.1
Reitan & Davison (1974)	Finger Tapping Test (FTT)	30.8
Benton & Hamsher (1976)	Multilingual Aphasia Examination	18.7
Buschke (1973)	Selective Reminding Test	17.0
Raven (1960)	Raven Progressive Matrices (RPM)	13.5 (an IQ equivalent that can be administered without special training – e.g. by a junior psychiatrist)
Kertesz (1979)	Western Aphasia Battery	12.2
Levin *et al* (1979)	Galveston Orientation and Amnesia Test (GOAT)	9.4
Annett (1967)	Handedness Inventory	8.1 (an established test for lateralisation)
Graham & Kendall (1960)	Graham–Kendall Memory for Designs Test	7.7
Berg (1948)	Wisconsin Card Sorting Test (WCST)	7.4
Banks (1970)	Signal Detection Memory Test (SDMT)	7.2
Warrington & James (1967)	Visual Retention Test (metric figures)	5.1

continued

Table 11.18 *continued*

Authors	Name of scale	Citations per year and comments
Moss *et al* (1998)	Psychiatric Assessment Schedule for Adults with a Developmental Disability (PAS–ADD) Checklist	5.0 (rapidly becoming a standard screening test for assessment of symptoms in learning disability – is couched in simple language so those without specialised knowledge can readily use the scales)
Thurstone (1944)	Hidden Figures Test	4.2
Armitage (1946)	Trail Making Test (TMT)	3.5
Ferris *et al* (1980)	Facial Recognition and Name –Face Association Test	3.3
Smith (1968)	Symbol Digit Modalities Test (SDMT)	3.3
Dixon (1988)	Metamemory in Adulthood (MIA)	3.2
Lingjaerde *et al* (1987)	UKU (Udvalg for Kliniske Undersolgelser) Side Effect Rating Scale	3.2 (mainly used for detecting adverse effects with antipsychotic drugs)
Holland (1980)	Communication Abilities in Daily Living	3.1

Acknowledgements

We thank Elena Garralda for advice and Sheila McKenzie for secretarial help in preparing this chapter.

References

Achenbach, T. M. (1978) The child behaviour profile: I. Boys aged 6–11. *Journal of Consulting and Clinical Psychology*, **46**, 478–488.

Achenbach, T. M. & Edelbrock, C. S. (1979) The child behaviour profile: II. Boys aged 12–16 and girls aged 6–11 and 12–16. *Journal of Consulting and Clinical Psychology*, **47**, 223–233.

Achenbach, T. M. & McConaughy, S. H. (1987*a*) Empirically-based assessment of child and adolescent psychopathology: practical applications. Newbury Park, CA: Sage.

Achenbach, T. M. & McConaughy, S. H. (1987*b*) Empirically based assessment of behavioural/emotional problems in 2 and 3 year old children. *Journal of Abnormal Child Psychology*, **15**, 629–650.

Adshead, F., Day Cody, D. & Pitt, B. (1992) BASDEC: a novel screening instrument for depression in elderly medical in-patients. *BMJ*, **305**, 397.

Affleck, J. W. & McGuire, R. J. (1984) The measurement of psychiatric rehabilitation status. A review of the needs and a new scale. *British Journal of Psychiatry*, **145**, 517–525.

213

Aitken, R. C. B. (1969) Measurement of feelings using visual analogue scales. *Proceedings of the Royal Society of Medicine*, **62**, 989.

Alderman, K. J., MacKay, C. J. & Lucas, E. G., *et al* (1983) Factor analysis and reliability studies of the Crown–Crisp experiential index (CCEI). *British Journal of Medical Psychology*, **56**, 329–345.

Alexopoulus, G. S., Adams, R. C., Young, R. C., *et al* (1988) Cornell scale for depression in dementia. *Biological Psychiatry*, **23**, 271–284.

Allen, N. H., Gordon, S., Hope, T., *et al* (1996) Manchester and Oxford Universities Scale for the Psychopathological Assessment of Dementia (MOUSEPAD). *British Journal of Psychiatry*, **169**, 293–307.

Altman, E. G., Hedeker, D. R., Janicak, P. G., *et al* (1994) The Clinician-Administered Rating-Scale for Mania (CARS–M) – development, reliability and validity. *Biological Psychiatry*, **36**, 124–134.

Amador, X. F., Strauss, D. H., Yale, S. A., *et al* (1993) Assessment of insight in psychosis. *American Journal of Psychiatry*, **150**, 873–879.

Aman, M. G., Singh, N. N., Stewart, A. W., *et al* (1985) The aberrant behavior checklist: a behavior rating scale for the assessment of treatment effects. *American Journal of Mental Deficiency*, **89**, 485–491.

Ambrosini, P. J., Metz, C., Prabucki, K., *et al* (1989) Videotape reliability of the third revised edition of the K–SADS. *Journal of the American Academy of Child and Adolescent Psychiatry*, **28**, 723–728.

American Psychiatric Association (1980) *Diagnostic and Statistical Manual of Mental Disorders* (3rd edn) (DSM–III). Washington, DC: APA.

Andreasen, N. C. (1979) Thought, language and communication disorders. I. Clinical assessment, definition of terms and evaluation of their reliability. *Archives of General Psychiatry*, **36**, 1315–1321.

Andreasen, N. C. (1982*a*) Negative symptoms in schizophrenia. *Archives of General Psychiatry*, **39**, 784–788.

Andreasen, N. C. (1982*b*) The scale for the assessment of negative symptoms (SANS). Iowa: University of Iowa.

Andreasen, N. C. (1984) The scale for the assessment of positive symptoms (SAPS). Iowa: University of Iowa.

Andreasen, N. C., Flaum, M. & Arndt, S. (1992) The comprehensive assessment of symptoms and history (CASH). *Archives of General Psychiatry*, **49**, 615–623.

Annett, M. (1967) The binomial distribution of right, mixed, and left handedness. *Quarterly Journal of Experimental Psychology*, **19**, 327–333.

Annis, H. M. (1986) A relapse prevention model for treatment of alcoholics. In *Treating Addictive Behaviors: Processes of Change* (eds W. R. Miller & N. Heather). New York: Plenum Press.

Aquilina, C. & Warner, J. (2004) *A Guide to Psychiatric Examination*. Knutsford, Cheshire: Pastest.

Armitage, S. G. (1946) An analysis of certain psychological tests used for the evaluation of brain injury. *Psychological Monographs*, **60**, 1–48.

Åsberg, M., Perris, C., Schalling, D., *et al* (1978) The comprehensive psychopathological rating scale (CPRS) – development and application of a psychiatric rating scale. *Acta Psychiatrica Scandinavica Supplementum*, **271**, 5–9.

Bandelow, B. (1995) Assessing the efficacy of treatments for panic disorder and agoraphobia 2: the panic and agoraphobia scale. *International Journal of Clinical Psychopharmacology*, **10**, 73–81.

Banks, W. P. (1970) Signal detection theory and memory. *Psychological Bulletin*, **74**, 81–99.

Barnes, T. R. (1989) A rating-scale for drug-induced akathisia. *British Journal of Psychiatry*, **154**, 672–676.

Baron, M., Asnis, L. & Gruen, R. (1981) The schedule for schizotypal personalities (SSP): a diagnostic interview for schizotypal features. *Psychiatry Research*, **4**, 213–228.

Barron, F. (1953) An ego-strength scale which predicts response to psychotherapy. *Journal of Consulting Psychology*, **17**, 327–378.

Barsky, A. J., Wyshak, G. & Klerman, G. L. (1990) The Somatosensory Amplification Scale and its relationship to hypochondriasis. *Journal of Psychiatric Research*, 24, 323–334.

Bech, P. (1993) *Rating Scales for Psychopathology, Health Status and Qualify of Life*. Berlin: Springer.

Beck, A. T., Ward, C. H., Mendelson, M., *et al* (1961) An inventory for measuring depression. *Archives of General Psychiatry*, **4**, 561–571.

Beck, A. T., Weissman, A., Lester, D., *et al* (1974a) The measurement of pessimism: the hopelessness scale. *Journal of Consulting and Clinical Psychology*, **42**, 861–865.

Beck, A. T., Schuyler, D. & Herman, J. (1974b) Development of suicidal intent scales. In *The Prediction of Suicide* (eds A. T. Beck, H. L. P. Resnik & D. J. Lettieri), pp. 45–56. Philadelphia: Charles Press Publishers.

Beck, A. T., Kovacs, M. & Weissman, A. (1979) Assessment of suicidal intention: the scale for suicide ideation. *Journal of Consulting and Clinical Psychology*, **47**, 343–352.

Beck, A. T., Brown, G., Steer, R. A., *et al* (1987) Differentiating anxiety and depression utilizing the cognition checklist. *Journal of Abnormal Psychology*, **96**, 179–183.

Beck, A. T., Epstein, N., Brown, G., *et al* (1988) An inventory for measuring clinical anxiety: psychometric properties. *Journal of Consulting and Clinical Psychology*, **56**, 893–897.

Beecher, H. K. (1959) *The Measurement of Subjective Responses (MSR)*. Oxford: Oxford University Press.

Bell, M. (1981) *Bell Object Relations Self-Report Scale*. West Haven, CT: Psychology Service, VA Medical Center.

Benton, A. L. & Hamsher, K. (1976) *Multilingual Aphasia Examination*. Iowa: University of Iowa.

Benton, A. L., Hamsher K., Varney, N. R., *et al* (1983) *Contributions to Neuropsychological Assessment*. New York: Oxford University Press.

Ben-Tovim, D. I. & Walker, M. K. (1991) The development of the Ben-Tovim Walker body attitudes questionnaire (BAQ), a new measure of women's attitudes towards their own bodies. *Psychological Medicine*, **21**, 775–784.

Berg, C. G., Rapoport, J. L. & Flament, M. (1986) The Leyton obsessional inventory – child version. *Journal of the American Academy of Child Psychiatry*, **25**, 84–91.

Berg, E. A. (1948) A simple objective test for measuring flexibility in thinking. *Journal of General Psychology*, **39**, 15–22.

Bernstein, E. M. & Putnam, F. W. (1986) Development, reliability, and validity of a dissociation scale. *Journal of Nervous and Mental Disease*, **174**, 727–735.

Berrios, G. E., Bulbena, A., Bakshi, N., *et al* (1992) Feelings of guilt in major depression. Conceptual and psychometric aspects. *British Journal of Psychiatry*, **160**, 781–787.

Birchwood, M., Smith, J., Cochrane, R., *et al* (1990) The Social Functioning Scale. The development and validation of a new scale of social adjustment for use in family intervention programmes with schizophrenic patients. *British Journal of Psychiatry*, **157**, 853–859.

Birchwood, M., Smith, J. & Drury, V. (1994) A self-report insight scale for psychosis: reliability, validity and sensitivity to change. *Acta Psychiatrica Scandinavica*, **89**, 62–67.

Birleson, P. (1981) The validity of depressive disorder in childhood and the development of a self-rating scale. *Journal of Child Psychology and Psychiatry*, **22**, 73–88.

Blessed, G., Tomlinson, B. E. & Roth, M. (1968) The association between quantitative measures of dementia and of senile change in the cerebral grey matter of elderly subjects. *British Journal of Psychiatry*, **114**, 797–811.

Brewin, C. R., Wing, J. K., Mangen, S., *et al* (1987) Principles and practice of measuring needs in the long-term mentally ill. *Psychological Medicine*, **17**, 971–981.

Brink, T. L., Yesavage, J. A., Lum, O., *et al* (1982) Screening tests for geriatric depression. *Clinical Gerontologist*, **1**, 37–43.

Broadbent, D. E., Cooper, P. F., Fitzgerald, P., *et al* (1982) The cognitive failures questionnaire (CFQ) and its correlates. *British Journal of Clinical Psychology*, **21**, 1–16.

Brodman, K., Erdnan, A. J., Lorge, I., *et al* (1949) The Cornell medical index. *JAMA*, **140**, 530–540.

Brown, G. & Harris, T. (1978) *The Social Origins of Depression: A Study of Psychiatric Disorders in Women.* London: Tavistock.

Brugha, T. S., Sturt, E., MacCarthy, B., *et al* (1987) The interview measure of social relationships: the description and evaluation of a survey instrument for assessing personal social resources. *Social Psychiatry*, **22**, 123–128.

Bucks, R. S., Ashworth, D. I., Wilcock, G. K. (1996) Assessment of activities of daily living in dementia: development of the Bristol Activities of Daily Living Scale. *Age and Ageing*, **25**, 113–120.

Buglass, D. & Horton, J. (1974) A scale for predicting subsequent suicidal behaviour. *British Journal of Psychiatry*, **124**, 573–578.

Bunney, W. E. & Hamburg, D. A. (1963) Methods for reliable longitudinal observation of behaviour. *Archives of General Psychiatry*, **9**, 280–294.

Burnam, M. A., Karno, M., Hough, R. L., *et al* (1983) The Spanish diagnostic interview schedule. *Archives of General Psychiatry*, **40**, 1189–1196.

Buschke, H. (1973) Selective reminding for analyses of memory and learning. *Journal of Verbal Learning and Verbal Behavior*, **12**, 543–550.

Buss, A. H. & Durkee, A. (1957) An inventory for assessing different kinds of hostility. *Journal of Consulting Psychology*, **21**, 343–348.

Carey, W. B. (1970) A simplified method of measuring infant temperament. *Journal of Pediatrics*, **77**, 188–194.

Carney, M. W., Roth, M. & Garside, R. F. (1965) The diagnosis of depressive syndromes and the prediction of ECT response. *British Journal Psychiatry*, **111**, 659–674.

Carskadon, M. A. (1986) ASDC task force on excessive sleepiness guidelines for multiple sleep latency test (MSLT). *Sleep*, **9**, 519–524.

Castaneda, A., McCandless, B. & Palermo, D. (1956) The children's form of the manifest anxiety scale. *Child Development*, **27**, 317–326.

Chalder, T., Berelowitz, G., Pawlikowska, T., *et al* (1993) Development of a fatigue scale. *Journal of Psychosomatic Research*, **37**, 147–153.

Chambless, D. L., Caputo, G. C., Bright, P., *et al* (1984) Assessment of fear in agoraphobics: the body sensations questionnaire and the agoraphobic cognitions questionnaire. *Journal of Consulting and Clinical Psychology*, **52**, 1090–1097.

Chambless, D. L., Caputo, G. C., Jasin, S. E., *et al* (1985) The mobility inventory for agoraphobia. *Behaviour Research and Therapy*, **23**, 35–44.

Chaney, E., O'Leary, M. & Marlatt, G. A. (1978) Skill training with alcoholics. *Journal of Consulting and Clinical Psychology*, **46**, 1092–1104.

Chick, J. (1980) Alcohol dependence: methodological issues in its measurement; reliability of the criteria. *British Journal of Addiction*, **75**, 175–186.

Clare, A. W. & Cains, V. E. (1978) Design, development and use of a standardised interview to assess social maladjustment and dysfunction in community studies. *Psychological Medicine*, **8**, 589–604.

Claridge, G. & Broks, P. (1984) Schizotypy and hemisphere function – 1: theoretical considerations and the measurement of schizotypy. *Personality and Individual Differences*, **5**, 633–648.

Cohen, C. & Sokolowsky, J. (1979) Clinical use of network analysis for psychiatric and aged populations. *Community Mental Health Journal*, **15**, 203–213.

Cohen-Mansfield, J., Marx, M. & Rosenthal, A. S. (1989) A description of agitation in a nursing home. *Journal of Gerontology*, **44**, M77–M84.

Conners, C. K. (1969) A teacher rating scale for use in drug studies with children. *American Journal of Psychiatry*, **126**, 884–888.

Connor, K. M., Davidson, J. R. T., Churchill, E., *et al* (2000) Psychometric properties of the Social Phobia Inventory (SPIN). New self rating scale. *British Journal of Psychiatry*, **176**, 379–386.

Cooper, J. (1970) The Leyton obsessional inventory. *Psychological Medicine*, 1, 48–64.

Cooper, P. J., Tawor, M. J., Cooper, Z., *et al* (1987) The development and evaluation of the body shape questionnaire. *International Journal of Eating Disorders*, 6, 485–494.

Cooper, Z. & Fairburn, C. (1987) The eating disorder examination: a semi-structure interview for the assessment of the specific psychopathology of eating disorders. *International Journal of Eating Disorders*, 6, 1–8.

Conte, H., Plutchik, R., Karasu, T., *et al* (1980) A self-report borderline scale: discriminative validity and preliminary norms. *Journal of Nervous and Mental Disease*, 168, 428–435.

Copeland, J. R. M., Kelleher, M. J., Kellett, J. M., *et al* (1976) A semi-structured clinical interview for the assessment of diagnosis and mental state in the elderly. I. Development and reliability. *Psychological Medicine*, 6, 439–449.

Copeland, J. R. M., Dewey, M. E. & Griffiths-Jones, H. M. (1986) A computerized psychiatric diagnostic system and case nomenclature for elderly subjects – GMS and AGECAT. *Psychological Medicine*, 16, 89–99.

Costello, A. J., Edelbrock, C. S., Dulcan, M. K., *et al* (1984) Development and testing of the NIMH diagnostic interview schedule for children in a clinic population: final report. Rockville, MD: Centre for Epidemiological Studies – National Institute for Mental Health.

Costello, C. G. & Comfrey, A. L. (1967) Scales for measuring depression and anxiety. *Journal of Psychology*, 66, 303–313.

Cox, J. & Holden, J. (2003) *Perinatal Mental Health: A Guide to the Edinburgh Postnatal Depression Scale*. London: Gaskell.

Cox, J. L., Holden, J. M. & Sagovsky, R. (1987) Detection of postnatal depression. Development of the 10-item Edinburgh Postnatal Depression Scale. *British Journal of Psychiatry*, 150, 782–786.

Crandall, C. S., Preisler, J. J. & Aussprung, J. (1992) Measuring life event stress in the lives of college students: the undergraduate stress questionnaire (USQ). *Journal of Behavioral Medicine*, 15, 627–662.

Crown, S. & Crisp, A. H. (1966) A short clinical diagnostic self-rating scale for psychoneurotic patients. The Middlesex Hospital Questionnaire (M.H.Q.). *British Journal of Psychiatry*, 112, 917–923.

Crowne, D. P. & Marlowe, D. (1960) A new scale of social desirability independent of psychopathology. *Journal of Consulting and Clinical Psychology*, 24, 349–354.

Cummings, J. L., Mega, M., Gray, K., *et al* (1994) The Neuropsychiatric Inventory: comprehensive assessment of psychopathology in dementia. *Neurology*, 44, 2308–2314.

Davidson, J. R. T. & Miner, C. M. (1997) Brief social phobia scale: a psychometric evaluation. *Psychological Medicine*, 27, 161–166.

Davidson, J. R. T., Book, S. W., Colket, J. T., *et al* (1997). Assessment of a new self-rating scale for posttraumatic stress disorder. *Psychological Medicine*, 27, 153–160.

Derogatis, L. R. (1976) *Scoring and Procedures Manual for PAIS*. Baltimore: Clinical Psychometric Research.

Derogatis, L. R. (1978) Derogatis Sexual Functioning Inventory (DSFI) (revised). Baltimore: Clinical Psychometric Research.

Derogatis, L. R., Lipman, R. S., Covi, L., *et al* (1973) The SCL-90: an outpatient psychiatric rating scale (SCL-90). *Psychopharmacology Bulletin*, 9, 13–28.

Derogatis, L. R., Lipman, R. S., Rickels, K., *et al* (1974) The Hopkins symptom checklist (HSCL): a self-report symptom inventory. *Behavioral Science*, 19, 1–15.

Ditommaso, E. & Spinner, B. (1993) The development and initial validation of the social and emotional loneliness scale for adults (SELSA). *Personality and Individual Differences*, 14, 127–134.

Dixon, R. A., Hultsch, D. F. & Hetzog, C. (1988) The metamemory in adulthood (MIA) questionnaire. *Psychopharmacology Bulletin*, 24, 671–688.

Dolan, M. & Doyle, M. (2000) Violence risk prediction: Clinical and actuarial measures and the role of the Psychopathy Checklist. *British Journal of Psychiatry*, 177, 303–311.

Doll, E. A. (1965) *Vineland Social Maturity Scale: Manual of Directions* (revised). Minneapolis: American Guidance Service.

Dupuy, H. J. (1984) The psychological general well-being (PGWB) index. In *Assessment of Quality of Life in Clinical Trials of Cardiovascular Therapies* (eds L. W. Chambers & H. J. Dupuy), pp. 170–183. New York: Le Jacq.

Elliott, C. D., Murray, D. J. & Pearson, L. S. (1983) British ability scales – revised (BAS–R). Windsor: NFER–Nelson.

Ellis, B. W., Johns, M. W., Lancaster, R., *et al* (1981) The St Mary's Hospital sleep questionnaire: a study of reliability. *Sleep*, **4**, 93–97.

Endicott, J. & Spitzer, R. L. (1972) Current and past psychopathology scales (CAPPS): rationale, reliability and validity. *Archives of General Psychiatry*, **27**, 678–687.

Endicott, J. & Spitzer. R. L. (1978) A diagnostic interview: the schedule for affective disorders and schizophrenia (SADS). *Archives of General Psychiatry*, **35**, 837–844.

Endicott, J., Spitzer, R. L., Fleiss, J. L., *et al* (1976) The global assessment scale: a procedure for measuring overall severity of psychiatric disturbance. *Archives of General Psychiatry*, **33**, 766–771.

Endler, N. S., Hunt, J. N. & Rosenstein, A. J. (1962) The stimulus response inventory. *Psychological Monographs*, **76**, 1–33.

Eysenck, H. J. (1971) Personality and sexual adjustment. *British Journal of Psychiatry*, **118**, 593–608.

Ferris, S. H., Crook, T., Clarke, E., *et al* (1980) Facial recognition memory deficits in normal ageing and senile dementia. *Journal of Gerontology*, **35**, 707–714.

Fichter, M. M., Elton, M., Engel, K., *et al* (1989) The structured interview for anorexia and bulimia nervosa (SIAB): development and characteristics of a (semi-) standardised instrument. In *Bulimia Nervosa: Basic Research, Diagnosis and Therapy* (ed. M. M. Fichter), pp. 57–70. Chichester: Wiley.

Fjordbak, T. & Fjordbak, B. S. (2005) WAIS–III norms for working-age adults: A benchmark for conducting vocational, career, and employment-related evaluations. *Psychological Reports*, **96**, 9–16.

Foa, E. B., Kozak, M. J., Salkovskis, P. M., *et al* (1998) The validation of a new obsessive-compulsive disorder scale: The obsessive-compulsive inventory. *Psychological Assessment*, **10**, 206–214.

Foa, E. B., Huppert, J. D., Leiberg, S., *et al* (2002) The Obsessive–Compulsive Inventory: development and validation of a short version. *Psychological Assessment*, **14**, 485–496.

Folstein, M. F., Folstein, S. E. & McHugh, P. R. (1975) "Mini-Mental State": a practical method for grading the cognitive state of patients for the clinician. *Journal of Psychiatric Research*, **12**, 189–198.

Frenken, J. & Vennix, P. (1981) *Sexual Experience Scales Manual*. Lisse: Swets & Zeitlinger.

Fukuda, K., Straus, S. E., Hickie, I., *et al* (1994) The Chronic Fatigue Syndrome – a comprehensive approach to its definition and study. *Annals of Internal Medicine*, **121**, 953–959.

Galissi, J. P., Frierson, H. T. & Sharer, R. (1981) Behavior of high, moderate and low test anxious students during an actual test situation. *Journal of Consulting and Clinical Psychology*, **49**, 51–62.

Garner, D. M. & Garfinkel, P. E. (1979) The eating attitudes test: an index of the symptoms of anorexia nervosa. *Psychological Medicine*, **9**, 273–279.

Garner, D. M., Olmstead, M. P. & Polivy, J. (1983) Development and validation of a multi-dimensional eating disorder inventory (EDI) for anorexia nervosa and bulimia. *International Journal of Eating Disorders*, **2**, 15–34.

Gelder, M. G. & Marks, I. M. (1966) Severe agoraphobia: a controlled trial of behaviour therapy. *British Journal of Psychiatry*, **112**, 309–319.

Gelinas, I. & Gauthier, L. (1999) Development of a functional measure for persons with Alzheimers disease: the Disability Assessment for Dementia. *American Journal of Occupational Therapy*, **53**, 471–481.

Glass, C. R., Merzulli, T. V., Biever, J. L., *et al* (1982) Cognitive assessment of social anxiety: development and validation of a self-statements questionnaire. *Cognitive Therapy and Research*, **6**, 37–55.

Goldberg, D. P. (1972) *The Detection of Psychiatric Illness by Questionnaire (GHQ)*, Maudsley Monograph 21. London: Oxford University Press.

Goldberg, D. P., Cooper, B., Eastwood, M. R., *et al* (1970) A standardised psychiatric interview for use in community surveys. *British Journal of Preventative and Social Medicine*, **24**, 18–23.

Golombok, S. & Rust, J. (1985) The Golombok–Rust inventory of sexual satisfaction (GRISS). *British Journal of Clinical Psychology*, **24**, 63–64.

Goodglass, H. & Kaplan, E. (1972) Assessment of aphasia and related disorders. Philadelphia: Lea & Febiger.

Goodman, W. K., Price, L. H., Rasmussen, S. A., *et al* (1989a) The Yale–Brown obsessive compulsive scale. *Archives of General Psychiatry*, **46**, 1006–1011.

Goodman, W. K., Price, L. H., Rasmussen, S. A., *et al* (1989b) The Yale–Brown obsessive compulsive scale 2. *Archives of General Psychiatry*, **46**, 1012–1016.

Gormally, J., Black, S., Daston, S., *et al* (1982) The assessment of binge eating severity among obese persons. *Addictive Behaviors*, **7**, 47–55.

Gossop, M., Darke, S., Griffiths, P., *et al* (1995) The Severity of Dependence Scale (SDS): psychometric properties of the SDS in English and Australian samples of heroin, cocaine and amphetamine users. *Addiction*, **90**, 607–614.

Gottfries, C. G., Brane, G., Gullberg, B., *et al* (1982a) A new rating scale for dementia syndromes 1. *Archives of Gerontology and Geriatrics*, **1**, 311–330.

Gottfries, C. G., Brane, G. & Steen, G. (1982b) A new rating scale for dementia syndromes. *Gerontology*, **28** (suppl. 2), 20–31.

Graham, F. K. & Kendall, B. S. (1960) Memory-for designs-test: revised general manual. *Perceptual and Motor Skills* (suppl. 2) **11**, 147–148.

Greene, J. G., Smith, R., Gardiner, M., *et al* (1982) Measuring behavioural disturbances of elderly demented patients in the community and its effects on relatives: a factor analytic study. *Age and Ageing*, **11**, 121–126.

Gross, M., Lewis, E. & Nagareijan, M. A. (1973) An improved quantitative system for assessing acute alcohol psychoses and related states (TSA and SSA). In *Alcohol Intoxication and Withdrawal Experimental Studies* (ed. M. M. Gross), pp. 365–376. New York: Plenum Press.

Guilleminault, C. (1982) *Sleeping and Waking Disorders: Indications and Techniques*. California: Addison–Wesley.

Gunderson, J., Kolb, J. & Austin, V. (1981) The diagnostic interview for borderline patients. *American Journal of Psychiatry*, **138**, 896–903.

Gurland, B. J., Yorkston, N. J., Stone, A. R., *et al* (1972) The structured and scaled interview to assess maladjustment (SSIAM). 1. Description, rationale and development. *Archives of General Psychiatry*, **27**, 259–264.

Hachinski, V. C., Iliff, L. D., Zihka, E., *et al* (1975) Cerebral blood flow in dementia. *Archives of Neurology*, **32**, 632–637.

Halikas, J. A., Kuhn, K. L., Crosby, R., *et al* (1991) The measurement of craving in cocaine paitents using the Minnesota cocaine craving scale. *Comprehensive Psychiatry*, **32**, 22–27.

Hall, K. S., Hendrie, H. C., Birttain, H. M., *et al* (1993) The development of a dementia screening interview in two distinct languages. *International Journal of Methods in Psychiatric Research*, **3**, 1–28.

Halmi, K. (1985) Rating scales in the eating disorders. *Psychopharmacology Bulletin*, **21**, 1001–1003.

Halmi, K. A., Falk, J. R. & Schwartz, E. (1981) Binge-eating and vomiting: a survey of a college population. *Psychological Medicine*, **11**, 697–706.

Hamilton, M. (1959) The assessment of anxiety states by rating. *British Journal of Medical Psychology*, **32**, 50–55.

Hamilton, M. (1960) A rating scale for depression. *Journal of Neurology, Neurosurgery and Psychiatry*, **23**, 56–62.

Handelsman, L., Cochrane, K. J., Aronson, M. J., *et al* (1987) Two new rating scales for opiate withdrawal. *American Journal of Drug and Alcohol Abuse*, **13**, 293–308.

Hansson, S. L., Röjvall, A. S., Rastam, M., *et al* (2005) Psychiatric telephone interview with parents for screening of childhood autism – tics, attention-deficit hyperactivity disorder and other comorbidities (A–TAC): Preliminary reliability and validity. *British Journal of Psychiatry*, **187**, 262–267.

Harding, T. W., Arango, M. V. & Baltazar, J. (1980) Mental disorders in primary health care. *Psychological Medicine*, **10**, 231–241.

Hare, R. D. (1980) A research scale for the assessment of psychopathy in criminal populations. *Personality and Individual Differences*, **1**, 111–119.

Hare, R. D. (1991) *The Hare Psychopathy Checklist–Revised*. Toronto, Ontario: Multi-Health Systems.

Harris, D. B. (1963) *Children's Drawings as Measures of Intellectual Maturity*. New York: Harcourt, Brace and World.

Hathaway, S. R. & McKinley, J. C. (1967) *Minnesota Multiphasic Personality Inventory: Manual for Administration and Scoring*. New York: Psychological Corporation.

Hawkins, R. C. & Clement, P. F. (1980) Development and construct validation of a self-report measure of binge eating tendencies. *Addictive Behaviors*, **5**, 219–226.

Helmes, E., Csapo, K. G. & Short, J. A. (1987) Standardization and validation of the multidimensional observation scale for elderly subjects (MOSES). *Journal of Gerontology*, **42**, 395–405.

Helzer, J. E. & Robins, L. N. (1981) Renard Diagnostic Interview. *Archives of General Psychiatry*, **38**, 393–398.

Henderson, M. & Freeman, C. P. (1987) A self-rating scale for bulimia. The "BITE". *British Journal of Psychiatry*, **150**, 18–24.

Henderson, S., Duncan-Jones, P., Byrne, D. G., *et al* (1980) Measuring social relationships: the interview schedule for social interaction. *Psychological Medicine*, **10**, 1–12.

Herjanic, B. & Campbell, W. (1977) Differentiating psychiatrically disturbed children on the basis of a structured interview. *Journal of Abnormal Child Psychology*, **5**, 127–134.

Hersch, E. I. (1979) Development and application of the extended scale for dementia. *Journal of American Geriatrics Society*, **27**, 348–354.

Hoddes, E., Dement, W. C. & Zarcone, V. (1972*a*) The development and use of the Stanford sleepiness scale (SSS). *Psychophysiology*, **9**, 150.

Hoddes, E., Zarcone, V. & Dement, W. C. (1972*b*) Cross-validation of the Stanford sleepiness scale (SSS). *Sleep Research*, **1**, 91.

Hodges, K., Kline, J., Stern, L., *et al* (1982) The development of a child assessment interview for research and clinical use. *Journal of Abnormal Child Psychology*, **10**, 173–189.

Hodgson, R. J. & Rachman, S. J. (1977) Obsessional-compulsive complaints. *Behaviour Research and Therapy*, **15**, 389–395.

Hodkinson, H. M. (1972) Evaluation of a mental test score for assessment of mental impairment in the elderly. *Age and Ageing*, **1**, 233–238.

Holland, A. L. (1980) *Communicative Abilities in Daily Living: A Test of Functional Communication for Aphasic Adults*. Baltimore: University Park Press.

Holmes, J., Lawson, D., Langley, K., *et al* (2004) The Child Attention-Deficit Hyperactivity Disorder Teacher Telephone Interview (CHATTI): reliability and validity. *British Journal of Psychiatry*, **184**, 74–78.

Holmes, T. H. & Rahe, R. H. (1967) The social readjustment rating scale. *Journal of Psychosomatic Research*, **11**, 213–218.

Holmes, N., Shah, A. & Wing, L. (1982) The disability assessment schedule: A brief screening device for use with the mentally retarded (DAS). *Psychological Medicine*, **12**, 879–890.

Honigfeld, G. & Klett, C. J. (1965) The nurses' observation scale for inpatient evaluation: a new scale for measuring improvement in chronic schizophrenia. *Journal of Clinical Psychology*, **21**, 65–71.

Hoon, E. F., Hoon, P. W. & Wincze, J. P. (1976) The SAI: an inventory for the measurement of female sexual arousability. *Archives of Sexual Behaviour*, **5**, 291–300.

Hope, T. & Fairburn, C. G. (1992) The present behavioural examination (PBE): the development of an interview to measure current behavioural abnormalities. *Psychological Medicine*, **22**, 223–230.

Horn, J. L., Wanberg, K. & Adams, S. G. (1974) Diagnosis of alcoholism. *Quarterly Journal of Studies on Alcohol*, **35**, 147–175.

Horowitz, L. M., Rosenburg, S. E., Baer, B. A., *et al* (1988) Inventory of personal problems: psychometric properties and clinical applications. *Journal of Consulting and Clinical Psychology*, **56**, 885–892.

Hughes, C. P., Berg, L., Danziger, W. L., *et al* (1982) A new clinical scale for the staging of dementia. *British Journal of Psychiatry*, **140**, 566–572.

Hurry, J. & Sturt, E. (1981) Social performance in a population sample – relation to psychiatric symptoms. In *What is a Case – The Problem of Definition in Psychiatric Community Surveys* (eds J. K. Wing, P. Bebbington & L. N. Robins), pp. 217–222. London: Grant McIntyre.

Hyler, S. E. & Reider, R. O. (1987) *PDQ–R: Personality Diagnostic Questionnaire – Revised*. New York: New York State Psychiatric Institute.

Hyler, S. E., Reider, R. O., Spitzer, R. L., *et al* (1982) *Personality Diagnostic Questionnaire (PDQ)*. New York: New York State Psychiatric Institute.

Inouye, S. K., van Dyck, C. H., Spitzer, R. L., *et al* (1990) Clarifying confusion: the confusion assessment method. *Annals of Internal Medicine*, **113**, 941–948.

Jarman, B. (1983) Identification of underprivileged areas. *BMJ*, **286**, 1705–1709.

Jenkins, G., Hale, R., Papassatasiou, M., *et al* (2002) Suicide rate 22 years after parasuicide: cohort study. *British Medical Journal*, **325**, 1155.

Jenkins, R., Maurs, A. H. & Belsey, E. (1981) The background, design and use of a short interview to assess social stress and support in research and clinical settings. *Social Science and Medicine*, **15**, 195–203.

Johnson, C. (1985) Initial consultation for patients with bulimia and anorexia nervosa. In *Handbook of Psychotherapy for Anorexia Nervosa and Bulimia* (eds D. Garner & P. Garfinkel), pp. 19–51. New York: Guilford Press.

Jorm, A. F. & Jacomb, P. A. (1989) The informant questionnaire on cognitive decline in the elderly (IQCODE): socio-demographic correlates, reliability, validity and some norms. *Psychological Medicine*, **19**, 1015–1022.

Jorm, A. F., MacKinnon, A. S., Henderson, A. S. (1995) Psychogeriatric Assessment Scales. A multidimensional alternative to categorical diagnosis of dementia and depression in the elderly. *Psychological Medicine*, **25**, 447–460.

Kandel, D. B. & Davies, M. (1982) Epidemiology of depressive mood in adolescents. *Archives of General Psychiatry*, **39**, 1205–1217.

Kanner, A. D., Coyne, J. C., Schaefer, C., *et al* (1981) Comparison of two modes of stress management: daily hassles and uplifts versus major life events. *Journal of Behavioral Medicine*, **4**, 1–39.

Katz, M. M. & Lyerly, S. B. (1963) Methods for measuring adjustment and social behaviour in the community: 1 Rationale, description, discriminative validity and scale development. *Psychological Reports*, **13** (suppl. 4), 503–555.

Katz, S., Ford, A. B., Moskowitch, R. W., *et al* (1963) Studies of illness in the aged: the index of ADL. *JAMA*, **185**, 914–919.

Katzman, R., Brown, T., Fuld, P., *et al* (1983) Validation of a short orientation-memory-concentration test of cognitive impairment. *American Journal of Psychiatry*, **140**, 734–739.

Keane, T. M., Cadell, J. M. & Taylor, K. L. (1988) Mississippi scale for combat-related posttraumatic stress disorder: three studies in reliability and validity. *Journal of Consulting and Clinical Psychology*, **56**, 85–90.

Kellner, R. (1987) A symptom questionnaire. *Journal of Clinical Psychiatry*, **48**, 268.

Kellner, R. & Sheffield, B. F. (1973) A self-rating scale of distress. *Psychological Medicine*, **3**, 88–100.

Kendell, R. & Jablensky, A. (2003) Distinguishing between the validity and utility of psychiatric diagnoses. *American Journal of Psychiatry*, **160**, 4–12.

Kendler, K. S., Glazer, W. M. & Morgenstern, H. (1983) Dimensions of delusional experience. *American Journal of Psychiatry*, **140**, 466–469.

Kendrick, D. C., Gibson, A. J. & Moyes, I. C. A. (1979) The revised Kendrick battery: clinical studies. *British Journal of Social and Clinical Psychology*, **18**, 329–340.

Kertesz, A. (1979) *Aphasia and Associated Disorders*. New York: Grune & Stratton.

Knopman, D. S., Knapp, M. J., Gracon, S. I., *et al* (1994) The Clinician Interview-Based Impression (CIBI): a clinicians' global change rating scale in Alzheimer's disease. *Neurology*, **44**, 2315–2321.

Kopelman, M., Wilson, B. & Baddeley, A. (1990) *The Autobiographical Memory Interview (AMI)*. Bury St Edmunds: Thames Valley Test Company.

Kovacs, M. (1985) The children's depression inventory. *Psychopharmacology Bulletin*, **21**, 995–998.

Kreitman, N. & Foster, J. (1991) The construction and selection of predictive scales, with special reference to parasuicide. *British Journal of Psychiatry*, **159**, 185–192.

Kuriansky, J. & Gurland, B. J. (1976) The performance test of activities of daily living. *International Journal of Aging and Human Development*, **7**, 343–352.

Larsen, D. L., Attkisson, C. C., Hargreaves, W. A., *et al* (1979) Assessment of client/patient satisfaction: development of a general scale. *Evaluation and Programme Planning*, **2**, 197–207.

Lawton, M. P. (1975) The Philadelphia geriatric center morale scale: a revision. *Journal of Gerontology*, **30**, 85–89.

Lawton, M. P. (1988*a*) Instrumental activities of daily living (IADL) scale: original observer-rated version. *Psychopharmacology Bulletin*, **24**, 785–787.

Lawton, M. P. (1988*b*) Instrumental activities of daily living (IADL) scale: self-rated version. *Psychopharmacology Bulletin*, **24**, 789–791.

Lawton, M. P. & Brody, E. M. (1969) Assessment of older people: self-maintaining and instrumental activities of daily living. *Gerontologist*, **9**, 179–186.

Lawton, M. P., Moss, M., Fulcomer, M., *et al* (1982) A research and service oriented multilevel assessment instrument. *Journal of Gerontology*, **37**, 91–99.

Lefkowitz, M. M. & Tesing, E. P. (1980) Assessment of childhood depression. *Journal of Consulting and Clinical Psychology*, **48**, 43–50.

Levenstein, S., Prantera, C., Varvo, V., *et al* (1993) Development of the perceived stress questionnaire: a new tool for psychosomatic research. *Journal of Psychosomatic Research*, **37**, 19–32.

Levin, H. S., O'Donnell, V. M., Grossman, R. G., *et al* (1979) The Galveston orientation and amnesia test: a practical scale to assess cognition after head injury. *Journal of Nervous and Mental Disease*, **167**, 675–684.

Lewis, G., Pelosi, A. J., Araya, R., *et al* (1992) Measuring psychiatric disorder in the community: a standardized assessment for use by lay interviewers. *Psychological Medicine*, **22**, 465–486.

Lingjaerde, O., Ahlfors, U. G., Bech, P., *et al* (1987) The UKU side effect rating scale: a new comprehensive rating scale for psychotropic drugs and a cross-sectional study of side effects in neuroleptic-treated patients. *Acta Psychiatrica Scandinavica Supplementum*, **334**, 1–100..

Linn, M. W., Sculthorpe, W. B., Evje, M., *et al* (1969) A social dysfunction rating scale. *Journal of Psychiatric Research*, **6**, 299–306.

Litman, G. K., Stapleton, J., Oppenheim, A. N., *et al* (1983) An instrument for measuring coping behaviours in hospitalised alcoholics: implications for relapse prevention treatment. *British Journal of Addiction*, **78**, 269–276.

Litman, G. K., Stapleton, J., Oppenheim, A. N., *et al* (1984) The relationship between coping behaviours, their effectiveness and alcoholism relapse and survival. *British Journal of Addiction*, **79**, 283–291.

Livesley, W. J. (2001) Commentary on reconceptualizing personality disorder categories using trait dimensions. *Journal of Personality*, **69**, 277–286.

Logsdon, R. G. & Gibbons, I. E. (1999) Quality of life in Alzheimer's disease: patient and caregiver reports. *Journal of Mental Health and Ageing*, **5**, 21–32.

Lopiccolo, J. & Steger, J. C. (1974) The sexual interaction inventory; a new instrument for the assessment of sexual dysfunction. *Archives of Sexual Behaviour*, **3**, 585–596.

Loranger, A. W., Susman, V. L., Oldham, J. M., *et al* (1985) *Personality Disorder Examination (PDE): A Structured Interview for DSM–III–R and ICD–9 Personality Disorders – WHO/ ADAMHA Pilot Version*. New York: New York Hospital, Cornell Medical Center.

Lorr, M. & Youniss, J. (1983) *The Interpersonal Style Inventory*. Los Angeles: Western Psychological Services.

Lorr, M., McNair, D. M., Michaux, W. W., *et al* (1962) Frequency of treatment and change in psychotherapy. *Journal of Abnormal and Social Psychology*, **64**, 281–292.

Lubin, B. (1965) Adjective checklists for measurement of depression. *Archives of General Psychiatry*, **12**, 57–62.

Luborsky, L. (1962) Clinicians' judgements of mental health: a proposed scale. *Archives of General Psychiatry*, **7**, 407–417.

Mann, A. H., Jenkins, R., Cutting, J. C., *et al* (1981) The development and use of a standardized assessment of abnormal personality. *Psychological Medicine*, **11**, 839–847.

Margolin, G., Talovic, S. & Weinstein, C. D. (1983) Areas of change questionnaire: a practical guide to marital assessment. *Journal of Consulting and Clinical Psychology*, **51**, 920–931.

Markova, I. S. & Berrios, G. E. (1992) The assessment of insight in clinical psychiatry: a new scale. *Acta Psychiatrica Scandinavica*, **86**, 159–164.

Marks, I. M. & Mathews, A. M. (1979) Brief standard self-rating scale for phobic patients. *Behaviour Research and Therapy*, **17**, 263–267.

Marmar, C. R., Horowitz, M. J., Weiss, D. S., *et al* (1986) Development of the therapeutic rating system. In *The Psychotherapeutic Process: A Research Handbook* (eds L. S. Greenberg & W. M. Pinsof), pp. 367–390. New York: Guilford Press.

Marshall, M., Lockwood, A., Bradley, C., *et al* (2000) Unpublished rating scales: A major source of bias in randomised controlled trials of treatments for schizophrenia. *British Journal of Psychiatry*, **176**, 249–252.

Matson, J. L., Gardner, W. I., Coe, D. A., *et al* (1991) A scale for evaluating emotional disorders in severely and profoundly mentally retarded persons. Development of the Diagnostic Assessment for the Severely Handicapped (DASH) scale. *British Journal of Psychiatry*, **159**, 404–409.

Mayfield, D., McLeod, G. & Hall, P. (1974) The CAGE questionnaire: validation of a new alcoholism screening instrument. *American Journal of Psychiatry*, **131**, 1121–1123.

McFarlane, A. H., Neale, K. A., Normal, G. R., *et al* (1981) Methodological issues in developing a scale to measure social support. *Schizophrenia Bulletin*, **7**, 90–100.

McGuffin, P., Farmer, A. E. & Harvey, I. (1991) A polydiagnostic application of operational criteria in studies of psychotic illness: development and reliability of the OPCRIT system. *Archives of General Psychiatry*, **48**, 764–770.

McLennan, A. T., Buborsky, L., O'Brien, C. P., *et al* (1980) An improved evaluation instrument for substance abuse patients: the addiction severity index. *Journal of Nervous and Mental Disease*, **168**, 26–33.

McNair, D. M. & Lorr, M. (1964) An analysis of mood in neurotics. *Journal of Abnormal and Social Psychology*, **69**, 620–627.

Meer, B. & Baker, J. A. (1966) The Stockton geriatric rating scale. *Journal of Gerontology*, **21**, 392–403.

Melzack, R. (1987) The short-form McGill pain questionnaire (SF–MPQ). *Pain*, **30**, 191–197.

Millon, T. (1981) *Disorders of Personality: Axis II*. New York: Wiley.

Mohs, R. C., Rosen, W. G. & Davies, K. L. (1983) The Alzheimer's disease assessment scale: an instrument for assessing treatment efficacy. *Psychopharmacology Bulletin*, **19**, 448–449.

Monahan, J., Steadman, H. J., Silver, E., *et al* (2001) *Rethinking Risk Assessment: The MacArthur Study of Mental Disorder and Violence*. Oxford: Oxford University Press.

Montgomery, S. A. & Åsberg, M. (1979) A new depression scale designed to be sensitive to change. *British Journal of Psychiatry*, **134**, 382–389.

Moos, R. H. (1974) *The Ward Atmosphere Scale Manual*. Palo Alto, CA: Consulting Psychologists Press.

Morey, L. C., Waugh, P. & Blashfield, R. K. (1985) MMPI scales for DSM–III disorders: their derivation and correlates. *Journal of Personality Assessment*, **49**, 245–251.

Morgan, H. G. & Russell, G. F. M. (1975) Value of family background and clinical features as predictors of long-term outcome in anorexia nervosa: four year follow up study of 41 patients. *Psychological Medicine*, **5**, 355–371.

Morosini, P. L. & Magliano, L. (2000) Development of reliability and acceptability of a new version of the DSM–IV Social and Functioning Assessment Scale (SOFAS) to assess routine social function. *Acta Psychiatrica Scandinavica*, **101**, 323–329.

Moss, S., Prosser, H., Costello, H., *et al* (1998). Reliability and validity of the PAS–ADD checklist for detecting psychiatric disorders in adults with intellectual disability. *Journal of Intellectual Disability Research*, **42**, 173–183.

Motto, J. A., Heilbron, D. C. & Juster, J. P. (1985) Development of a clinical instrument to estimate suicide risk. *American Journal of Psychiatry*, **142**, 680–686.

Nelson, H. E. (1976) A modified card sorting test sensitive to frontal lobe defects. *Cortex*, **12**, 313–324.

Nelson, H. E. (1982) *National Adult Reading Test (NART) for the Assessment of Premorbid Intelligence in Patients with Dementia: Test Manual*. Windsor: NFER–Nelson.

Neugarten, B. L., Havighurst, R. J. & Tobin, S. S. (1961) The measurement of life satisfaction. *Journal of Gerontology*, **16**, 134–143.

Nichols, H. & Molinder, I. (1984) *Manual for the Multiphasic Sex Inventory* (MSI). Tacoma, WA: Crime and Victims Psychology Specialists.

Olson, D. H., Bell, R. & Portner, J. (1978) *The Family Adaptability and Cohesion Evaluation Scale (FACES)*. St Paul, MN: Family Social Science, University of Minnesota.

Overall, J. E. & Gorham, D. R. (1962) The brief psychiatric rating scale. *Psychological Reports*, **10**, 799–812.

Pallis, D. J., Barrraclough, B. M., Levey, A. B., *et al* (1982) Estimating suicide risk among attempted suicides: 1. The development of new clinical scales. *British Journal of Psychiatry*, **141**, 37–44.

Palmstierna, T. & Wistedt, B. (1987) Staff observation and aggression scale, SOAS: presentation and evaluation. *Acta Psychiatrica Scandinavica*, **76**, 657–673.

Parker, G., Tupling, H. & Brown, L. B. (1979) Parental bonding instrument (PBI). *British Journal of Medical Psychology*, **52**, 1–10.

Parloff, M. B., Kelman, H. C. & Frank, J. D. (1954) Comfort, effectiveness and self-awareness as criteria of improvement in psychotherapy. *American Journal of Psychiatry*, **111**, 343–351.

Parrott, A. C. & Hindmarch, J. (1978) Factor analysis of a sleep evaluation questionnaire (SEQ). *Psychological Medicine*, **8**, 325–329.

Patel, V. & Hope, R. A. (1992) A rating scale for aggressive behaviour in the elderly – the RAGE. *Psychological Medicine*, **22**, 211–221.

Pattie, A. H. & Gilleard, C. J. (1979) *Manual of the Clifton Assessment Procedures for the Elderly* (CAPE). Kent: Hodder & Stoughton.

Paykel, E. S., Prusoff, B. A., Uhlenhuth, E. H., *et al* (1971) Scaling of life events. *Archives of General Psychiatry*, **25**, 340–347.

Pfeiffer, E. (1975) A short portable mental status questionnaire for the assessment of organic brain deficit in elderly patients. *Journal of the American Geriatrics Society*, **23**, 433–441.

Pfohl, B., Stangl, D. & Zimmerman, M. (1983) *Structured Interview for DSM–III Personality.* Iowa: Department of Psychiatry, University of Iowa.

Phelan, M., Slade, M., Thornicroft, G., *et al* (1995) The Camberwell Assessment of Need: the validity and reliability of an instrument to assess the needs of people with severe mental illness. *British Journal of Psychiatry*, **167**, 589–595.

Pilowsky, I. & Spence, N. D. (1975) Patterns of illness behaviour in patients with intractable pain. *Journal of Psychosomatic Research*, **19**, 279–287.

Platt, S., Weymann, A., Hirsch, S., *et al* (1980) The social behaviour assessment schedule (SBAS): rationale, contents, scoring and reliability of a new interview schedule. *Social Psychiatry*, **15**, 43–55.

Plutchik, R., Conte, H., Lieberman, M., *et al* (1970) Reliability and validity of a scale for assessing the functioning of geriatric patients. *Journal of the American Geriatrics Society*, **18**, 491–500.

Plutchik, R., Van-Praaq, H. M., Conte, H. R., *et al* (1989) Correlates of suicide and violence risk: 1. The suicide risk measure. *Comprehensive Psychiatry*, **30**, 296–302.

Power, M. J., Champion, L. A. & Aris, S. J. (1988) The development of a measure of social support: the significant others (SOS) scale. *British Journal of Clinical Psychology*, **27**, 349–358.

Poznanski, E. O., Cook, S. C. & Carroll, B. J. (1979) A depression rating scale for children. *Pediatrics*, **64**, 442–450.

Puig-Antich, J. & Chambers, W. (1978) *The Schedule for Affective Disorders and Schizophrenia for School-Age Children.* New York: New York State Psychiatric Institute.

Puig-Antich, J., Orvaschel, H. & Tabrizi, M. A., *et al* (1980) *The Schedule for Affective Disorders and Schizophrenia for School-Age Children–Epidemiologic Version* (3rd edn). New York: New York State Psychiatric Institute & Yale University School of Medicine.

Quay, H. C. & Peterson, D. R. (1975) *Manual for the Behavior Problem Checklist.* Miami, FL: University of Miami.

Qureshi, K. N. & Hodkinson, H. M. (1974) Evaluation of a ten-question mental test in the institutionalised elderly. *Age and Ageing*, **3**, 152–157.

Raistrick, D., Dunbar, G. & Davidson, R. (1983) Development of a questionnaire to measure alcohol dependence. *British Journal of Addiction*, **78**, 89–96.

Raskin, A. & Crook, T. (1988) Relative's assessment of global symptomatology (RAGS). *Psychopharmacology Bulletin*, **24**, 759–763.

Raskin, A., Schulterbrandt, J., Reatig, N., *et al* (1969) Replication of factors of psychopathology in interview, ward behaviour and self report ratings of hospitalised depressives. *Journal of Nervous and Mental Disease*, **148**, 87–98.

Raven, J. C. (1960) *Guide to the Standard Progressive Matrices.* London: H. K. Lewis.

Reisberg, B. (1988) Functional assessment staging. *Psychopharmacology Bulletin*, **24**, 653–659.

Reisberg, B. & Ferris, S. (1988) Brief cognitive rating scale (BCRS). *Psychopharmacology Bulletin*, **24**, 629–636.

Reisberg, B., Ferris, S. H., De Leon, M. J., *et al* (1982) The global deterioration scale for assessment of primary degenerative dementia. *American Journal of Psychiatry*, **139**, 1136–1139.

Reitan, R. M. & Davison, L. A. (1974) *Clinical Neuropsychology: Current Status and Application.* New York: Hemisphere.

Remington, M. & Tyrer, P. (1979) The social functioning schedule – a brief semi-structured interview. *Social Psychiatry*, **14**, 151–157.

Reynolds, C. R. & Richmond, B. O. (1978) What I think and feel: a revised measure of children's manifest anxiety. *Journal of Abnormal Child Psychology*, **6**, 271–280.

Reynolds, W. M., Anderson, G. & Bartell, N. (1985) Measuring depression in childhood. *Journal of Abnormal Child Psychology*, **13**, 513–526.

Richman, N. & Graham, P. (1971) A behavioural screening questionnaire for use with three-year-old children: preliminary findings. *Journal of Child Psychology and Psychiatry*, **12**, 5–33.

Robins, L. N., Helzer, J. E., Croughan, J., *et al* (1981) National Institute of Mental Health diagnostic interview schedule: its history, characteristics and validity. *Archives of General Psychiatry*, **38**, 381–389.

Robins, L. N., Wing, J., Wittchen, H. U., *et al* (1988) An epidemiologic instrument suitable for use in conjunction with different diagnostic systems and in different cultures. *Archives of General Psychiatry*, **45**, 1069–1077.

Robinson, R. G., Parikh, R. M., Lipsey, J. R., *et al* (1993) Pathological laughing and crying following stroke: validation of a measurement scale and a double-blind treatment study. *American Journal of Psychiatry*, **150**, 286–293.

Robson, P. (1989) Development of a new self-report questionnaire to measure self-esteem. *Psychological Medicine*, **19**, 513–518.

Rosenbaum, M. (1980) A schedule of assessing self-control behaviors: preliminary findings. *Behavior Therapy*, **11**, 109–121.

Roth, M., Huppert, F. A., Tym, E., *et al* (1988) *The Cambridge Examination for Mental Disorders of the Elderly (CAMDEX)*. Cambridge: Cambridge University Press.

Ruggeri, M. & Dall'Agnola, R. (1993) The development and use of the Verona Expectations for Care Scale (VECS) and the Verona Service Satisfaction Scale (VSSS) for measuring expectations and satisfaction with community-based psychiatric services in patients, relatives and professionals. *Psychological Medicine*, **23**, 511–523.

Russell, D., Peolau, L. A. & Ferguson, M. L. (1978) Developing a measure of loneliness. *Journal of Personality Assessment*, **42**, 290–294.

Rutter, M. (1967) A children's behaviour questionnaire for completion by teachers: preliminary findings. *Journal of Child Psychology and Psychiatry*, **8**, 1–11.

Salkovskis, P. M., Rimes, K. A., Warwick, H. M. C., *et al* (2002) The Health Anxiety Inventory: development and validation of scales for the measurement of health anxiety and hypochondriasis. *Psychological Medicine*, **32**, 843–853.

Sanavio, E. (1988) Obsessions and compulsions: the Padua inventory. *Behaviour Research and Therapy*, **26**, 169–177.

Sarason, I. G., Levine, H. M., Basham, H. M., *et al* (1983) Assessing social support: the social support questionnaire. *Journal of Personality and Social Psychology*, **44**, 127–139.

Saunders, J. B., Aasland, O. G., Babor, T. F., *et al* (1993) Development of the Alcohol Use Disorders Identification Test (AUDIT): WHO collaborative project on early detection of persons with harmful alcohol consumption II. *Addiction*, **88**, 791–804.

Scheier, M. F. & Carver, C. S. (1985) Optimism, coping and health: assessment and implications of generalised outcome expectancies. *Health Psychology*, **4**, 219–247.

Schooler, N., Hogarty, G. & Weissman, M. M. (1979) Social adjustment scale 11 (SAS 11). In *Resource Material for Community Mental Health Program Evaluators* (ed. W. A. Hargreaves), pp. 290–302. Washington, D.C.: US Department of Health, Education and Welfare.

Schwartz, G. E. (1983) Development and validation of the geriatric evaluation by relative's rating (GERRI). *Psychological Reports*, **53**, 479–488.

Schwartz, R. M. & Gottman, K. M. (1976) Towards a task analysis of assertive behaviour. *Journal of Consulting and Clinical Psychology*, **44**, 910–920.

Sclan, S. G. & Saillon, A. (1996) The behaviour pathology in Alzheimer's disease rating scale. Reliability and analysis of symptom category scores. *International Journal of Geriatric Psychiatry*, **11**, 819–839.

Seligman, M. E. P., Abramson, L. Y., Semmel, A., *et al* (1979) Depressive attributional style. *Journal of Abnormal Psychology*, **88**, 242–247.

Selzer, M. L. (1971) The Michigan alcoholism screening test: the quest for a new diagnostic instrument. *American Journal of Psychiatry*, **127**, 1653–1658.

Sensky, T., Turkington, D., Kingdon, D., *et al* (2000). A randomized controlled trial of cognitive–behavioral therapy for persistent symptoms in schizophrenia resistant to medication. *Archives of General Psychiatry*, **57**, 165–172.

Shader, R. I., Harmatz, J. S. & Salzman, C. (1974) A new scale for clinical assessment in geriatric populations: Sandoz clinical assessment–geriatric (SCAG). *Journal of the American Geriatrics Society*, **22**, 107–113.

Shipley, K., Hilborn, B., Hansell, A., *et al* (2000) Patient satisfaction: a valid measure of quality of care in a psychiatric service. *Acta Psychiatrica Scandinavica*, **101**, 330–333.

Simpson, G. M. (1988) Tardive dyskinesia rating scale (TDRS). *Psychopharmacology Bulletin*, **24**, 803–806.

Skinner, H. A. & Allen, B. A. (1983) Alcohol dependence scale, measurement and validation. *Journal of Abnormal Psychology*, **91**, 199–209.

Skinner, H. A. & Goldberg, A. (1986) Evidence for a drug dependence syndrome among narcotic users. *British Journal of Addiction*, **81**, 479–484.

Slade, P. D. & Russell, G. F. M. (1973) Awareness of body dimensions in anorexia nervosa – cross sectional and longitudinal studies. *Psychological Medicine*, **3**, 188–199.

Slade, P. D. & Dewey, M. E. (1986) Development and preliminary validation of SCANS: a screening instrument for identifying individuals at risk of developing anorexia and bulimia nervosa. *International Journal of Eating Disorders*, **5**, 517–538.

Slade, P. D., Dewey, M. E., Newton, T., *et al* (1990) Development and preliminary validation of the body satisisfaction scale (BSS). *Psychology and Health*, **4**, 213–220.

Smith, A. (1968) The symbol digit modalities test: a neuropsychologic test for economic screening of learning and other cerebral disorders. *Learning Disorders*, **3**, 83–91.

Smith, M. C. & Thelen, M. H. (1984) Development and validation of a test for bulimia. *Journal of Consulting and Clinical Psychology*, **52**, 863–872.

Smith, S. G. T., Touquet, R. G. M., Wright, S., *et al* (1996) Detection of alcohol misusing patients in accident and emergency departments: The Paddington alcohol test (PAT). *Journal of Accident & Emergency Medicine*, **13**, 308–312.

Snaith, R. P., Ahmed, S. N., Mehta, S., *et al* (1971) Assessment of the severity of primary depressive illness: the Wakefield self assessment depression inventory. *Psychological Medicine*, **1**, 143–149.

Snaith, R. P., Bridge, G. W. & Hamilton, M. (1976) The Leeds scales for the self-assessment of anxiety and depression. *British Journal of Psychiatry*, **128**, 156–165.

Snaith, R. P., Constantopoulos, A. A., Jardine, M. Y., *et al* (1978) A clinical scale for the self-assessment of irritability. *British Journal of Psychiatry*, **132**, 164–171.

Snaith, R. P., Baugh, S. J., Clayden, A. D., *et al* (1982) The Clinical Anxiety Scale: an instrument derived from the Hamilton Anxiety Scale. *British Journal of Psychiatry*, **141**, 518–523.

Solomon, P. R., Hirschoff, A., Kelly, B., *et al* (1998) A 7 minute neurocognitive screening battery highly sensitive to Alzheimer's disease. *Archives of Neurology*, **55**, 349–355.

Sorgi, P., Ratey, J., Knoedler, D. W., *et al* (1991) Rating aggression in the clinical setting a retrospective adaptation of the Overt Aggression Scale: preliminary results. *Journal of Neuropsychiatry*, **3**, 552–556.

Spanier, G. B. (1987) Measuring dyadic adjustment: new scales for assessing the quality of marriage and similar dyads. *Journal of Marriage and the Family*, **17**, 485–493.

Spiegel, R., Brunner, C., Phil, L., *et al* (1991) A new behavioral assessment scale for geriatric out- and in-patients: the NOSGER (nurses' observation scale for geriatric patients). *Journal of the American Geriatrics Society*, **39**, 339–347.

Spielberger, C. D., Gorsuch, R. L., Luchene, R., *et al* (1983) *Manual for the State–Trait Anxiety Inventory*. Palo Alto, CA: Consulting Psychologists Press.

Spielberger, C. D., Johnson, E. H., Russell, S. F., *et al* (1985) The experience and expression of anger: construction and validation of an anger expression scale. In *Anger and Hostility in Cardiovascular and Behavioural Disorders* (eds M. A. Chesney & R. H. Rosenman), pp. 5–30. Washington: Hemisphere.

Spitzer, R. L, Fleiss, J. L., Endicott, J., *et al* (1967) Mental status schedule: properties of factor-analytically derived scales (MSS). *Archives of General Psychiatry*, **16**, 479–493.

Spitzer, R. L., Endicott, J., Fleiss, J. L., *et al* (1970) The psychiatric status schedules: a technique for evaluating psychopathology and impairment in role functioning. *Archives of General Psychiatry*, **23**, 41–55.

Spitzer, R. L., Williams, J. B. W., Gibbon, M., *et al* (1990a) *Structured Clinical Interview for DSM–III–R – Non-Patient Edition* (SCID–NP, Version 1.0). Washington, DC: American Psychiatric Press.

Spitzer, R. L., Williams, J. B. W., Gibbon, M., *et al* (1990*b*) *Structured Clinical Interview for DSM–III–R – Patient Edition* (SCID–P, Version 1.0). Washington, DC: American Psychiatric Press.

Spitzer, R. L., Williams, J. B. W., Gibbon, M., *et al* (1990*c*) *Structured Clinical Interview for DSM–III–R Personality Disorders* (SCID–II, Version 1.0). Washington, DC: American Psychiatric Press.

Spitzer, R. L., Williams, J. B. W., Gibbon, M., *et al* (1990*d*) *Structured Clinical Interview for DSM–III–R – Patient Edition with Psychotic Screen* (SCID–PW/PSYCHOTIC SCREEN, Version 1.0). Washington, DC: American Psychiatric Press.

Steinberg, M., Rounsaville, B. & Cicchetti, D. V. (1990) Structured clinical interview for DSM–III–R dissociative disorders: preliminary report on a new diagnostic instrument. *American Journal of Psychiatry*, **147**, 76–82.

Steiner, M., Haskett, R. F. & Carroll, B. J. (1980) Premenstrual tension syndrome: the development of research diagnostic criteria and new rating scales. *Acta Psychiatrica Scandinavica*, **62**, 177–190.

Strauss, J. S. & Harder, D. W. (1981) The case record rating scale: a method for rating symptoms and social function data from case records. *Psychiatry Research*, **4**, 333–345.

Stunkard, A. J. & Messick, S. (1985) The three-factor eating questionnaire to measure dietary restraint, disinhibition and hunger. *Journal of Psychosomatic Research*, **29**, 71–83.

Sutherland, G., Edwards, G., Taylor, C., *et al* (1986) The measurement of opiate dependence. *British Journal of Addiction*, **81**, 485–494.

Sunderland, T., Alterman, I. S., Yount, D., *et al* (1988) A new scale for the assessment of depressed mood in demented patients. *American Journal of Psychiatry*, **145**, 955–959.

Tantam, D. (1988) Lifelong eccentricity and social isolation. II: Asperger's syndrome or schizoid personality disorder? *British Journal of Psychiatry*, **153**, 783–791.

Taylor, J. A. (1953) A personality scale of manifest anxiety. *Journal of Abnormal and Social Psychology*, **48**, 285–290.

Teasdale, G. & Jennett, B. (1974) Assessment of coma and impaired consciousness. *Lancet*, **ii**, 81–84.

Teng, E. L. & Chui, H. C. (1987) The modified mini-mental state (3MS) examination. *Journal of Clinical Psychiatry*, **48**, 314–318.

Tennant, C. & Andrews, G. (1976) A scale to measure the stress of life events. *Australian and New Zealand Journal of Psychiatry*, **10**, 27–32.

Teri, L., Truax, P., Logsdon, R., *et al* (1992) Assessment of behavioural problems in dementia: the revised memory and behaviour checklist. *Psychology and Aging*, **7**, 622–631.

Thurstone, L. L. (1944) *A Factorial Study of Perception*. Chicago: University of Chicago Press.

Trzepacz, P. T., Baker, R. W. & Greenhouse, J. (1988) A symptom rating scale for delirium. *Psychiatry Research*, **23**, 89–97.

Tuckman, J. & Youngman, W. F. (1968) A scale for assessing suicide risk of attempted suicides. *Journal of Clinical Psychology*, **24**, 17–19.

Tyrer, P. (1990) Personality disorder and social functioning. In: *Measuring Human Problems: a Practical Guide* (eds D. F. Peck & C. M. Shapiro), pp. 119–142. Chichester: Wiley.

Tyrer, P. (2001) The case for cothymia: mixed anxiety and depression as a single diagnosis. *British Journal of Psychiatry*, **179**, 191–193.

Tyrer, P. & Alexander, J. (1979) Classification of personality disorder. *British Journal of Psychiatry*, **135**, 163–167.

Tyrer, P. & Casey, P. (eds) (1993) *Social Function in Psychiatry: The Hidden Axis of Classification Exposed*. Petersfield: Wrightson Biomedical.

Tyrer, P., Owen, R. T. & Cicchetti, D. V. (1984) Brief anxiety scale. *Journal of Neurology, Neurosurgery and Psychiatry*, **47**, 970–975.

Tyrer, P., Murphy, S. & Riley, P. (1990) The Benzodiazepine Withdrawal Symptom Questionnaire. *Journal of Affective Disorders*, **19**, 53–61.

Tyrer, P., Jones, V., Thompson, S., *et al* (2003) Service variation in baseline variables and prediction of risk in a randomised controlled trial of psychological treatment in repeated parasuicide: the POPMACT study. *International Journal of Social Psychiatry*, **49**, 58–69.

Tyrer, P., Nur, U., Crawford, M., *et al* (2005) The Social Functioning Questionnaire: a rapid and robust measure of perceived functioning. *International Journal of Social Psychiatry*, 51: 265–275.

Ullman, R. K., Sleator, E. K. & Sprague, R. L. (1984) A new rating scale for diagnosis and monitoring of ADD children (ACTeRS). *Psychopharmacology Bulletin*, **19**, 160–164.

Van Strien, T., Frijters, J. E. R., Bergers, G. P. A., *et al* (1986) Dutch eating behaviour questionnaire for assessment of restrained, emotional and external eating behaviour. *International Journal of Eating Disorders*, **5**, 295–315.

Vaughan, C. F. & Leff, J. P. (1976) The measurement of expressed emotion in families of psychiatric patients. *British Journal of Social and Clinical Psychology*, **15**, 157–165.

Ward, M. F., Wender, P. H. & Reimherr, F. W. (1993) The Wender Utah rating scale: an aid in the retrospective diagnosis of childhood attention deficit hyperactivity disorder. *American Journal of Psychiatry*, **150**, 885–890.

Ware, J. E. & Sherbourne, C. D. (1992) The MOS 36 item short form health survey: conceptual framework and item selection. *Medical Care*, **30**, 473–483.

Warrington, E. K. & James, M. (1967) Disorders of visual perception in patients with localized cerebral lesions. *Neuropsychologica*, **5**, 253–266.

Washton, A. M., Stone, N. S. & Hendrickson, E. C. (1988) Cocaine abuse. In *Assessment of Addictive Behaviours* (eds D. M. Donovan & G. A. Marlatt). London: Hutchinson.

Watson, D. & Friend, R. (1969) Measurement of social-evaluative anxiety. *Journal of Consulting and Clinical Psychology*, **33**, 448–457.

Wechsler, D. (1945) A standardized memory scale for clinical use. *Journal of Psychology*, **19**, 87–95.

Wechsler, D. (1949) *Manual for the Wechsler Intelligence Scale for Children*. New York: Psychological Corporation.

Wechsler, D. (1958) *The Measurement and Appraisal of Adult Intelligence* (4th edn). Baltimore: Williams & Wilkins.

Weissman, M. M. & Bothwell, S. (1976) Assessment of social adjustment by patient self-report. *Archives of General Psychiatry*, **33**, 1111–1115.

Wells, C. E. (1979) Pseudo-dementia. *American Journal of Psychiatry*, **136**, 895–900.

Wilhelm, K. & Parker, G. (1988) The development of a measure of intimate bonds. *Psychological Medicine*, **18**, 225–234.

Wilkinson, I. M. & Graham-White, J. (1980) Psychogeriatric dependency rating scales (PGDRS): a method of assessment for use by nurses. *British Journal of Psychiatry*, **137**, 558–565.

Wing, J. K., Cooper, J. E. & Sartorius, N. (1974) *Measurement and Classification of Psychiatric Symptoms: An Instruction Manual for the PSE and Catego Program*. London: Cambridge University Press.

Wing, J. K., Babor, T., Brugha, T., *et al* (1990) SCAN – Schedules for clinical assessment in neuropsychiatry. *Archives of General Psychiatry*, **47**, 589–593.

Wing, L. & Gould, J. (1978) Systematic recording of behaviours and skills of retarded and psychotic children. *Journal of Autism and Childhood Schizophrenia*, **8**, 79–97.

Wolpe, J. & Lang, P. J. (1964) A fear survey schedule for use in behaviour therapy (FSS). *Behaviour Research and Therapy*, **2**, 27–30.

Wykes, T. & Sturt, E. (1986) The measurement of social behaviour in psychiatric patients: an assessment of the reliability and validity of the SBS schedule. *British Journal of Psychiatry*, **148**, 1–11.

Young, R. C., Biggs, J. T., Ziegler, V. E., *et al* (1978) A rating scale for mania: reliability, validity and sensitivity. *British Journal of Psychiatry*, **133**, 429–435.

Yudofsky, S. C. (1986) The overt aggression scale for the objective rating of verbal and physical aggression. *American Journal of Psychiatry*, **143**, 35–39.

Zahl, D. L. & Hawton, K. (2004) Repetition of deliberate self-harm and subsequent suicide risk: long-term follow-up study of 11 583 patients. *British Journal of Psychiatry*, **185**, 70–75.

Zatz, S. & Chassin, L. (1983) Cognitions of test-anxious children. *Journal of Consulting and Clinical Psychology*, **51**, 526–534.

Zigmond, A. S. & Snaith, R. P. (1983) The hospital anxiety and depression scale. *Acta Psychiatrica Scandinavica*, **67**, 361–370.

Zuckerman, M. (1960) The development of an affect adjective checklist for the management of anxiety. *Journal of Consulting Psychology*, **24**, 457–462.

Zung, W. W. K. (1965) A self-rating depression scale. *Archives of General Psychiatry*, **12**, 63–70.

Zung, W. W. K. (1971) A rating instrument for anxiety disorders. *Psychosomatics*, **12**, 371–379.

Part IV

Special areas of research

CHAPTER 12

Research in child and adolescent psychiatry

Atif Rahman and Richard Harrington

The basic principles of research in child and adolescent psychiatry are identical to those in other areas of medicine. They include all of the standard features of scientific research, such as defining the research question, refining testable hypotheses, designing an appropriate investigation, collecting and analysing the data, and writing up the project. However, child and adolescent psychiatry and related disciplines pose special demands and challenges for researchers. The breadth of the field is huge. Child and adolescent psychiatry includes the study of highly heterogeneous populations, ranging from infants to young adults. People in contact with these groups, such as parents, teachers, siblings and peers, are often also studied. This means that researchers must usually be familiar with many different research methods. Moreover, since it is now widely believed that psychopathology in young people involves the interplay of biological, psychological and social factors over time, the approach taken must be developmental and focused on how these evolving factors lead to psychiatric disorder.

But what exactly is a developmental approach to psychopathology? In this chapter we shall begin by describing the hallmarks of developmental research approaches. We shall then describe some of the key conceptual and methodological issues that have to be dealt with when researching the development and treatment of psychopathology among the young. Finally we shall review some of the current research areas in child psychiatry.

Developmental approaches to psychopathology

During the past two decades developmental psychopathology, which is the study of the origins and course of individual patterns of behavioural maladaptation, has emerged as a new science. It brings together and integrates a variety of disciplines, including epidemiology, genetics, psychiatry, psychology, the neurosciences, and sociology. There are many features of a developmental approach to psychopathology that could make it important, but the defining features can be reduced to three key issues (Rutter & Sroufe, 2000).

Causal processes

The first is the understanding of causal processes. It is now widely understood that most psychiatric illnesses do not result from single linear causes. Individual risk factors are seldom powerful. More often, psychopathology arises from the complex interplay of multiple risk and protective factors, some genetic and others environmental. For example, research on depression in adolescents has shown that genetic effects are likely to act through multiple mechanisms, many of which are indirect (Silberg *et al*, 1999). In some cases genetic factors act by increasing the person's vulnerability to adverse life events, an example of gene–environment interaction. In others genes appear to increase the liability to depressing life events, such as falling out with friends, an example of active gene–environment correlation (Silberg *et al*, 1999).

Processes of development

A second central concept, which is at the core of much developmental research, is an understanding of the processes of development, including the emergence of patterns of adaptation and maladaptation over time. Developmental analyses tend therefore to be progressive, with one step leading to another. It is recognised that the mechanisms involved in causation may entail dynamic processes over time, with several routes to the same outcome. For example, research on the childhood precursors of self-harm in adult life suggests that there may be at least two distinct pathways (Harrington *et al*, 1994): one through persistent depression and the other through antisocial behaviour. Continuities of psychopathology can take the form of direct persistence of the same problem (homotypic continuity), for example when an antisocial child becomes an antisocial teenager. Sometimes, however, psychopathology in childhood can be followed by a different form of psychopathology in adolescence or adult life (heterotypic continuity). For example, behavioural problems are a strong risk factor for subsequent depression (Angold *et al*, 1999).

Even when there is continuity of the same form of psychopathology, it does not necessarily follow that the continuities are a result of autonomous unfolding of pathological processes. There is evidence that continuities of some kinds of psychopathology over development depend to an important extent on causal chain processes in which there is an evolving interaction between individual personal dispositions and social circumstances. For example, the adult outcomes of girls brought up in children's homes appear to be mediated to a significant degree by their experiences in late adolescence (Fig. 12.1). Girls who become pregnant and then live with a partner who has significant problems are much more likely to become depressed than those who do not (Quinton *et al*, 1984).

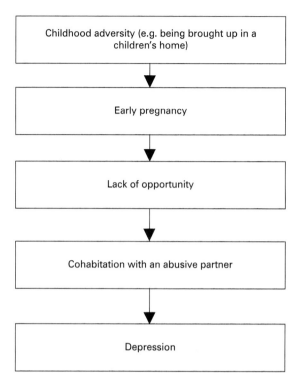

Fig. 12.1 Causal chain linking childhood adversity to later depression in women.

Normality and pathology

A third key concern has been the links between normality and pathology. Much causal research in psychiatry has been based on the idea that diagnostic categories represent some kind of reality or 'truth' distinct from normal behaviour. By contrast, many developmental psychopathological concepts are dimensional, with the need to take account of variations along dimensions.

Age effects in development and psychopathology

Another hallmark of developmental studies is a focus on age as a key issue both in designing research and in data analysis. It will be appreciated that age is an ambiguous variable that can refer to many different things (Rutter, 1989), such as cognitive level, biological maturation or the duration and type of experiences. It is, however, these very different aspects of age that can be used as natural experiments to test competing hypotheses about the causes of psychopathology. For example, the finding that the incidence of depressive disorders more than doubles during early adolescence has been used in epidemiological studies to examine potential correlates of this increase, such as hormone levels, depressive cognitions and life events. Alternatively, disorders can be divided according to their age at onset. Conduct disorders that start in childhood tend to have a worse outcome in adult life than those starting in adolescence (Moffitt *et al*, 2002).

Conceptual issues in developmental research

Defining disorder

Ideally, a diagnosis should identify disorders with the same underlying aetiology, the same course and the same response to treatment. However, even in general medicine such an ideal is seldom achieved. Many of the most common problems, such as heart disease, have multiple causes. Moreover, a single 'medical' cause, such as smoking, may lead to many different disorders, each with different consequences in terms of morbidity and treatment.

Similar issues apply in child and adolescent psychiatry. Most disorders have a multifactorial causation and most risk factors can lead to several different types of disorder. Accordingly, the diagnosis and classification of child psychopathology has increasingly focused on the presenting features of the disorder rather than its aetiology. With a few exceptions, (e.g. post-traumatic stress disorder) diagnoses tell us about the symptoms and signs of a disorder, but not necessarily about its causes or treatment, which must be considered separately.

The main current diagnostic schemes used in research are the 10th revision of the *International Classification of Diseases* (ICD–10) and the 4th edition of the *Diagnostic and Statistical Manual of Mental Disorders* (DSM–IV). Although the schemes differ in many ways, their overall classifications are very similar. ICD–10 has a clinical version (World Health Organization, 1992), which gives broad prototypic descriptions of disorders, and a research version (World Health Organization, 1993) that lists clearly defined diagnostic criteria. DSM contains only specified diagnostic criteria (American Psychiatric Association, 1994).

Both ICD–10 and DSM–IV classify psychopathology into categories. Although it is likely that most psychopathology in children is based on continuously distributed underlying liability, categorical systems have several merits. First, most clinical decisions are categorical in nature, so even if a dimensional approach were used it would be necessary to define categories using cut-off points. Second, diagnostic categories provide a simple summary of a large amount of information.

The establishment of lists of diagnostic criteria has been a major step forward because these lists have improved agreement among clinicians and investigators. Nevertheless, when using these schemes in research work a number of issues should be borne in mind. First, diagnostic criteria are no more than a consensus of current concepts in a field that is changing rapidly. It is certain that our diagnostic schemes will change substantially in the future. Second, many children who are significantly impaired by psychiatric problems do not meet diagnostic criteria. Equally, it is quite common to find children who meet the symptomatic criteria for a psychiatric diagnosis but are not significantly affected their symptoms and are not impaired. Indeed, when psychiatric disorders are diagnosed using symptom criteria alone, the rate of so-called disorders becomes implausibly high. Hence it is important that judgement is used when applying the criteria. The criteria were never meant to be applied rigidly in a cookbook fashion.

Comorbidity

There is a great deal of overlap between different types of diagnosis in children and adolescents (Angold *et al*, 1999). For example, around one-fifth of young people with major depression also have a conduct disorder, and about a third have an anxiety disorder. This comorbidity between supposedly separate diagnostic categories is important for several reasons. First, it can create diagnostic difficulties. For example, there is a great deal of overlap between the symptoms of attention-deficit disorder and mania (e.g. overactivity, distractibility), with the result that manic disorders may be overdiagnosed among young children. Second, unless comorbidity is assessed and controlled for in some way, what seem to be the correlates of one disorder may in fact be those of another. However, comorbidity is not always a problem: it can be exploited to understand the aetiology of child psychiatric disorder. For example, hyperkinetic conduct disorder may represent a more severe form of conduct disorder.

Multi-axial diagnosis

Most children with psychiatric problems have multiple difficulties. For example, a child with a behavioural problem may also have mental retardation and live in a home where there is much family discord. No single diagnostic term can describe all of these difficulties, yet it is often important to record all of them in research studies. The multi-axial diagnostic scheme was devised to deal with this issue.

The Axes that are used are shown in Table 12.1. A diagnosis in this scheme records something about a child's problems on all six Axes, even if one or more of them are negative. For instance, the diagnosis could be hyperkinetic syndrome (Axis I) leading to moderate social disability (Axis VI) in a child with mild mental retardation (Axis III), who suffers from epilepsy (Axis IV) and who comes from a family characterised by discord

Table 12.1 ICD–10 multi-axial diagnosis

Axis	Features
I	Clinical psychiatric syndrome
II	Specific disorders of psychological development
III	Intellectual level
IV	Associated medical conditions
V	Associated abnormal psychosocial situations
VI	Global assessment of disability

(Axis V). The child's reading problems can be explained by their mental retardation; there is no specific reading retardation (Axis II).

Choosing an instrument to measure psychopathology in young people

Methods of assessment and diagnosis in child psychopathology have progressed rapidly over the past 20 years. There are now at least six structured interviews and dozens of questionnaires of known reliability to choose from. Since these have recently been reviewed in specialised books (Shaffer *et al*, 1999), textbooks (Rutter & Taylor, 2002) and journal articles (McClellan & Werry, 2000) we will not review them in detail here. Instead, we will outline the key questions that need to be considered when choosing an interview or questionnaire.

What exactly will be measured?

The first and most important issue is to define the research question precisely and then to decide exactly what needs to be measured in order to answer that question. It cannot be assumed, for example, that all structured psychiatric interviews (see below) assess all psychopathological constructs with equal accuracy. Researchers should select a measure because it best suits the demands of the study, not because it is what everyone else uses. Occasionally this will mean developing a new measure. However, it can take a long time to develop and test new measures and editors of journals are quite rightly sceptical about studies that are based on measures of unknown reliability and validity.

How should it be measured?

The next question is how best to measure the psychopathological construct or constructs under investigation. There are three types of measures: structured interviews, rating scales and observational assessments.

Interviews are most often used in child psychiatric research to make diagnoses. They are particularly helpful when it is necessary to probe the participant's responses to clarify their meaning (though not all interviews can do this – see below), as is often the case with relatively rare phenomena such as psychotic symptoms or obsessions. Interviews are also used when it necessary to establish temporal sequences, which is difficult to do by a self-report questionnaire.

It usually takes at least an hour to complete a structured interview and such interviews often require that the interviewer is trained. By contrast, behaviour rating scales are often quite quick and seldom require that the administrator has training. They can therefore provide an economic means for obtaining information on emotional and behavioural problems in large population surveys. Other applications include measuring change in treatment studies and screening for high-risk cases who require interview in epidemiological surveys.

At present observational assessments are seldom used to measure psychopathology in children and adolescents. Their main use is to measure family life and relationships. However, observational ratings are used to assess autism through a series of semi-structured opportunities or 'presses' for play or social interaction (Lord *et al*, 1989). They can also be employed to assess the outcomes of behavioural disorders in pre-adolescents (Patterson, 1982).

What is the developmental stage of the participant?

There are developmental changes in children's abilities both to experience and to report almost all types of psychopathology. Children are capable of recognizing their own emotional states from as young as two years (Kagan, 1989) and during the preschool years they start to differentiate the basic emotions and to understand their meaning (Kovacs, 1986). However, even if they experience repeated failure, preschool children are not easily discouraged and they only rarely show evidence of negative cognitions such as learned helplessness (Rholes *et al*, 1980). With the onset of concrete operational thinking (age range 7–11 years) the child begins to discover what is consistent in the course of any change or transformation (Piaget, 1970). Egocentrism declines. The child starts to develop self-consciousness and to evaluate his own competence by comparison with others (Dweck & Elliot, 1983). Self is perceived more in psychological than physical terms and concepts such as guilt and shame become prominent. Enduring and relatively stable negative attributions about the self therefore become possible. In addition, children begin to understand the implications of certain kinds of adverse events. It is at around this age, for example, that most children can understand that death is permanent (Lansdown, 1992). At the same time the child's emotional vocabulary expands, and children start to make fine-grain distinctions between emotions such as sadness and anger.

The type of interview or rating scale chosen will therefore depend crucially on the developmental stage of the participant. Although it is difficult to make generalisations, as a general rule most children under the age of 10 years find it hard to complete a structured diagnostic interview or questionnaire. Much the same applies to adolescents with an IQ of less than 50. In such cases it is usually necessary to obtain diagnostic information from a parent or teacher.

The quickest way to judge whether an instrument is suitable for the developmental stage of participants in research is to pilot it with a small sample. For questionnaires the investigator should try to establish not only whether the child can read the questions out loud but also whether he or she can understand the content. Problems with reading comprehension are very common in samples of children with psychiatric problems, particularly in children with conduct disorder (Rutter *et al*, 1970).

Similar principles apply to interviews. It should not be assumed, for instance, that all children can understand concepts such as 'concentration'. The investigator should ensure that the child understands the idea (e.g. the investigator should ask 'do you know what it means to concentrate?').

Several measures have been developed to assess psychopathology in children aged 4–9 years, including the use of cartoons (Valla *et al*, 1994) or puppets (Ablow *et al*, 1999). Early studies have produced promising results, but these methods are highly specialised and the results can be difficult to interpret.

Which kind of psychopathology?

Child psychopathology rating scales can be divided into those that assess most or all types of psychopathology and those that assess just one construct. Most of the diagnostic interviews assess a wide range of types of psychopathology. There are also many questionnaires that assess a broad range of psychopathology, although in general their symptomatic coverage is less extensive than the interviews.

There are now specific diagnostic interviews and ratings scales for most forms of psychopathology in young people, including conduct problems, hyperactivity, anxiety, phobias and depression. These will be briefly described in the sections that follow. At this stage the following points are worth noting. First, as described earlier, there is a great deal of overlap between different kinds of psychopathology, so if the goal is a comprehensive evaluation of the child's psychopathology, then choose a broad scale. Second, however, broad scales seldom have enough specific items on a construct to enable full differentiation and description of that construct. Third, many of the broad scales were originally designed for large epidemiological studies and therefore work best as screening or descriptive instruments. They are not generally very good as repeated measures of change in clinical trials.

Which sources of information?

One of the most consistent findings from research on most types of psychopathology among young people is that the level of agreement between different sources of information (e.g. parent, teacher, child, direct observations) seldom exceeds 0.4. Indeed, the source of information often accounts for as much or more variation in the level of psychopathology as substantive risk factors such as social class, family problems, etc. In deciding from whom information should be collected, the following issues should be borne in mind. First, low levels of agreement between informants are not simply a result of error or informant biases but also occur because the way children behave and how they feel changes according to the situation. For example, some forms of childhood anxiety such as social inhibition do not occur when the child is with the parent and can only be observed in the presence of a stranger (Kagan, 1989). Hyperactive and inattentive behaviours also vary across different settings, but when they are pervasive usually have a worse outcome. Second, parents and teachers are often unaware of 'internal' symptoms such as sadness and negative thinking. Therefore reports from older children and adolescents are essential. Third, when it is necessary to have multiple sources of information (e.g. parent and teacher reports on disruptive behaviour), a strategy for dealing with discrepancies should be devised. The best way of doing this is to analyse and present data from different sources separately. However, it is sometimes necessary to combine data from different sources (for example when the presence or absence of a diagnosis determines entry into a clinical trial). In such cases it is quite common to use some kind of 'best estimate' technique. For example, priority could be given to any positive account of psychopathology, on the grounds that it is more likely that discrepancies between sources arise because one informant does not know about a problem than that the other has manufactured it.

What resources are available?

In any study it is important to consider carefully the resources available to complete the measures. How much time is available to complete the measures? More is not always better. Many studies in child and adolescent psychiatry would be improved by having half the number of measures and twice the number of participants. Remember also that although most children and parents are happy to take part in research, they can find the completion of large numbers of questionnaires onerous.

Diagnostic interviews

Respondent- and investigator-based interviews

In respondent-based interviews carefully worded and ordered questions are read to the informant as they are written. There is little or no probing of the informant's responses, and the informant must decide on a reply without help from the interviewer (hence the term 'respondent-based'). Such interviews rely on the respondent having the same understanding of the concept being studied as the investigator. By contrast, in investigator-based interviews it is the interviewer who makes the final decision about whether or not a rating is made. To do this he or she is expected to probe the participant's responses to decide whether a particular phenomenon is present. The phenomenon would usually be defined in detail in a manual devised by the investigator (hence the term 'investigator-based').

These different types of interviews have different strengths and weaknesses. Respondent-based interviews are potentially cheaper to use than investigator-based interviews because the interviewers need not be clinicians. The rigidity and structure of respondent-based interviews also make them easier to computerise and mean that they can be used by non-mental health professionals for purposes such as screening. Their very rigidity also means, however, that the interviewee's responses cannot be probed to see if they understand the question. By contrast, in an investigator-based interview the question can be rephrased to help the interviewee to understand it. Investigator-based interviews also offer more opportunities to investigate symptoms outside the range of standard enquiry.

General diagnostic interviews

Table 12.2 shows the main characteristics of a selection of diagnostic interviews. All will give diagnoses using DSM–IV criteria (American Psychiatric Association, 1994) but it is wise to check whether they can also give ICD–10 (World Health Organization, 1996) diagnoses. The most widely used respondent-based interview in the USA is the Diagnostic Interview Schedule for Children (Shaffer *et al*, 2000). In the UK another highly structured interview has been developed: the Development and Well-Being Assessment (DAWBA; Goodman *et al*, 2000). This was used in the Office of National Statistics national survey of mental health in children and adolescents (Meltzer *et al*, 2000) and therefore extensive normative data are available. Another advantage of the DAWBA is that clinical vignettes based on the interview can be re-rated by a clinician, which is particularly helpful when making rare but difficult diagnoses such as obsessive–compulsive disorder or psychosis.

The investigator-based interviews all tend to cover the same types of psychopathology. The best known are the Child and Adolescent Psychiatric Assessment (CAPA; Angold *et al*, 1995) and the Kiddie Schedule for Affective Disorders and Schizophrenia (K–SADS; Puig-Antich & Chambers, 1978). The CAPA is one of a family of instruments that assess psychopathology, impairment, service use, family problems and traumatic events. The full version provides a very detailed coverage of psychopathology and impairment, but there is also a shorter version available. The CAPA is most often used in genetic and epidemiological studies, and was the main

Table 12.2 Selected diagnostic interviews for general assessment (see also Chapter 11)

Name	Reference	Main characteristics
NIMH Diagnostic Interview Schedule for children (NIMH DISC–IV)	Shaffer *et al* (2000)	Highly structured, respondent based; lay interviewer; computer scored; approximately 3000 questions; ages 9–17; youth and parent versions; 70–105 min for completion
Development and Well-Being Assessment (DAWBA)	Goodman *et al* (2000)	Structured, interview supplemented with open-ended questions; lay interviewer, but vignettes can be scored by a clinician; ages 5–16
Child and Adolescent Psychiatric Assessment (CAPA)	Angold *et al* (1995)	Structured, interviewer based; clinician; primarily rates previous 3 months
Diagnostic Interview for Children and Adolescents (DICA)	Herjanic & Reich (1982)	Highly structured, respondent based; 267–311 items; for ages 6–17; 60–90 min for completion; computer scored; lay interviewer or clinician; current episode assessed; not for schizophrenia or Axis II
Kiddie–Schedule for Affective Disorders and Schizophrenia (K–SADS)	Puig-Antich & Chambers (1978)	Semi-structured, interviewer based; over 200 items; for ages 6–17 years; 45–120 min for completion; clinician rated; rates schizophrenia; not for Axis II

instrument in a landmark epidemiological survey, the Smoky Mountain Study (Costello *et al*, 1996). The K–SADS is less structured than the CAPA. It is often employed in research studies of treatment but has also been used in epidemiology. The Diagnostic Interview for Children and Adolescents (DICA; Herjanic & Reich, 1982) was initially a respondent-based interview but is now investigator-based. It has a wide range of applications.

Specific diagnostic interviews

It should be borne in mind that most of these general diagnostic interviews do not cover some rare but important diagnoses such as autism. The Autism Diagnostic Interview–Revised (ADI–R) is an investigator-based interview for caregivers that will generate both DSM–IV and ICD–10 diagnoses of autism and related disorders (Lord *et al*, 1994). Administration of the interview requires prior training. The Autism Diagnostic Observation Schedule (ADOS) was developed as a companion to the ADI and contains a series of 'presses' (planned social occasions) for social interaction, communication and play. Specific diagnostic interviews may also be helpful when a disorder that is covered by one of the general assessments requires additional coverage (Table 12.3). Thus, for example, there are specific

Table 12.3 Selected diagnostic interviews for specific disorders

Name	Reference	Disorder	Main characteristics
Autism Diagnostic Interview–Revised (ADI–R)	Lord *et al* (1994)	Autistic disorder	Semi-structured, interviewer based; several hours for completion; experienced clinician
Autism Diagnostic Observation Schedule (ADOS)	Lord *et al* (1989)	Autistic disorder	Contains 'presses' for social interaction, communication and play
Children's Depression Rating Scale–Revised (CDRS–R)	Poznanski *et al* (1985)	Depression	Semi-structured, interviewer based; 17 items including 3 observed items; for ages 6–12; 30 min for completion; clinician rated
Anxiety Disorder Interview Schedule for Children (ADIS–C)	Silverman & Nelles(1988)	Anxiety disorders	Structured, interviewer based; questions scored on 3- to 9-point scale; assessment of primarily anxiety but also other disorders

interview-based rating scales for depression (Poznanski *et al*, 1985) and for anxiety (Silverman & Nelles, 1988) in young people. Such scales are often used to measure change during treatment trials.

Rating scales and questionnaires

These resemble the highly structured interviews in having predefined questions and limited response options. However, questionnaires usually obtain less-detailed information about symptoms. The format is less complex and one question is followed by the next without any contingencies. Because of their simplicity, symptom questionnaires are often self-administered.

Rating scales and questionnaires can assess a broad range of behavioural and emotional problems or can be directed towards more specific areas of pathology, such as disruptive behavioural disturbances, anxiety and mood disorders, and pervasive developmental disorders. Within these categories, further differentiation can be made by broad and narrow scales. Broader scales are preferable if comprehensive evaluation of the child's functioning is desired, whereas narrower scales are preferred if differentiation between sub-categories of behaviour/emotion is primarily required. The choice of a particular scale will depend on the research question and the time and resources available.

General rating scales for behaviour and emotion

Over the past decade, many scales have been developed that provide a simple, reliable and efficient method for surveying large populations. Some of these are best suited for use in two-stage studies to screen for those suitable for more detailed assessment with diagnostic interviews in the second stage (Rutter *et al*, 1970; Goodman, 1997). Others, such as the Child Behaviour Checklist (Achenbach & Edelbrock, 1983), are intended to be part of an empirically based diagnostic system.

Although most rating scales rely on adult informants, there has been a move towards viewing older children and adolescents as reliable informants on their own behaviour; therefore there has been an increase in the development of parallel rating scales for different informants. A representative sample of these scales with their salient features is shown in Table 12.4. As is the case for most rating scales, these measures are scored in terms of empirically derived scales rather than categorical syndromes. They ask the informant (parent, teacher or child) to rate the presence, frequency and/or severity of the behaviour problems. Most scales are able to distinguish between diagnostic groups, although, as mentioned above, rating scales generally do not provide sufficient information for determining diagnostic status. Some scales are particularly well suited for use in younger age-groups (e.g. the MacArthur Health and Behaviour Questionnaire; Ablow *et al*, 1999).

Table 12.4 Selected rating scales for general behaviour and emotional problems

Name	Reference	Main characteristics
Child Behaviour Checklist (CBCL)	Achenbach & Edelbrock (1983)	Parent versions for ages 2–3 and 4–18 years; teacher version for 5–18 years; self-report version for adolescents aged 11–18; 99–118 items; 10–15 min for completion; emotional and behavioural problems, social and academic competence
Revised Conners Rating scales (CPRS–R)	Conners *et al* (1998*a*,*b*)	Teacher and parent versions; ages 3–17 years, 38–57 items; 10–15 min for completion; behavioural and emotional problems, hyperactivity/impulsivity, social problems, psychosomatic problems
Rutter A and B Scales	Rutter *et al* (1970)	Parent (A) and teacher (B) versions; ages 7–16, 10–15 min for completion; behavioural and emotional problems
Strength and Difficulties Questionnaire (SDQ)	Goodman (1997)	Parent scale (teacher and child versions available); 25 items; ages 4–16; rates behaviour, emotions and relationships; useful as a screening instrument

245

Specific rating scales

There are also a large number of rating scales designed to assess specific behavioural or emotional problems in young people. These include questionnaires designed to assess hyperactivity (Conners, 1990), fears (Ollendick, 1983), anxiety (Reynolds & Richmond, 1978) and depression (Kovacs, 1981; Angold *et al*, 1995).

Types of developmental research

Developmental research can be divided into three overlapping areas (Wallace *et al*, 1997): normal and abnormal development, epidemiological studies and clinical and health delivery research.

Normal and abnormal development

Over the past 10 years one of the major developments in the study of individual differences in children's behaviour has come from sophisticated quantitative analysis of data from studies designed to assess the effects of genetic background and the environment (twin and adoptee studies). Early studies concentrated on quantifying the strength of genetic influences and showed that genetic effects play a part in many different types of psychopathology (Rutter *et al*, 1999). Quantitative genetic research has therefore now moved beyond the question of whether genetic factors are important to issues such as the mode of operation of genetic risk factors, the best way to define psychiatric phenotypes and the extent to which genetic factors can explain continuities and discontinuities over development.

The other major development in genetics has been the use of molecular genetic techniques to analyse the human genome. For neurodevelopmental disorders such as attention–deficit disorder and autism, in which genetic influences are likely to play a role, molecular genetic research could provide important leads about the biological mechanisms. Of course, this type of research will take a long time. Nevertheless, molecular genetic findings may eventually have important implications for prevention and intervention and may also be helpful in the development of new pharmacological treatments or in enhancing the effectiveness of existing treatments. For example, although we know that methylphenidate is an effective treatment for hyperkinetic syndrome, some children fail to respond (Spencer et al, 2000). Findings from molecular genetic analyses could help to predict those who are most likely to benefit (so-called pharmacogenetics).

Longitudinal research designs have been a key feature of studies in developmental psychopathology. They have shown that there are both continuities and discontinuities in the onset and persistence of psychiatric symptoms and disorder. They have also helped us to understand that the links between early problems and later psychiatric disorder may be indirect and may depend on other mediating variables. There are three main longitudinal designs. Prospective longitudinal studies collect detailed measures from the outset and then follow the sample prospectively, sometimes for long periods. Such designs are, however, very expensive and are rarely suitable for psychiatric trainees. 'Catch-up' longitudinal studies take as their starting point a group of participants for whom data have already been collected, usually for some other purpose. These data might comprise case records (Robins, 1966) or computerised data sheets (Harrington *et al*, 1990). The sample is then followed up later in life. Catch-up designs are usually much cheaper then prospective designs and have the considerable advantage that it is not necessary to wait for long periods before assessing the outcome of interest. Their main disadvantage is that the baseline data are often of unknown reliability and are usually less extensive than the investigators would wish. Follow-back designs start with a sample that has been ascertained at the point of outcome and then follow it back to a pre-existing data set. For example, Zeitlin (1986) studied adults who had attended the same psychiatric hospital both as children and as adults. One of the great advantages of this type of study is that the investigator need not collect any new data. A disadvantage is that studies with this design cannot study escape from risk.

There is a strong association between mental health problems in young people and parental difficulties of one kind or another. In part this is probably a reflection of genetic factors. However, it is likely that parental mental illness and parenting difficulties also have an environmental effect. Surprisingly little is known about these processes. For example, although the association between maternal depression and poor developmental and psychiatric outcomes in offspring has been documented on numerous occasions, the precise mechanisms remain largely unknown. Much more research is needed.

Epidemiological studies

The principles of epidemiological research are described in Chapter 5. Child psychiatric epidemiology started in the mid-1960s with the British Isle of Wight studies (Rutter, 1966; Rutter *et al*, 1970, 1976). In many ways these studies provided a model for future research. They employed a two-stage design in which a large sample was screened with questionnaires, which were followed by in-depth interview-based assessments of those who were positive by screening and a random sample of those who screened negative. Information was obtained from multiple sources, including the parents, teachers and the children themselves (which was unusual at the time).

Since the Isle of Wight studies there have been numerous cross-sectional and prevalence surveys around the world (Offord *et al*, 1989; Costello *et al*, 1996; Meltzer *et al*, 2000). It might be thought, therefore, that there is little scope for further work, but in fact there are many unresolved issues. The first concerns the definition of a case of psychiatric illness. One of the most striking findings from almost all epidemiological surveys conducted to date is how high the rates of psychopathology are in children and adolescents, with rates in most cross-sectional surveys of between 10% and 20%. In longitudinal surveys the proportion of 'cases' becomes even higher, so that by the end of adolescence more than half of the young people have been found to 'need' treatment at one point or another (Angold *et al*, 2000). Clearly these extremely high rates raise questions as to how exactly cases are being defined in these studies. In many studies 'caseness' has been defined by impairment in social role functioning. If emotional or behavioural symptoms are substantially affecting a child's life, then it does seem reasonable to classify the problem as a disorder. However, it remains unclear as to how far the impairments described in many epidemiological studies are a consequence or a cause of the child's symptoms. The concept of impairment requires much more investigation.

A related issue concerns the ways that need is defined in epidemiological studies. To date need for treatment has usually been defined as having a psychiatric illness and not being in contact with a service. However, such definitions of need take no account of whether the young person and family would agree to treatment, and even if they did, whether treatment would work (Harrington *et al*, 1999). New definitions of the need for treatment are required.

Another important issue concerns the methods used to collect data about mental health problems in children. Modern technology has made it possible for many diagnostic procedures to be computerised, and several questionnaires and diagnostic interviews now have computerised versions. Computerised interviewing has some advantages (see above) but much more information is needed on its merits and demerits.

Clinical and health delivery research

Over the past decade there has been substantial progress in the development and evaluation of new treatments. There is growing evidence that psychological treatments are effective for a wide range of psychiatric disorders in children and adolescents, including depression (Harrington *et al*, 1998*a,b*), anxiety (Kendall *et al*, 1997), oppositional behaviour in pre-adolescents (Scott *et al*, 2001*a,b*) and conduct disorder in adolescents (Henggeler *et al*, 1986). The evidence base for pharmacological treatments has also grown considerably. Relatively large randomised trials have found beneficial effects in several disorders, including attention-deficit disorder (MTA Cooperative Group, 1999), anxiety (Research Unit on Pediatric Psychopharmacology Anxiety Study Group, 2001), obsessive–compulsive disorder (March *et al*, 1998) and depression (Keller, 1999; Keller *et al*, 2001). Progress is also being made in the evaluation of the ways in which services should be delivered (Harrington *et al*, 1999; Henggeler *et al*, 1999), in the development of clinical outcome measures (Gowers *et al*, 1999) and in the assessment of cost-effectiveness (Byford *et al*, 1999; Scott *et al*, 2001*b*).

Nevertheless much more remains to be done. More work is needed across the range of treatments on effectiveness, with particular emphasis on longer term outcomes and the management of specific problems. There is also a need for studies that examine whether treatments work in clinical practice and whether they have an impact on important outcomes such as school attendance or delinquency. New larger trials will therefore be required (Harrington *et al*, 2002). These could include studies on the relative merits of different service delivery settings (primary care, special care, special clinics, school) as well as modes of service delivery (direct intervention *v.* parent training and responsiveness to the needs of different communities and ethnic groups). Studies are needed to improve the recognition of mental health problems such as depression in primary care.

We also need to know whether treatments work in specific groups of children and adolescents. These include 'hard-to-place adolescents', children in social services care, children who have been abused, and children and adolescents with challenging and/or persistent self-injurious behaviour.

Conclusions

Developmental research presents many challenges but also great prospects. There is a deepening appreciation of the importance of developmental factors in many psychiatric disorders. Recent advances in genetics, sociology and psychology have set the scene for major advances in our understanding of many psychiatric disorders in children and adolescents. At the same time there are many opportunities for research into treatment and the best ways of delivering services.

References

Ablow, J. C., Measelle, J. R., Kraemer, H. C., *et al* (1999) The MacArthur three city outcome study: evaluating multi-informant measures of young children's symptomatology. *Journal of the American Academy of Child and Adolescent Psychiatry*, **38**, 1580–1590.

Achenbach, T. M. & Edelbrock, C. S. (1983) *Manual for the Child Behaviour Checklist and Revised Profile*. Burlington, VT: University of Vermont, Department of Psychiatry.

American Psychiatric Association (1994) *Diagnostic and Statistical Manual of Mental Disorders* (4th edn) (DSM–IV). Washington, DC: American Psychiatric Association.

Angold, A., Costello, E. J., Messer, S. C., *et al* (1995) The development of a short questionnaire for use in epidemiological studies of depression in children and adolescents. *International Journal of Methods in Psychiatric Research*, **5**, 237–249.

Angold, A., Prendergast, M., Cox, A., *et al* (1995) The Child and Adolescent Psychiatric Assessment (CAPA). *Psychological Medicine*, **25**, 739–753.

Angold, A., Costello, E. J. & Erkanli, A. (1999) Comorbidity. *Journal of Child Psychology and Psychiatry*, **40**, 57–87.

Angold, A., Costello, E. J., Burns, B. J., *et al* (2000) Effectiveness of nonresidential specialty mental health services for children and adolescents in the "real world". *Journal of the American Academy of Child and Adolescent Psychiatry*, **39**, 154–160.

Byford, S., Harrington, R., Torgerson, D., *et al* (1999) Cost-effectiveness analysis of a home-based social work intervention for children and adolescents who have deliberately poisoned themselves. Results of a randomized controlled trial. *British Journal of Psychiatry*, **174**, 56–62.

Conners, C. K., Parker, J. D. A., Sitarenios, G., *et al* (1998a) The Revised Conners' Parent Rating Scale (CPRS–R): factor structure, reliability, and criterion validity. *Journal of Abnormal Child Psychology*, **26**, 257–268.

Conners, C. K., Sitarenios, G., Parker, J. D. A., *et al* (1998b) Revision and restandardization of the Conners Teaching Rating Scale (CTRS–R): factor structure, reliability, and criterion validity. *Journal of Abnormal Child Psychology*, **26**, 279–291.

Costello, E. J., Angold, A., Burns, B. J., *et al* (1996) The Great Smoky Mountains Study of Youth. Goals, design, methods, and the prevalence of DSM–III–R disorders. *Archives of General Psychiatry*, **53**, 1129–1136.

Dweck, C. & Elliot, E. (1983) Achievement motivation. In *Handbook of Child Psychology*, Vol. 4. *Social and Personality Development* (eds P. Mussen & M. Hetherington), pp. 643–691. New York: Wiley.

Goodman, R. (1997) The strengths and difficulties questionnaire: a research note. *Journal of Child Psychology and Psychiatry*, **38**, 581–586.

Goodman, R., Ford, T., Richards, H., *et al* (2000) The Development and Well-Being Assessment: description and initial validation of an integrated assessment of child and adolescent psychopathology. *Journal of Child Psychology and Psychiatry*, **41**, 645–655.

Gowers, S. G., Harrington, R. C., Whitton, A., *et al* (1999) Brief scale for measuring the outcomes of emotional and behavioural disorders in children. Health of the Nation Outcome Scales for Children and Adolescents (HoNOSCA). *British Journal of Psychiatry*, **174**, 413–416.

Harrington, R. C., Fudge, H., Rutter, M., *et al* (1990) Adult outcomes of childhood and adolescent depression: I. Psychiatric status. *Archives of General Psychiatry*, **47**, 465–473.

Harrington, R. C., Bredenkamp, D., Groothues, C., *et al* (1994) Adult outcomes of childhood and adolescent depression. III. Links with suicidal behaviours. *Journal of Child Psychology and Psychiatry*, **35**, 1380–1391.

Harrington, R., Whittaker, J. & Shoebridge, P. (1998a) Psychological treatment of depression in children and adolescents. A review of treatment research. *British Journal of Psychiatry*, **173**, 291–298.

Harrington, R. C., Kerfoot, M., Dyer, E., *et al* (1998b) Randomized trial of a home based family intervention for children who have deliberately poisoned themselves. *Journal of the American Academy of Child and Adolescent Psychiatry*, **37**, 512–518.

Harrington, R. C., Kerfoot, M. & Verduyn, C. (1999) Developing needs-led child and adult mental health services. Issues and prospects. *European Child and Adolescent Psychiatry*, **8**, 1–10.

Harrington, R., Cartwright-Hatton, S. & Stein, A. (2002) Annotation: randomised trials. *Journal of Child Psychology and Psychiatry*, **43**, 695–704.

Henggeler, S. W., Schoenwald, S. K., Borduin, C. M., *et al* (1986) Multisystemic treatment of juvenile offenders: Effects on adolescent behaviour and family interaction. *Developmental Psychology*, **22**, 132–141.

Henggeler, S. W., Rowland, M. D., Randall, J., *et al* (1999) Home-based multisystemic therapy as an alternative to the hospitalization of youths in psychiatric crisis: clinical outcomes. *Journal of the American Academy of Child and Adolescent Psychiatry*, **38**, 1331–1339.

Herjanic, B. & Reich, W. (1982) Development of a structured psychiatric interview for children. Part 1: Agreement between parent and child on individual symptoms. *Journal of Abnormal Child Psychology*, **10**, 307–324.

Kagan, J. (1989) *Unstable Ideas*. Cambridge, MA: Harvard University Press.

Keller, M. B. (1999) The long-term treatment of depression. *Journal of Clinical Psychiatry*, **60** (suppl. 17), 41–45.

Keller, M. B., Ryan, N. D., Strober, M., *et al* (2001) Efficacy of paroxetine in the treatment of adolescent major depression: a randomized, controlled trial. *Journal of the American Academy of Child and Adolescent Psychiatry*, **40**, 762–772.

Kendall, P. C., Flannery-Schroeder, E., Panichelli-Mindel, S. M., *et al* (1997) Therapy for youths with anxiety disorders: a second randomized clinical trial. *Journal of Consulting and Clinical Psychology*, **65**, 366–380.

Kovacs, M. (1981) Rating scales to assess depression in school aged children. *Acta Paedopsychiatrica*, **46**, 305–315.

Kovacs, M. (1986) A developmental perspective on methods and measures in the assessment of depressive disorders: the clinical interview. In *Depression in Young People: Developmental and Clinical Perspectives* (eds M. Rutter, C. E. Izard & R. B. Read), pp. 435–465. New York: Guilford Press.

Lansdown, R. (1992) The child's concept of death. In *Bereaved Children* (ed. C. Kaplan), pp. 2–6. London: Association of Child Psychology and Psychiatry.

Lord, C., Rutter, M. & Le Couteur, A. (1989) Autism Diagnostic Observation Schedule. A standardized observation of communicative and social behaviour. *Journal of Autism and Developmental Disorders*, **19**, 185–212.

Lord, C., Rutter, M. & Le Couteur, A. (1994) Autism Diagnostic Interview–Revised: a revised version of a diagnostic interview for caregivers of individuals with possible pervasive developmental disorders. *Journal of Autism and Developmental Disorders*, **24**, 659–685.

March, J. S., Biederman, J., Wolkow, R., *et al* (1998) Sertraline in children and adolescents with obsessive–compulsive disorder: a multicenter randomized controlled trial. *JAMA*, **280**, 1752–1756.

McClellan, J. M. & Werry, J. S. (2000) Research psychiatric diagnostic interviews for children and adolescents. *Journal of the American Academy of Child and Adolescent Psychiatry*, **39**, 19–27.

Meltzer, H., Gatward, R., Goodman, R., *et al* (2000) *Mental Health of Children and Adolescents in Great Britain*. London: TSO (The Stationery Office).

Moffitt, T. E., Caspi, A., Harrington, H., *et al* (2002) Males on the life-course persistent and adolescence-limited antisocial pathways: follow-up at age 26 years. *Development and Psychopathology*, **14**, 179–207.

MTA Cooperative Group (1999) A 14-month randomized clinical trial of treatment strategies for attention-deficit/hyperactivity disorder. *Archives of General Psychiatry*, **56**, 1073–1086.

Offord, D. R., Boyle, M. H. & Racine, Y. A. (1989) Ontario Child Health Study: correlates of disorder. *Journal of the American Academy of Child and Adolescent Psychiatry*, **28**, 856–864.

Ollendick, T. H. (1983) Reliability and validity of the revised fear survey schedule for children (FSSC–R). *Behaviour Research and Therapy*, **21**, 685–692.

Patterson, G. R. (1982) *Coercive Family Process*. Eugene, OR: Castalia.

Piaget, J. (1970) Piaget's theory. In *Carmichael's Manual of Child Psychology*, Vol. 1 (ed. P. H. Mussen), pp. 703–732. New York: Wiley.

Poznanski, E. O., Freman, L. N. & Mokros, H. B. (1985) Children's depression rating scale–revised. *Psychopharmacology Bulletin*, **21**, 979–989.

Puig-Antich, J. & Chambers, W. (1978) *The Schedule for Affective Disorders and Schizophrenia for School-Aged Children*. New York, NY: New York State Psychiatric Institute.

Quinton, D., Rutter, M. & Liddle, C. (1984) Institutional rearing, parenting difficulties and marital support. *Psychological Medicine*, **14**, 107–124.

Research Unit on Pediatric Psychopharmacology Anxiety Study Group (2001) Fluvoxamine for the treatment of anxiety disorders in children and adolescents. *New England Journal of Medicine*, **344**, 1279–1285.

Reynolds, C. R. & Richmond, B. O. (1978) What I think and feel: a revised version of the children's manifest anxiety. *Journal of Abnormal Child Psychology*, **6**, 271–280.

Rholes, W., Blackwell, J., Jordan, C., *et al* (1980) A developmental study of learned helplessness. *Developmental Psychology*, **16**, 616–624.

Robins, L. N. (1966) *Deviant Children Grown Up: A Sociological and Psychiatric Study of Sociopathic Personality*. Baltimore: Williams & Wilkins.

Rutter, M. (1966) *Children of Sick Parents: An Environmental and Psychiatric Study*. London: Oxford University Press.

Rutter, M. (1989) Age as an ambiguous variable in developmental research: some epidemiological considerations from developmental psychopathology. *International Journal of Behavioral Development*, **12**, 1–34.

Rutter, M. & Sroufe, L. A. (2000) Developmental psychopathology: concepts and challenges. *Development and Psychopathology*, **12**, 265–296.

Rutter, M. & Taylor, E. (eds) (2002) *Child and Adolescent Psychiatry: Modern Approaches* (4th edn). Oxford: Blackwell Scientific.

Rutter, M., Tizard, J. & Whitmore, K. (eds) (1970) *Education, Health and Behaviour*. London: Longmans.

Rutter, M., Graham, P., Chadwick, O. F., *et al* (1976) Adolescent turmoil: fact or fiction? *Journal of Child Psychology and Psychiatry*, **17**, 35–56.

Rutter, M., Silberg, J., O'Connor, T., *et al* (1999) Genetics and child psychiatry. II. Empirical research findings. *Journal of Child Psychology and Psychiatry*, **40**, 19–55.

Scott, S., Spender, Q., Doolan, M., *et al* (2001*a*) Multicentre controlled trial of parenting groups for childhood antisocial behaviour in clinical practice. *BMJ*, **323**, 194–197.

Scott, S., Knapp, M., Henderson, J., *et al* (2001*b*) Financial cost of social exclusion: follow up study of antisocial children into adulthood. *BMJ*, **323**, 191–197.

Shaffer, D., Lucas, C. P. & Richters, J. E. (eds) (1999) *Diagnostic Assessment in Child and Adolescent Psychopathology*. New York: Guilford Press.

Shaffer, D., Fisher, P., Lucas, C., *et al* (2000) NIMH Diagnostic Interview Schedule for Children version IV (NIMH DISC–IV). Description, differences from previous versions, and reliability of some common diagnoses. *Journal of the American Academy of Child and Adolescent Psychiatry*, **39**, 28–38.

Silberg, J., Pickles, A., Rutter, M., *et al* (1999) The influence of genetic factors and life stress on depression among adolescent girls. *Archives of General Psychiatry*, **56**, 225–232.

Silverman, W. K. & Nelles, W. B. (1988) The Anxiety Disorders Interview Schedule for Children. *Journal of the American Academy of Child and Adolescent Psychiatry*, **27**, 772–778.

Spencer, T., Biederman, J. & Wilens, T. (2000) Pharmacotherapy of attention deficit hyperactivity disorder. *Child and Adolescent Psychiatric Clinics of North America*, **9**, 77–97.

Valla, J., Bergeron, L., Berube, H., *et al* (1994) A structured pictorial questionnaire to assess DSM–III–R-based diagnoses in children (6–11 years): development, validity, and reliability. *Journal of Abnormal Child Psychology*, **22**, 403–423.

Wallace, S. A., Crown, J. M., Berger, M., *et al* (1997) Child and adolescent mental health. In *Health Care Needs Assessment. The Epidemiologically Based Needs Assessment Reviews* (eds A. Stevens & J. Raftery), pp. 55–127. Oxford: Radcliffe Medical Press.

World Health Organization (1992) *The ICD–10 Classification of Mental and Behavioural Disorders: Clinical Descriptions and Diagnostic Guidelines*. Geneva: WHO.

World Health Organization (1993) *The ICD–10 Classification of Mental and Behavioural Disorders: Diagnostic Criteria for Research*. Geneva: WHO.

World Health Organization (1996) *Multiaxial Classification of Child and Adolescent Psychiatric Disorders*. Cambridge: Cambridge University Press.

Zeitlin, H. (1986) *The Natural History of Psychiatric Disorder in Children*. Oxford: Oxford University Press.

CHAPTER 13

Research in the psychiatry of learning disability

Walter Muir and Susie Gibbs

The UK is unusual in having learning disability as a fully recognised psychiatric specialty. This is not generally the situation in other countries, where the psychiatric problems that people with learning disability experience are catered for by a variety of services or by generalists. Although this may be appropriate for people with very mild or borderline learning disability there are many special considerations for those with significant cognitive impairment that can influence and alter psychiatric practice. Research is vital if we are to understand and act on these, but compared with other disciplines it is perhaps fair to say that the psychiatry of learning disability has suffered markedly in the past from both an undervalued and under-resourced research base.

Learning disability encompasses a huge domain and the potential for useful research into its causes, its comorbidities and the amelioration of associated problems is vast. This potential, for a variety of historical reasons, has not yet been fully realised. Our hospitals were large and our specialty small, and there were often grossly simplistic administrative divisions into people who had 'challenging behaviours' and those with 'special needs' that tended to impart false homogeneities. Learning disability (or more commonly the former usage – mental handicap) was frequently regarded as a disorder in itself, and that the term alone was all that was needed to define a person. Hindsight always permits such 20/20 vision and in fact there were very many important studies by specialty psychiatrists over the decades. However, the closure of our institutions seems to have been accompanied by a rapidly increasing interest in learning disability, offering great research opportunities for the interested psychiatrist. The increased interest is also reflected by the large recent jump in the impact factor of the leading specialty British journal, the *Journal of Intellectual Disability Research*, from 0.8 in 1997 to 2.22 in 2002 (ISI Journal Citation Reports).

The sheer breadth of the field is exemplified by the coverage of the latest edition of *Seminars in the Psychiatry of Learning Disability* (Fraser & Kerr, 2003). Psychiatrists in the speciality are expected to be familiar with the presentations of cognitive impairment in people of all ages from infancy through to the very elderly. They should be conversant in the assessment and management of psychiatric, psychological and, very often, general medical associates (epilepsy included) of learning disability and also how these interact with each other – disability most often exists in multiple domains, physical and sensory as well as cognitive. Treatment modalities from pharmacotherapy through behavioural therapies to the various psychotherapies (including cognitive–behavioural therapy) all have their place, and a thorough understanding of communication strategies and impairments is needed to facilitate our interactions with the person. Learning disability is possibly the area of psychiatry that requires the greatest multidisciplinary approach – not only within the health professions but also across the wider field of social services and education. All these areas are covered in the *Seminars* volume, which should be considered as a companion to this chapter. Other comprehensive summaries of the psychiatry of learning disability are also available (Muir, 2004).

What then is useful for the trainee (or indeed trained) psychiatrist in learning disability to know? This chapter is divided into three sections. First is an overview of possible research areas. The range of the subject means that these can only give brief and necessarily selective descriptions of the possible areas for research in learning disability. The references throughout have been chosen not necessarily for their research primacy but more often for their useful summaries and pointers to the original literature. Second, a description is given of various psychometric and diagnostic tools that the researcher may find useful. Some might see in the opening pages a possible bias towards biological research, and especially in those conditions known to have genetic origins. A defence is that these are increasingly important areas not only because of the knowledge they generate about the causes of learning disability but also in their rapidly increasing percentage contribution, in developed countries at least, to the totality of conditions that have learning disability as a component. The quantitative methods used particularly in biological research in learning disability are, in many ways, intrinsically similar to those in general psychiatry and are found elsewhere in this volume. Qualitative methods are increasingly being recognised as valuable in research with people with learning disability across a number of specialties. Thus our final focus is on the special issues involved in applying these methods to learning disability research. This section is more expansive than the others but includes vital points in working with people with learning disability that are applicable to all research areas. It uses as an example work conducted by one of the authors (S.G.) while a trainee.

The concept of learning disability and its relation to psychiatry

In the UK the term learning disability implies that a person has a group of features – the childhood onset of a persistent and significantly lowered IQ compared with the general population (usually less than 70) with associated problems in social adaptation. Elsewhere (particularly in North America) the equivalent term is often 'mental retardation'. Although 2–3% of any population may be predicted to have an IQ in the learning disability range, practical prevalence figures for learning disability itself are less, owing to the additional diagnostic requirement for adaptive problems. Psychiatrists are involved with both children and adults with learning disability in the assessment, treatment and management of additional psychiatric or behavioural problems. Very often still there is no separation between child and adult psychiatric services, with the same psychiatrist involved with both – partly a consequence of our former hospitals for people with learning disability at one time providing support for individuals of all ages. The role of the psychiatrist has changed considerably from being a general physician of the broadest sort to a much more focused role. However, there are still considerable differences from the role of general adult psychiatrists – notably an involvement in assessing and treating behavioural disorders that are not a consequence of psychiatric illness, the direct management of epilepsy (which occurs in over 20% of our patients) and in providing and developing services for people with autistic-spectrum disorders. Although these additional responsibilities may change in the future, for many psychiatrists they are part of their current clinical remit and widen the research scope considerably.

Research areas

Categorisation of research into specific areas is often artificial in practice but does help understanding by systematising the coverage of the field. Four divisions can roughly be made (Table 13.1). Selected aspects of each area are discussed in greater detail below.

Biological research

Research into the origins of learning disability: a search for proximate causes

Learning disability is not a disorder; it is a descriptor of sustained cognitive and social adaptive outcomes arising in children and usually a result of underlying developmental disturbance of the central nervous system. Some of the cognitive features will be common to all people with a learning disability and often studies have simply grouped people on the basis of the intellectual impairment. On one level this can be readily justified since there are so many conditions that are associated with cognitive impairment that it would be impractical to subdivide them when examining very general issues that affect people with learning disability, especially in education and social research. After all we all share a common humanity and there is no merit in further increasing the social segregation of people with learning

Table 13.1 Research areas of interest to the psychiatrist in learning disability

Research area	Notes
Biological research	
Proximate cause	Both genetic and non-genetic causes and the definition and study of developmental and behavioural syndromes
Cognitive associates	Developmental psychology across the life span and research into how to maximise cognitive potential
Psychiatric associates	Abnormal psychology of learning disability – psychiatric disorders and behavioural outcomes
Medical associates	Common medical associates, including physical and sensory impairments, communication problems and medical disorders such as epilepsy
Epidemiological, societal and educational research	
Prevalence and incidence of associated conditions	Subsumes additional research into psychiatric and medical outcomes as well as learning disability in these conditions
Social and educational needs	Includes research into inclusion and integration
Societal views and the place of the person in society	Ethical principles governing the place and status of the person with learning disability in society, the changing moral and humanistic frameworks
Perceived needs and perceived role in society of people with learning disability themselves	
The law in relation to learning disability	Issues around consent, capability and capacity; how the legal framework, including criminal justice and mental health legislation, is devised and affects people with learning disability
Interventions	
Educational	Aimed at maximising the cognitive potential
Pharmacotherapy	Clinical trials of medications used in treating the psychiatric and medical associates of learning disability (e.g. drug treatments for psychoses; anti-epileptic therapies)
Behavioural theories	Research into methods of reducing unwanted or socially maladaptive behaviours and enhancing behavioural strengths
Psychotherapy	Cognitive–behavioural therapy as well as psychodynamic psychotherapies
Services	
Existing and future educational, health and social care services	Subsumes psychiatric services for people with learning disability and the role of the psychiatrist
Longitudinal health and social support	Transition issues such as starting school, adolescence, moving to adult services, and ageing
Cross-boundary research	Multidisciplinary approaches to the person's social and health needs

disability by creating unneeded sub-specialties. However, when it comes to our understanding of the origins, course and treatments for the innate problems experienced by people with learning disability, then knowledge of proximate causes is a necessary prerequisite. Causes of learning disability need not be single or simple – environmental factors interact with genetic and sociocultural inheritance in us all – but it is clear not only that learning disability is the outcome of a huge range of circumstances, but also that the specific cognitive profiles of deficits and strengths differ as well as the temporal developmental series for the disability.

Thus 'learning disability' is akin to 'mental illness'. We can quite validly examine the effects of using such social and administrative labels on people, especially when looking at their place in society, the stigmas associated with them and so on. For those working in medicine, an important example would be the ways that people with learning disability experience, and are treated within, general healthcare settings.

Such studies are not designed to address the intrinsic (biologically driven) difficulties of the person themselves. Yet even when the feature to be studied is largely biologically determined, inappropriate grouping still occurs and may be a reason for the lack of consistently reproducible results in treatment and intervention studies. 'Lumping together' has been especially true in studies of interventions. It is true that most current studies will distinguish between people with well-defined clinical syndromes (Down's syndrome for example), but the remaining non-syndromic group is tacitly but probably incorrectly assumed to be homogeneous. For example, most studies into treatments for self-injurious behaviour have not stratified their groups other than on degree of learning disability. Even here, however, there are merits in addressing subgroups where self-injury is especially common. For instance, small-scale studies have indicated significant differences not only in the presentation but also in the time course of the self-injury associated with the well known (if rare) Lesch–Nyhan syndrome compared with that seen in other conditions associated with learning disability such as autism (Hall *et al*, 2001).

Syndromes and learning disability

Although our knowledge is rapidly advancing, we still do not know the underlying or proximate cause of the learning disability in most cases. Such information is certainly not purely academic. Where the cause has been found, the most common is trisomy of chromosome 21, which leads to Down's syndrome, which still occurs in around 1 in 700 newborn babies. (Although in some countries the numbers of newborn babies with Down's syndrome are declining, in others, such as Switzerland, the rate is constant, an association with the increasing average age at which mothers have their first child (Mutter *et al*, 2002).) Identification of the trisomy has definite prognostic implications for both the child and adult, with an increasingly well-defined set of medical and cognitive associates. Thus we know that very common medical outcomes include congenital abnormalities of the cardiovascular and gastrointestinal systems, which are usually surgically remediable, that stature will be small, that sensory impairments and autoimmune disorders are frequent; the list is extensive, although no feature is invariably associated.

In addition to predicting on average a moderate degree of learning disability, we know that depression is more common in women with Down's syndrome and for all the risk of early dementia of the Alzheimer's type is greatly increased. Thus we can raise our threshold of awareness for the detection of depression and dementia; the former is treatable, careful forward planning can ameliorate the effects of the latter. Genetically the number of genes in trisomy is large (over 200) and this has limited attempts to link the outcomes to the genotype. However, advances in the mapping of the human genome mean that the task no longer seems impossible and partial duplications show that most of the key clinical features seem to be associated with a smaller subset of genes (Epstein, 2002). Eliciting the interplay between genetics and environment for the clinical associates of Down's syndrome that suggest premature ageing (the early onset dementia) and features that indicate failure of autoimmune surveillance (including the endocrinopathies and the increased incidence of haematological malignancy) will greatly increase our understanding of these in the general population. There is already a large body of work on the various manifestations of Down's syndrome, but there remain large gaps in our knowledge and a focus (like much of previous learning disability research) on childhood populations. The cognitive correlates of normal (and aberrant) ageing in Down's syndrome, especially through the late teenage and early adult years, are relatively understudied.

For some disorders the severity of the cognitive impairment can be reduced. The classic example is phenylketonuria, where dietary control of phenylalanine intake can greatly reduce the amount of cognitive damage, so that in most cases severe learning disability is now highly unusual (Cederbaum, 2002). The importance of knowledge of underlying causes is perhaps even more obvious in situations where environmental agents are at work. Fetal alcohol syndrome is a relatively recent example which was only recognised by a cluster of birth defects since 1973. It is estimated to have been present in between 0.5 and 2 per 1000 births in the US in the past two decades (May & Gossage, 2001). Hence many individuals will now be adults, providing an important opportunity to study both cross-sectional and longitudinal effects on cognition and behaviour. The case of fetal alcohol syndrome also points to another emergent phenomenon – many specific conditions that underlie mild learning disability can be defined. The older maxim that most cases were a result of multifactorial and polygenic inheritance from parents (who themselves were more likely to have a mild learning disability) has been shown to be more restricted than previously thought.

Genetic syndromes

The classical genetic condition associated with learning disability is, of course, trisomy 21, which results in Down's syndrome. This is still common in newborn babies and illustrates the usefulness of defining a given aetiology for the learning disability in order to generate prognostic (and ultimately therapeutic) considerations. There has probably been as much research into the medical and psychiatric associates of Down's syndrome as all the other aetiologies for learning disability put together, and yet there is still a huge amount to be done. Over 1100 different syndromes with an inherited basis and with learning disability as a component are listed in the Online Mendelian Inheritance in Man (httpp://www.ncbi.nlm.nih.gov/omim/) This is likely to be a significant underestimate and it is of interest that some of the most recent discoveries have been of conditions that are not extremely rare.

There are a very large number of other genetic syndromes associated with learning disability. The sex chromosome aneuploidies, Klinefelter's syndrome (XXY) and the triple X syndrome between them occur in around 1 in 500 births and are associated with a decrease in average IQ and thus an increase in the numbers of people who will also have mild learning disability. In spite of their frequency, their effects have been relatively understudied.

X-linked conditions

Those who work with people with learning disability are usually struck by the preponderance of men. Most of this is the result of the inheritance of X-linked conditions, a vast number of which remain to be discovered and defined. The main division is into those that are associated with other physical changes – syndromic X-linked mental retardation disorders (MRXS); and those where the learning disability is the only clinically apparent feature – non-syndromic X-linked mental retardation disorders (MRX). 'Non-syndromic' is perhaps a rather unfortunate choice and readily misinterpreted as suggesting that the basis of learning disability does not lie in a physical process. The MRX disorders are heritable and the number defined both on the basis of genetic linkage analysis and through direct evidence for genetic mutations is now large (Chelly & Mandel, 2001).

The classical X-linked syndromic condition is the fragile X syndrome. This is a relatively common condition (1 in 4000 men; 1 in 8000 women) which has inconsistent physical features but mild-to-moderate cognitive impairment in men. Although children with learning disability are now screened routinely for this condition, it still remains undiagnosed in a large percentage of adults. Again the natural history of the condition is open for exploration, especially of cognitive and behavioural outcomes. There has been a surge of recent research into the neurobiology of the condition in model systems (Oostra & Willemsen, 2003). When this is paralleled by careful clinical studies across the life span, then the two requisites (detailed clinical and biological understanding) are in place that allow us to devise rational therapeutic interventions. This dual approach is needed for all the conditions that are associated with learning disability if we are to move away from a situation of therapeutic nihilism.

The variation in the clinical outcome can be studied over time in any one individual but there is also variation within a family in genetic conditions that are inherited. Staying with fragile X syndrome, it has been recently shown that boys with premutations (that is a sub-threshold expansion of the dynamic repeat) show subtle cognitive changes (Aziz *et al*, 2003). Women with the premutation also show a specific cognitive profile, with impairments in executive function which are now beginning to be related to regional brain activity by functional imaging (Tamm *et al*, 2002). Thus from learning disability we cross the border into non-global cognitive dysfunctions. In fact one key boundary condition that separates learning disability from normality is a statistical one based on the population distribution of a given set of psychological measures that comprise the IQ score. It is valid in defining a group of people that are significantly different from normal on these measures; it has utility at both conceptual and service definition levels, but an IQ score of 70 or less does not define a dichotomy. Learning disability shades into the contentious area of borderline learning disability and specific cognitive impairments that are found in people without learning disability. The cross-over zones have been very understudied, especially in relation to the prevalence of psychiatric morbidity in the borderline group. There is no reason to suppose that they may not also have syndromic and genetic associates, and certainly they would inform our understanding of cognitive processes in general.

Patterns of cognitive–behavioural disability within syndromes

Even where there is significant learning disability the profile of abilities is not uniformly depressed. These cognitive–behavioural profiles suggest areas of relative strengths as well as weaknesses, and an understanding of their nature can be used to maximise the potential of an individual. Williams syndrome is a case in point. This condition usually arises on the basis of a microdeletion of chromosomal material on the long arm of chromosome 7 that contains up to 16 genes. There is a characteristic facial pattern and often infantile hypercalcaemia and heart valve anomalies. Williams syndrome is not common (1 in 20 000 to 1 in 50 000 live births) but is of great interest because of the pattern of cognitive changes. IQ is highly variable (20–106) and three-quarters of people have IQ in the learning disability range (mean IQ is 58). The key cognitive features are a relative weakness in visuospatial constructive ability, with greater abilities in auditory rote memory and language (Mervis & Klein-Tasman, 2000). Children with Williams syndrome tend to focus on parts of objects rather than the whole, although visual perception seems completely normal. Thus there seems to be a pattern of deficits tending to the opposite of that seen in Down's syndrome, suggesting that the cognitive systems involved or invoked to compensate for disruption are different; without such detailed study such findings are hidden behind the average moderate degree of learning disability in both conditions. For most syndromes, however, we do not have such detailed knowledge either in cross-section or for temporal changes in the profiles, and this is an area of research that is likely to become increasingly important.

Changes over the life span

Behavioural changes in a syndrome over time are well illustrated by Rett's syndrome. This is again due to mutations in a gene (*MECP2*) on the X chromosome, and is almost exclusively expressed in females (males with the mutation have no compensatory X chromosome; they are usually very severely affected if they survive at all). After a period of apparently normal development there is a halt in development at around 6–28 months of life, followed by a rapid deterioration in motor and speech performance. There are subsequent age-related changes with a secondary plateau that lasts for many years followed by motor system deterioration in later life (Hagberg, 2002). Such a temporal progression of features, although very dramatic in Rett's syndrome, can be seen in many disorders, and is an area for further investigation with a lifespan approach to phenomenology and symptomatology. There does not need to be an assumption that the disorder itself is causing progressive change (though of course this could be the case). Some of the changes seen may reflect the body's attempt at a normal sequence of brain maturation in the face of a major mutational mechanism.

Behavioural phenotypes

This is usually now interpreted as meaning a consistent (across persons) cluster of behavioural symptoms that arise in association with learning disability and which is thought to be due to a common underlying biological (often genetic) causation. Classical examples that have been proposed include the association between severe self-mutilation seen in the Lesch–Nyhan syndrome through to the dementia that affects so many people with Down's syndrome at a relatively early age. However, it is the classifying and predictive value that is perhaps the most important – that is, when the symptom cluster is shown to predict the existence of an underlying consistent biological disorder. For example, the overeating behaviour (due to a lack of satiety mechanisms) that is the main presenting feature of the Prader–Willi syndrome is now known consistently to be due to inactivation of a set of genes on the long arm of chromosome 15. The definition of the behavioural pattern as well as the mild learning disability and minor dysmorphic features came first; the understanding of the genetic underpinnings came later (Dimitropoulos *et al*, 2000; Nicholls & Knepper, 2001). Other aspects of behaviour and cognition can be added. It has been known for some time that affective disorder is common among adults with Prader–Willi syndrome, but recently the psychotic form of affective disorder has been shown to be possibly associated with a specific chromosome 15 genetic subtype (uniparental disomy; Boer *et al*, 2002). This requires replication but illustrates the power of defining groups of clinically consistent behavioural symptoms in association with learning disability as a means of identifying valid clinical syndromes that can be studied at a deeper biological level. Williams syndrome is another good example – there is a characteristic social behavioural pattern (overfriendly in approaching others, socially anxious, highly excitable and distractible) in association with a mild or borderline learning disability and subtle dysmorphic features (Mervis & Klein-Tasman, 2000). This syndrome has now been shown to be due to microdeletions on Chromosome 7 (Tassabehji, 2003) and the social features in particular have attracted psychological interpretations based on 'theory of mind' explanations. There is obviously considerable power in the behavioural phenotype concept that can usefully be further explored (O'Brien, 2002).

The cognitive and behavioural associates of learning disability

This is a huge area, in which a great deal of work has been done but also remains to be done. An alternative name for the discipline of psychiatry was (is) abnormal psychology, and no more so is this appropriate than in the cognitive and behavioural consequences associated with a learning disability. Psychiatrists in learning disability not only have the role of diagnosing and treating psychiatric disorders in people with learning disability but also are in a special position to work with our clinical psychology colleagues in the management of the various cognitive and behavioural changes that may cause problems for the person and others. Understanding how such changes arise is a necessary prerequisite of designing rational interventions that limit their consequences. Cognition has many domains. Speech and language development are often impaired in people with learning disability and yet an ability to communicate (and hopefully to understand) is the essence of psychiatry. There is much to be learned from the study of language development and also language usage. There are distinctively different developmental patterns in Williams syndrome as opposed to Down's syndrome for instance; in the early years the vocabulary use is similar in extent for both conditions, but later children with Williams syndrome markedly outpace those with Down's syndrome, eventually often developing an apparently vocabulary-rich speech (Tassabehji, 2003). The 'cluttered' speech patterns associated with full fragile X syndrome are different again, and there are indications that a milder but similar clinical profile exists in boys that carry the premutation; this may provide direct insights into how knowledge of aberrant cognitive events in people with learning disability can help us understand similar outcomes in those without learning disability (Aziz *et al*, 2003). In people who have limited, or absent speech, oral language equivalents may come into play – signing systems and body language. Where does this fit with psychiatry? Very often it is with the misinterpretation of such altered communication strategies as behavioural disturbances. Much more work is required to explore the relationship between communication and behaviours in learning disability. A particularly distressing but useful example is the interpretation and management of self-injury. Except in people with very mild learning disability this is not usually a product of the same dynamic factors as in the general population. A relatively recent review of published work in this area from 1964 to 2000 revealed almost 400 research articles (Kahng *et al*, 2002). Most of the participants were male and had severe or profound learning disability. The tendency is towards reward-based interventions based on behavioural psychology and learning theory, although there are some punishment-based approaches that still persist. In spite of the volume of research, the problem represents a continuing major challenge and both behavioural and pharmacological investigations have a place in the future.

Psychiatric and medical associates of learning disability

Psychiatric disorders

The concept of behavioural phenotypes overlaps with comorbidities when psychiatric disorders are considered. There are many – the dementia associated with Down's syndrome has been mentioned above. Compared with people without Down's syndrome (including those with learning disability) it is common and of early onset. In fact it may be the most common single associate of presenile dementia. Since Down's syndrome is usually easily distinguished and is a relatively frequent cause of learning disability, there probably have been as many studies of the associated dementia as of all the other comorbidities combined. However, there is still a tremendous amount that can be done. The diagnosis is still difficult in many cases, especially when the degree of learning disability is severe, or where there are confounding alternative diagnoses (depression, bereavement reactions, endocrine disturbances, etc.). There has been considerable difficulty in identifying dementia in its earliest stages, but very early decline in memory can now be detected and followed to see if it is a true predictor of clinical dementia (Krinsky-McHale *et al*, 2002). We are at the beginning of treatment studies – there is no reason *per se* why a person with Down's syndrome should not be given the possible benefits of anticholinesterase drugs, and such studies need to be properly conducted with detailed longitudinal psychometric testing and clinical monitoring if we are to learn from them. The health and social implications of early-onset dementia are important. There is a need to study the current models of care delivery and how these can be improved. The rate of decline in the illness can be dramatic and its specific association with myoclonic epilepsy remains unexplained and a predictor of a more sinister course.

Schizophrenia

Another psychiatric disorder that is overrepresented in those with learning disability is schizophrenia. Although psychosis associated with learning disability has been long known (Kraepelin's 'propfschizophrenie'), it is only relatively recently that interest has been renewed. This was in part because of the idea that people with learning disability lacked the cognitive structures that were considered essential to psychosis – schizophrenia in particular was thought to require such complex psychological schemata for its development that it could not exist in those with a learning disability. It is now known, however, that the rate of schizophrenia in people with learning disability is threefold that seen in the general population (Doody *et al*, 1998) and there seems no reason to assume that people with more severe learning disability are not also susceptible. There is still much to be done in delineating the clinical features and associates of this condition. The greatly increased prevalence of both schizophrenia and dual diagnosis in families of affected individuals can be interpreted as implying a genetic basis. Some of this may be due to known associates of dual diagnosis such as the velocardiofacial syndrome (Murphy & Owen, 2001), but the condition is likely to be heterogeneous and other causative factors must exist.

Affective disorders

Women with Down's syndrome are at increased risk of major depression, especially in their fourth and fifth decades (Cooper & Collacott, 1994). The cause of this is not known, but the concept of depressive equivalents for people with learning disability (although controversial), where symptoms and signs other than those seen in the general population signify a depressive illness, is worth exploring further. Underdiagnosis is a major risk for people with learning disability, with psychiatric disorder often being misinterpreted as a behavioural disturbance. The related concept of 'diagnostic overshadowing' refers to the adoption of one diagnosis as being prevalent to the exclusion of other valid diagnoses in the person (Jopp & Keys, 2001). It is less common today (but not absent), especially in the community setting, to assume that all the person's problems arise out of the learning disability *per se*.

Physical comorbidities

An understanding of non-psychiatric medical conditions is especially important to the psychiatrist in learning disability. They can often influence and mimic the presence of psychiatric illness, in addition to causing considerable distress and difficulties for the person themselves. Endocrine disorders are common in association with Down's syndrome, but can mimic both depressive illness and dementia. Congenital heart disease is also very common, but outcomes in adults have been underinvestigated and there are early reports that secondary vascular lesions (including arterio-venous stenosis) may increase the risk of cerebrovascular cognitive changes. The prevalence and study of such complications in adults with Down's syndrome and how they affect cognitive performance is obviously an important area for future work. Other syndromes also have longitudinal medical outcomes – the premature ovarian failure that is common in women who are carriers of fragile X diathesis is an example (Allingham-Hawkins *et al*, 1999). The premutation also seems to confer a specific set of cognitive anomalies. However, perhaps the most common and well-described medical associate of a very wide range of people with learning disability is epilepsy, the frequency of which increases with the severity of the cognitive impairment (as do speech disorders and cerebral palsy (Arvio & Sillanpaa, 2003)). The psychiatric and behavioural presentations of epilepsy are especially important sources of misdiagnosis in people with learning disability, in whom complex multiform epilepsies are relatively frequent (e.g. complex partial, simple partial and grand mal epilepsy can occur in the same person). The newer anti-epileptic medications can have psychiatric effects (in addition to their mood-stabilising properties) and an important area for the future would be to systematically study the desired and unwanted effects of mono- and polypharmacy with the newer agents in the control of complex epilepsy in our patients. Among psychiatrists, those specialising in learning disability are almost unique in that they are often still required to be the main therapists dealing with the person's epilepsy. This offers the opportunity to study the interaction of neurology and psychiatry directly.

Other important conditions

Although the diagnosed prevalence has recently increased markedly in people without learning disability, this does not alter the fact that autism remains a major associate of intellectual impairment (Fombonne, 1999). There has been much research into the psychological correlates of autism in children, but less in adults. However, the stability of the condition cannot be assumed and longitudinal data are needed. The behavioural correlates of autism in people with learning disability are many and include the well-known difficulties with imaginative cognitions and abstractions, communication and social difficulties, repetitive stereotypic behaviours and apparent behavioural rigidity. There has been very little work on defining how psychiatric illness affects people with autism and learning disability in spite of there being no evidence that they are protected against it. As with learning disability, autism is probably the name we give to the cognitive and behavioural outcome of a variety of underlying conditions. A currently interesting area for research is the delineation of syndromic conditions that seem to be associated with autism to a greater degree than expected by chance. The link between autism and fragile X syndrome is still controversial, but there may be a specific subgroup of children with fragile X syndrome that develop typical autism (Rogers *et al*, 2001).

Epidemiological, societal and educational research

At first glance these areas may seem remote from the activities of the psychiatrist. However, with the increasing drive towards closer integration of health, social and educational services, the boundaries have become much less distinct and interdisciplinary research involving the psychiatrist in learning disability is increasingly important. Two simple examples might make this clear. The impact is likely to be especially important in studies that define the best possible services for people with learning disability. The prevalence of certain psychiatric disorders (conduct disorder, anxiety disorder, hyperkinesis and the various pervasive developmental disorders) among children with learning disability seems extremely high compared with children without learning disability (Emerson, 2003). The reasons for this are not at all clear, but these psychiatric disorders certainly influence the inclusion of a child in mainstream schooling, an educational objective for many of their parents and increasingly also a service aim. Without studies that jointly involve educational services it is unlikely that we will make further progress in understanding or tackling these problems, or even in consistently recognising their presence. Minimisation of their impact on educational achievement will not be attained through psychiatric intervention alone. At the other end of the age range a whole new area is emerging as the life span for people with learning disability steadily increases, for it is not only with Down's syndrome that differential ageing can be seen. Older people with learning disability without Down's syndrome are also at increased risk of both psychiatric illness (including dementia) and physical morbidity (including a lifelong associate such as epilepsy and the occurrence of *de novo* problems). There is still much to do to estimate whether there are specifically increased risks above those seen in a general ageing population, but it is clear that multiple and interacting pathologies are common and can be difficult to treat.

For development and planning of effective support systems to meet such needs a similarly complex integrated network of social and health research is needed. Epidemiological considerations imply a continuing trend for the numbers of older people with learning disability to increase, and also an increase in the numbers within this cohort who have severe and profound learning disability. The previously apparent 'healthy survivor' effect may be time limited and it is to be expected that many more of the older population with learning disability will have identifiable organic bases to their condition. Syndromic ageing can throw up surprising findings. There has been relatively little research into older people with fragile X syndrome, but a study of certain male premutation carriers has shown there to be a sub-syndrome of parkinsonism and generalised brain atrophy (Hagerman *et al*, 2001) that is associated with specific neuroimaging findings (Jacquemont *et al*, 2003). This may be due to elevated mRNA but normal protein levels of the fragile X protein, and perhaps a different phenotype is to be expected in full mutation carriers. Further study of the two groups will yield much information on the long-term effects of altered brain function in fragile X syndrome and might give insight into the pathogenesis of certain neurological movement disorders and dementia. Thus again we see the cross-over effects into aspects of cognition and ageing in the general population of studying conditions associated with learning disability.

The place of people with learning disability in society

How we perceive this affects the way we treat people with learning disability within our society, and also directly and indirectly how we create a specific legal framework that addresses their needs and problems. In the past there has been an unnecessary marginalisation of the person with learning disability – not least into our former huge institutions. Although most people with learning disability did not live in these hospitals, the past decade has seen a shift to general living for many thousands of people with the most severe cognitive deficits and/or coexisting behavioural psychiatric and psychiatric disorders. It is probably fair to say that there has been an inordinate focus on the resettlement process itself without a corresponding large-scale effort to study the effects of this on the person with learning disability and society. The tacit assumption that it must be an improvement is largely based on empirical and observational evidence and has not been tested as it should, so follow-on work can be done to build on the de-institutionalisation process. The concept of 'community' is one that is not fulfilled for many with learning disability. There are continuing barriers to integration and to the related concept of community acceptance. Some of these seem to exist on a simple level – but are extremely important to people with learning disability. Logistical problems are still in evidence – travel (especially alone) and community access to facilities come high on the list. Community acceptance of the person with learning disability has also not been fully explored. Problems with this can manifest in many ways, from direct measures such as antipathy or rejection of community placements or through more passive resistance often related to poverty of social access or communication. Employment opportunities are still very limited for many people with learning disability, which can further increase social isolation while they are apparently living within the community. Many people with learning disability continue to have multiple health needs wherever they live. Primary healthcare also presents new challenges for many with learning disability. As the general practitioner is increasingly the primary carer, studies on how to improve communication with people with learning disability and how to increase the primary care professional's recognition of the various presentations of physical and mental disorders in this group are essential. The role of specialist learning disability screening services in primary care settings has recently been evaluated (Marshall *et al*, 2003), but there is a need for more work in this area and in secondary services.

Research: ethical issues, capability, consent and legislation for people with learning disability

This is a difficult and often controversial area. As in general psychiatry, concepts of learning disability during the first half of the past century centred in large part on eugenic research theories which culminated in widespread sterilisation policies and ultimately the genocidal activities during the 1940s. There has been an understandable concern that research should not take such directions again, but recent rapid advances, especially in genetic technologies, have again emerged as a source of worry (Muir, 2003). However, it is important that the psychiatrist in learning disability should advocate continued research into the problems experienced by individuals with learning disability – their sources and solutions cannot be simply extrapolated from the general population.

Legislation specific to people with learning disability differs not only around the world but also within a given country. Thus legislation in England and Wales differs from that in Scotland. From the researcher's point of view the relevant area is that of obtaining valid consent and estimating whether the person has the capacity to understand information in sufficient detail to give valid consent. In Scotland, the Incapable Adults (Scotland) Act 2000 deals with the issues regarding consent to research similarly to issues concerning consent to treatment, and it has helpfully clarified many formerly unclear issues that are still relegated to case law in England and Wales. It is designed to protect the individual's rights but also to prevent the disenfranchisement of many individuals with learning disability from participating in research by recognising that capacity is not an all or nothing concept. Furthermore, the inclusion of those who are not fully capable of giving informed consent is not totally debarred, and if the study is of great importance and is likely to benefit the individual (or group in the longer term) and cannot be done on any other group of individuals, then there is provision in the Act for the next of kin or an appointed welfare attorney to give proxy consent after approval by the appropriate research ethics committee. (In Scotland the Multicentre Research Ethics Committee (MREC) as a body examines all (health) research proposals concerning individuals with learning disability.) At present there are no such directives in English law and the direction these will take is unclear. Some European lawyers have emphasised that they see full personal informed consent as crucial and that proxy consent should not be permitted. This would mean that large numbers of people with severe learning disability and their underlying disorders could not be investigated, and it remains to be seen whether conflict will emerge between European and local legislatures.

The practicalities of helping the person to understand the study and give or refuse consent should be carefully considered. The involvement of people with learning disability themselves in the process of research (rather than just as participants) is often helpful, but there is a need to avoid tokenism. The authors have experience of the benefits of independent advisory groups of people with learning disability who have formed part of studies sponsored by the Joseph Rowntree Foundation (Stalker *et al*, 1999). Such groups may be brought together by relevant independent voluntary agencies (in the particular example this was Downs Syndrome Scotland). There is often an inordinate focus on written material, which may not be the best means for delivering information to this group. Audiotapes and/or pictorial information sheets and pictorial consent forms have been found useful, and the assistance of a speech and language therapist in their design is often helpful. In one study involving magnetic resonance imaging a videotape of the process, made with help from people with learning disability themselves, was found invaluable in allaying anxiety and helping individuals to make informed choices about participation (Sanderson *et al*, 1999). The person may use hand-signing (Makaton, Signalong, etc.) to assist communication and this should be respected using a translator if needed. The time taken for the person to understand the study should not be underestimated. The person may need to go over the study with carers or family as well as have several discussions with the investigators. However, with such help the authors have found that most people with at least mild learning disability are able to understand most research studies and give their consent to them in a valid way. People with learning disability have as much right to and concern about confidentiality as anyone else – they need to be reassured on this issue and also that if publication is envisaged then the information will not be presented in a way that can reveal their identity. Where the person does not object, it can also be useful to have their consent witnessed by an independent party, especially if they cannot fully write their own name.

Research into interventions used with people with learning disability

Although psychotropic medications of many forms are very widely prescribed to people with learning disability, there have been very few adequately controlled trials of their use in this group. The reasons for this can be surmised but are not fully clear. In addition to the treatment of specific co-existing psychiatric disorders, phenothiazines in particular have been widely used for the control of behavioural disorders and also in the treatment of disturbances of a psychotic nature in people with severe learning disability when the usual diagnostic systems cannot be easily applied. The different use of drugs compared with general psychiatry is not limited to the major tranquillizers. At present lithium is licensed in the UK for the treatment of aggression, and it is still occasionally used to reduce the rate of aggressive outbursts in people with severe learning disability. In many cases it is presumed (but often never fully clarified) that when lithium has an effect that the person has an underlying bipolar or recurrent unipolar affective disorder as the basis for the disturbances. It is doubtful whether such wide prescribing is useful, but there have been a dearth of adequate treatment studies in people with learning disability that are well-controlled and very few that are double-blind and cross-over in design. A Cochrane review found only one tiny (four participants with results on only two!) randomised controlled trial of antipsychotic medication in people with learning disability and schizophrenia (Duggan & Brylewski, 2001). There have also been concerns about the numbers of participants studied. The power of the study necessary to generate significant results seems not to have been an important criterion in conducting most research in this area – small case series abound. Significant problems arise when comparing one study with another, which would allow meta-analyses to be performed to overcome some of the problems arising from numerical inadequacy. The Diagnostic Criteria for Learning Disability (DC–LD; Royal College of Psychiatrists, 2001) have been produced to try and achieve some consistency in diagnostic ratings in learning disability research.

Another important factor that has limited research (and will continue to do so if not addressed) is the problem of obtaining valid consent from the participants. Well-designed clinical trials are also expensive to carry out properly and usually need to be multicentre in design – often funding for such studies can only be provided by a large donor, the Medical Research Council for example, or more commonly the pharmaceutical industry. The consent and especially indemnity issues are not inconsiderable and may be one reason for shying away from this area of research. However, it is vitally important that we make efforts in this direction rather than continuing to rely on extrapolations of treatment response from the general population to those with learning disability.

One interesting recent study that has tried to circumvent some of the methodological shortcomings looked at the use of risperidone in reducing difficult behaviours (not psychiatric disorders but temper tantrums, aggression and self-injury – all of which are common in people with severe learning disability) in children from 5 to 17 years with autism (McCracken *et al*, 2002). The study bears examination for its methodology in addition to its findings because it is a multisite placebo-controlled double-blind study – all features that are standard for clinical trials in most medical conditions but are unfortunately rare for conditions associated with learning disability. The limitation compared with standard clinical trials was in the relatively small numbers (101 children) studied, but even this number is large compared with most learning disability research. The instruments used to measure change would be familiar to most working in the learning disability field – the Aberrant Behaviour Checklist (Aman & Singh, 1985) and the Clinical Global Impressions Scale (Guy, 1976). Although there were concerns about the long-term effects of atypical neuroleptic prescribing in children, the findings with regards to reducing the behavioural disturbances were robust and positive. Although there have been other sizeable trials employing good trial design to investigate medication response in people with learning disability, these have been largely restricted to the control of epilepsy (e.g. Crawford *et al*, 2001). In addition to treatment studies of psychiatric, behavioural and physical disorders, another emerging area for research is the use of anticholinesterase in the maintenance of cognitive function in dementia. It is well known that Down's syndrome confers a consistent and high risk for presenile dementia in the population with learning disability and there are several treatment studies underway at present to investigate the response.

Research into health services for people with learning disability

This is an important research area at this time of change for people with learning disability. There are various topics – the conflict over generic versus specialist services at all ages; the transitions of life; the move from children's to adult services which involves the change from the paediatrician-centred model to the multidisciplinary model coordinated by the general practitioner; and the increasingly specific role of the psychiatrist in learning disability. There is an increasing need for an integrated lifespan approach to the development of health services to overcome the trauma engendered by such transitions (Cuskelly *et al*, 2002). Traditionally the learning disability psychiatrist has played the role of the learning disability hospital generalist – looking after all the health (and often social) needs of the individual with learning disability. Now there is a focus on the management of psychiatric disorders within the setting of the multidisciplinary team.

There is a need for research into the effects on psychiatrists of this change as well as the effects on the person with learning disability and also other health professionals. The number of in-patient beds for learning disability has fallen precipitously and we now tend to focus on those with the most challenging needs, both psychiatrically and behaviourally, and how to manage these with more limited access to in-patient treatment and assessment facilities. There has been little work on how such changes have affected the psychiatric profession. Much change is driven by government policy decisions and working parties which are not always clearly backed up by research evidence. There is a clear need for an evidence-based approach to such initiatives. In England and Wales there exists the Healthcare Commission (since 2004), National Service Frameworks and the Commission for Social Care Inspection (since 2004); in Scotland there is the Care Commission for Scotland (since 2002 for non-NHS agencies) and the Mental Welfare Commission for Scotland (for NHS) which are all heavily involved in regulating and overseeing the changes. There is a key role for psychiatric learning disability service research within these frameworks. One example where service development may benefit from a research base is in the unique role (among psychiatrists) of the learning disability specialist in the management of epilepsy (Bowley & Kerr, 2000). Up to two-fifths of our patients may have epilepsy – often complex. The past few years have seen the development of many specialist epilepsy services for people with learning disability across the UK led by psychiatrists. Since learning disability is the classical neurodevelopmental disorder, the interphase between neurology, genetics and psychiatry is likely to increase markedly in the near future and services will have to incorporate all these disciplines within their ambit.

Psychometric tools in learning disability research

Levels of cognition and communication vary among people with learning disability and differ from the general population. Thus it is obvious that psychometric instruments that rely on gathering information from the person need either to be modified or to be created specifically for this population. A multitude of scales, tests and interviews have been validated in those with learning disability, but there is only space to consider broad areas and some representative tests here. It is usually essential to obtain the advice (and often the participation) of a clinical psychologist experienced in working with people with learning disability when designing studies that collect psychometric information about cognitive and behavioural parameters. The number of tests available is legion – but not all have been validated in those with learning disability, not all in adults, and not all in severe rather than mild learning disability. The sensitivity, selectivity, reliability and (often the most difficult to ascertain) validity of some tests are found to be wanting. Many tests originate from the USA and unless shown to be applicable their transfer to other cultures (and ethnic minorities within cultures) may be a problem. It is proposed here to cover briefly some selected areas and tests that the psychiatrist in learning disability may have to understand or make use of.

Assessing the spectrum of intellectual abilities

A significant degree of intellectual impairment (IQ < 70) is a necessary (but not sufficient) criterion for identifying learning disability in a person, and a large number of tests that purport to give global indications of IQ tests have been devised. Full testing is rightly the province of the educational and clinical psychologist, but there are shorter versions of most tests that can be useful rapid tools for use by the psychiatrist in learning disability.

Probably the most widely used set of full tests is that originating from Wechsler. There are now three main groups of tests based on the age of the person to whom they are applied. Their norms are regularly updated in surveys of large numbers of people, but unless specifically stated these are based in the USA. The Wechsler Preschool and Primary Scale Intelligence, version III (WPPSI–III UK) applies to children of 2 years 6 months to 7 years 3 months with norms from 800 children in the UK (Wechsler, 2004). There are two main test batteries – one for children up to 3 years 11 months and one for children from 4 years to 7 years 3 months. They differ in the subgroups of tests (the former has verbal, performance and full scale IQs, the latter adds processing speed). The Wechsler Intelligence Scale for Children – fourth edition (WISC–IV) applies from 6 to 16 years and has been recently updated (Williams et al, 2003). The full-scale IQ is derived from four main subgroups of tests – verbal comprehension, perceptual reasoning, working memory and processing speed. The scores on these can be used to give an estimate of profiles of ability within the full-scale IQ. This will supersede the 10-year-old WISC–III UK and it is expected that a UK version will be produced. The Wechsler Adult Intelligence Scale – third edition (WAIS–III UK; Wechsler, 1999a) is for people aged 16–89 years and is useful as it has been normalised in the UK population and has been recently revised. It also allows sub-test grouping based on the traditional verbal, performance and full-scale IQ scores or into the same four blocks as for the WISC–IV. The WAIS in its various versions has been in use for a long period and is reliable (0.98 for full-scale score), repeatable (0.96) and has very good interrater reliability. These large instruments take around 60–75 min to complete by an experienced psychologist. However, shortened versions of the WAIS are available which can give relatively rapid and reliable estimates of the full-scale IQ (e.g. Wechsler Abbreviated Scale of Intelligence (WASI; Wechsler, 1999*b*); the two sub-test forms of this can be administered in about 15 min). It should be noted that even the abbreviated form of the Wechsler test is recommended only to be used by clinical psychologists. However, there are other useful short IQ tests, such as the Quick Test which is based on receptive vocabulary (Mortimer & Bowen, 1999), that can be used by psychiatrists. The Wechsler is not the only large IQ battery. The Raven's Standard Progressive Matrices (Raven, 1998) are based on non-verbal material and are not related to culture as much as other tests. The Stanford–Binet Intelligence Scales are now in their fifth revision (SB–V; Roid, 2003) and are said to be useful from age 2 to over 90 years.

Instruments used to assess dementia

The Mini-Mental State Examination (MMSE; Folstein *et al*, 1975) remains the clinical touchstone for studies of dementia in the general population. However, its use in people with learning disability is limited and other rating scales have been devised. Both the Dementia Questionnaire for People with Mental Retardation (DMR) and the Dementia Scale for Down Syndrome (DSDS) have specificity and sensitivity. (Deb & Braganza, 1999). Although they are observer-rated scales, they have not as yet been shown to be less useful than neuropsychological test batteries. For more direct assessment some use the Severe Impairment Battery (Saxton *et al*, 1993), which is more useful in those with pre-existing very severe and profound learning disability. Adaptations of subsets of the Rivermead Behavioural Memory Tests which are used extensively in general populations are also used by some psychologists (Wilson *et al*, 2003). The latter two tests are also useful for measuring temporal changes as well as assisting in diagnosis.

Assessing behaviours

The second requirement for defining the presence of learning disability is that the person has some degree of socio-adaptive dysfunction. In addition to problems with such adaptive behaviours (including those of daily living) that are an intrinsic part of the person's learning disability and intellectual impairment (Schalock & Braddock, 1999), there may be a series of aberrant behaviours that do not occur in most people with an equivalent level of intellectual disability, constitute serious difficulties in socialisation and may be intense enough to be considered a behaviour disorder. There are a multitude of tests and scales for both these types of behaviours.

There are currently at least 15 separate scales for measuring adaptive behaviour. A typical scale for those aged 15–21 years is the Adaptive Behavior Assessment System (ABAS; Harrison & Oakland, 2000), which covers the AAMR and DSM–IV areas of adaptive skills. Many other systems are in common use; some like the ABAS only apply to children and adolescents (e.g. Adaptive Behavior Inventory – ABI) others such as the AAMR Adaptive Behavior Scales Residential/Community apply over 18 years. Also in current wide use are the full and subset versions of the Vineland Adaptive Behavior Scales – applicable to children and also to adults with learning disability. These are currently undergoing revision (Sparrow *et al*, 1984).

There are also numerous scales to assess current and temporal changes in specific aberrant behavioural domains. Perhaps the most commonly used in the UK is the Aberrant Behavior Checklist (ABC; Aman & Singh, 1985). The most recent version of this is the Aberrant Behavior Checklist Residential (ABC–1R). It is useful in both children and adults but is based on a factor analysis of persons in adolescent years or younger. There are five sub-scales covering irritability and agitation, lethargy and social withdrawal, stereotypic behaviour, hyperactivity and non-adherence, and inappropriate speech. The community version is the same except that the settings are simply listed as home, workplace, etc. It is simple to use and has formed the behavioural assessment tool for many studies of learning disability as well as being of practical clinical utility (Aman *et al*, 1995). The AAMR Aberrant Behavior Scales for those aged 18–80 years (ABS, Revised Residential and Community edition) take around 15–30 min to complete (Nihara *et al*, 1993) and there is a version especially for children.

Structured and semi-structured diagnostic instruments for learning disability research

Most of the older studies investigating psychiatric disorders in people with learning disability lacked good diagnostic interview tools with sufficient validity, sensitivity and stability to ensure that findings from different groups were directly comparable. However, there are now a series of instruments that can be used to obviate such difficulties. First there are those schedules that gather the information needed to make a reliable psychiatric diagnosis according to a structured diagnostic schema. In the case of learning disability these usually rely on interviews with key informants such as family members and carers as well as the person with learning disability themselves, and may also allow the review of case notes and other written material regarding the participant.

For those with mild learning disability the schedule for affective disorders and schizophrenia (Endicott & Spitzer, 1978) (especially its newer 'lifetime' variant) or other similar general psychiatry instruments are probably valid and have been used successfully to diagnose serious psychiatric disorders (Doody *et al*, 1998). Several schedules have been created that are for use specifically in people with learning disability. The Psychopathology Inventory for Mentally Retarded Adults (PIMRA) is useful for those over the age of 16 years with an IQ of 60–80 and is available in both self-report and informant versions (Senatore *et al*, 1985). In addition to a screening instrument for maladaptive behaviours, Steven Reiss in Ohio has also produced screening instruments for dual diagnosis in both adults (Reiss Screen) and children (Reiss Screen for Children's Dual Diagnosis). The latter can be helpful in diagnosing affective and anxiety disorders in this group (Reiss & Valenti-Hein, 1994). The Diagnostic Assessment for the Severely Handicapped (DASH–II; Matson, 1995) covers 13 psychiatric disorders with items partly based on the requirements of DSM–III–R; it may be especially useful in the diagnosis of schizophrenia in those with severe learning disability. (Unfortunately there is another test with the same acronym – DASH–II – which is also for the developmental assessment of students with severe disabilities. This is a useful initial assessment instrument for children with learning disability up to the age of 6 years (Dykes & Erin, 1999)). The Psychiatric Assessment Schedule for Adults with Developmental Disabilities (PAS–ADD) was the outcome of many years of work by members of the former Hester Adrian Research Centre led by Professor Steve Moss. Its revision included questions based on the Schedules for Clinical Assessment in Neuropsychiatry (SCAN) and it comes with a computer program to assist in creating diagnoses from the information (Costello *et al*, 1997). The most recent version, the mini PAS–ADD, is a shortened version that also has been shown to have reasonable validity (Prosser *et al*, 1998; Edwards, 2003).

The above are tools to collect information that is then used to make a diagnosis according to one or other schema. The PAS–ADD generates diagnoses according to the current ICD–10 system. The diagnostic criteria specified in the major classification systems (DSM–IV–R and ICD–10) are not without problems when applied to people with learning disability, especially those with severe disability. The Royal College of Psychiatrists has issued the Diagnostic Criteria for Learning Disability (DC–LD; Royal College of Psychiatrists, 2001), which especially takes into account diagnostic difficulties in moderate-to-severe learning disability, and should go some way to improving consistency and reliability. The DC–LD uses a hierarchical approach with a series of axes.

The DC–LD allows the incorporation of such previously hard-to-systematise disorders in people with learning disability as attention-deficit hyperactivity disorder, personality disorders and behavioural problems. The lack of a useful classification of behavioural problems in those with learning disability has been an especially obvious weakness of the current diagnostic systems. The DC–LD has the great merit of allowing such diagnoses to be made in adults with learning disability as well as children.

Qualitative and participatory research with people with learning disability

Qualitative methodologies explore the understanding, and describe the personal and social experiences of participants. They try to capture the meanings particular phenomena hold for participants. They usually (but not exclusively) involve attempts at comprehending the views or frames of reference of a small number of participants, rather than testing a preconceived hypothesis on a large sample. Removing the restriction of hypothesis testing creates the potential to uncover new and sometimes surprising information. Qualitative researchers recognise that there are many different ways of making sense of the world. Qualitative methodologies offer particularly useful approaches to complex or novel (and thus under-researched) areas (Jones, 1995; Smith, 1996). They often ask the question 'why?' Exploring context is all important, whereas quantitative approaches often study only one aspect in isolation. Although the roots of qualitative methods lie in social science, health researchers increasingly use these methods and publish the results in peer-reviewed journals. The methodologies are discussed in more detail in Chapter 6. This section will focus on their application to the psychiatry of learning disability. As a practical example, a qualitative study conducted by one of the authors (S.G.) during her psychiatric training illustrates why a particular methodology may be chosen and how it may be applied in research with people with learning disability.

Why should psychiatrists of learning disability consider qualitative methods?

The complex nature of the specialty

Learning disability psychiatry is full of complex issues – ethical dilemmas, attitudes, interactions between biological, psychological and social factors, and service provision in a multidisciplinary environment. Qualitative methods are ideally suited for the exploration of such issues, which often interest psychiatrists and can be of vital importance to their patients.

The relative lack of research in many areas

Learning disability psychiatry is understudied. Qualitative studies can provide a starting point for research, also permitting those with learning disability, their carers or professionals to describe their own experiences, set priorities and evolve ideas. The results can generate hypotheses for further qualitative or quantitative research.

The opportunity to give people with learning disability a voice

Involving lay people in research is a key goal for major funding and UK governmental organisations. They have insights and expertise unavailable to health professionals that can assist in setting research priorities (Entwistle *et al*, 1998). Today people with learning disability are increasingly considered reliable informants with valid opinions and a right to express them (Stalker, 1998). However, studies incorporating the views of people with learning disability remain relatively rare.

The insights gained from working closely with participants

Psychiatrists usually have little contact with people with learning disability outside the clinical sphere. Qualitative methods that involve working closely with participants result in insights into their lives and abilities that inform clinical practice. The qualitative researcher has to explicitly explore and acknowledge their influence on the research outcome. This adds a richness to the interpretation of the results and can be an illuminating experience for the researcher.

The limitations of quantitative methods

One limitation (of which learning disability psychiatrists are well aware) is the difficulty faced in applying the results of randomised controlled trials to clinical situations. Trials are often, of necessity, conducted under rather rigid constraints. This affects their applicability to people with learning disability, given the complex nature of their lives and multidisciplinary service provision. Qualitative research can help address the practical clinical realities for both clinicians and their patients and help apply quantitative research results to real-life situations. Qualitative research is also now becoming an established part of systematic reviews (Dixon-Woods & Fitzpatrick, 2001).

The use of qualitative methodologies in research relating to people with learning disability

The increased use of qualitative methods (also see Chapter 6) over the past decade is clear from Tables 13.2–13.4. A literature review of this period showed individual interviews, focus groups and observation to be the most common methodologies, either singly or in combination. Qualitative, 'open-ended' questions were also used in some questionnaires. Using different qualitative methodologies to address a question can yield different results (Carnaby, 1997). Therefore combining methodologies may add extra insights. The work of Espie and his colleagues (Espie *et al*, 1998, 2001) provides an interesting example of how qualitative and quantitative methods can complement each other. The Epilepsy Outcome Scale was developed using focus groups, followed by psychometric procedures to generate data on reliability, validity and component structure. Research akin to qualitative methodologies has also been used to explore historical facets of the life of people with learning disability (Atkinson *et al*, 1997).

Particular methodological and ethical issues relating to qualitative research with people with learning disability are summarised in Box 13.1. Communication with participants is at the heart of qualitative research, but

Table 13.2 Examples of qualitative research involving people with learning disability

Study	Qualitative methodology	Topic
Fraser & Fraser (2001)	Focus groups	Contribution of people with learning disability to focus groups on health promotion
Hart (1998, 1999)	Interviews	Experiences of people with learning disabilities in general hospitals and with consent to treatment
March (1991)	Interviews using questionnaires; quantitative and qualitative analysis	Conceptualisation of physical illness and its cause by people with learning disability
Kjellberg (2002)	Interviews	Participation and independence in everyday life
Richardson (2000)	Group discussion and observation	Participatory research into 'How we live'
March et al (1997)	Interviews	Participatory research into self-advocacy and families
Carnaby (1997)	Interviews/observation	Social service planning and evaluation
Cambridge & McCarthy (2001)	Focus groups	Social service planning and evaluation
Llewellyn (1995)	Observation and interviews	Views of parents with learning disability

Table 13.3 Qualitative studies with parents and family members of people with learning disability

Studies	Methodology	Topic
Shearn & Todd (1997)	Interviews	
Kearney & Griffin (2001)	Interviews	
Freedman & Boyer (2000)	Focus groups	Parental work, experiences, needs and support in caring for people with learning disability
Llewellyn et al (1999)	Postal questionnaire and interviews (qualitative/quantitative methods)	
Lehmann & Roberto (1996)	Interviews	Mothers' perceptions of the futures of their adolescents
Craig et al (2003)	Interviews	Parental views on gastrostomy

Table 13.4 Qualitative studies with health professionals

Studies	Methodology	Topic
Espie *et al* (1998, 2001)	Scale developed using focus groups and quantitative methods	Development of the Epilepsy Outcome Scale
Dovey & Webb (2000)	Qualitative and quantitative questionnaire	Perception of primary healthcare professionals of the provision of healthcare for people with learning disability
Thornton (1996)	Semi-structured focus groups	
Lindop & Read (2000)	Focus groups led to formulation of questionnaire, which was used for quantitative analysis	District nurses' and palliative care for people with learning disability

can be problematic with people with learning disability. This may be owing to the severity of the learning disability or specifically altered communication patterns, for example when autism coexists with learning disability. There is a need for creativity in designing methodologies that allow people's true opinions to be heard. Traditional interview and focus group approaches may need substantial adaptation or new ones should be designed from scratch. Several ways to improve communication with participants with learning disability are listed in Box 13.2. Information can also be sought from third parties. However, one must be careful not to discount a person with learning disability's account if it is thought not to be the objective 'truth'. It is often their personal perception of an experience that is important.

Inclusion of people with learning disability in the research process – participatory research

Medical researchers increasingly recognise the importance of using the knowledge, expertise and resources of the researched community, and in this they draw on developments in social science. Primary features of such 'participatory research' include collaboration, mutual education, and acting on results emerging from research questions relevant to the community (Macaulay *et al*, 1999). The value of narratives (patients' stories) and how these enrich evidence-based medicine has recently been highlighted (Greenhalgh & Hurwitz, 1999). The DIPEx database of patient experiences, for example, has been created as a research/teaching resource, and a route of dissemination for qualitative research (Herxheimer *et al*, 2000). This could be developed to include the experiences of people with learning disability.

Direct inclusion of people with learning disability in the research process has also increased, but is still largely in the social science and nursing fields. The related 'participatory', 'action' and 'emancipatory' research methods

---

Box 13.1 Some methodological and ethical issues in qualitative research with people with learning disability

- 'Gatekeepers' – researchers tend to rely on carers or staff to choose potential participants, which may result in bias
- Communication – particularly the difficulty in eliciting the feelings or perceptions of people with multiple or profound impairments
- Gaining informed consent – particularly from people with profound impairment
- Acquiescence – this is a tendency of some people with learning disability, perhaps because others control many aspects of their lives; this may hamper obtaining truly informed consent, or influence opinions expressed
- Intrusion into privacy – particularly when conducting research in people's homes
- Raising difficult emotional issues for participants – research is not therapy and participants may not have the opportunity to deal with emotions raised
- Raising expectations of continuing friendships – participants may misunderstand the role of the researcher and those with few opportunities for social interaction may be disappointed when they withdraw once the project is complete
- Time – extra time is needed to facilitate the inclusion of people with communication difficulties in research.

Based on authors' experience; see also Stalker (1998); Swain et al (1998); Kitzinger & Barbour (1999).

Box 13.2 Aids to communication with participants with learning disability

- Take time to get to know individuals before collecting the data
- Use photographs and drawings to supplement speech in interviews
- Use the person's preferred method of communication (e.g. symbols or signing) if there are speech and language difficulties
- Obtain advice from experienced speech and communication therapists when designing a project
- Use 'interpreters' or 'co-facilitators' who understand the person's communication
- Supplement interview data with observational/descriptive techniques.

Adapted in part from Stalker (1998) and Fraser & Fraser (2001).

---

have developed out of a number of qualitative methodologies and are now being used in research with people with learning disability. Walmsley & Johnson (2003) summarised these methods as 'research in which people with learning disability are active participants, not only as subjects but also as initiators, doers, writers and disseminators of research'. Some have found Zarb's (Zarb, 1992) criteria helpful in considering issues of participation (Box 13.3; Rodgers, 1999).

Some studies listed in Tables 13.2–13.4 explicitly used participatory methods. An early study (March, 1991) involved people with learning disability as co-researchers and included them as co-authors. Evaluations of services by people with learning disability have been described (Whittaker, 1997). Dissemination of research to people with learning disability is also important. The Norah Fry Research Centre makes research results available in a form accessible to people with learning disability through 'plain facts' sheets (http://www.bris.ac.uk/Depts/NorahFry/PlainFacts/index.html). Participatory research can pose considerable challenges to researchers, especially when pressurised to obtain funding, respond to research briefs and produce academic publications within limited time scales (Stalker, 1998). Involvement of people with learning disability in medical research is still usually restricted to those with good verbal communication skills and limited to answering the (non-disabled) professional's questions, rather than shaping the research and research agenda.

Example of participatory qualitative research

As an illustrative example of the qualitative research process, we use a study (by S.G.) of the experiences of adults with learning disability in local general medical hospitals (Gibbs, 2001). The idea originated from negative experiences reported by some patients with learning disability (or their carers) and the creation of a local general hospital liaison learning disability service (Brown & MacArthur, 1999). An initial literature search revealed that virtually no relevant research work had been published, other than some written from clinicians' personal experiences. This is probably not an uncommon situation in learning disability research. Thus there was no research base to assist in the design of a quantitative or structured qualitative study, even at the questionnaire level. The research question was therefore addressing the experiences of people in an area that was both under-researched and complex. A qualitative methodology seemed entirely

---

Box 13.3 Zarb's criteria for consideration of issues of participation (Zarb, 1992)

- Who controls what research will be carried out, and how it will be done?
- How far are disabled people involved in the research process?
- What opportunities are there for disabled people to criticise the research and influence future directions?

appropriate. Here we focus on the methodological issues relating to the participants with learning disability rather than their carers.

A focus group may be defined as a 'carefully planned discussion designed to obtain perceptions on a defined area of interest in a permissive and non-threatening environment' (Kreuger, 1994). Focus groups were chosen for this study for a number of reasons (Box 13.4). Four focus groups were formed with a total of 11 adults with mild-to-moderate learning disability who had experience of general hospitals in the previous year. Each group met twice in familiar surroundings. The researcher acted as group facilitator, aided by a 'co-facilitator' well known to the participants. As there was a lack of previous evidence, we wished results to reflect the priorities of participants, rather than imposing the issues that the researchers themselves felt to be important. We therefore deliberately chose an unstructured interview format for the groups, asking people to describe their experiences and comment on or discuss issues that arose. Subsequent groups were also asked for their views on issues raised in earlier groups. The discussions of the focus groups were recorded onto audiotapes.

It was important to be aware of the potential problems with focus groups, including silencing of those who disagree with the majority views and issues of confidentiality (Kitzinger, 1995). Two main disadvantages emerged from the use of focus groups in this study. Some participants appeared excessively suggestible and repeated stories told by others. This suggestibility is an intrinsic facet of many people with learning disability. Corroboration by a third party would be needed to distinguish repetition of the views of others from actual personal experiences. Second, it was impossible to ensure that very talkative members of groups with more

---

Box 13.4 Reasons for use of focus groups in study of experiences of adults with learning disability in general hospitals

- Especially suited to the study of attitudes and experiences
- Group discussions were felt to be less intimidating than individual interviews for people with learning disability who were used to such group settings in the care homes or day centres in which the focus groups took place
- The use of 'naturally occurring groups' can make the participants more relaxed and able to support each other, and prompt others to comment on experiences or views that they had already shared
- Group dynamics can encourage participation from people who initially may indicate they have nothing to say; focus groups can empower people who are reluctant to give negative feedback, or who feel that all problems result from their own inadequacies
- Focus groups do not discriminate against people who cannot read or write.

dominant social/relationship skills did not inhibit the expression of others in the group. The variability and impairment of social skills is a key feature in learning disability. There were noticeable differences in the communication patterns observed. The 'gatekeeper' effect (Box 13.1) may have affected the present study. We used carers or day-centre staff to identify participants for the project. They may have (deliberately or unconsciously) chosen people known to have had particularly positive or negative experiences. Also, it is a common and understandable practice in the UK for primary physicians, carers or family members to give sole or additional proxy permission for people with learning disability to take part in research. Ethics committees often require this. However, this is another potential source of bias – in the study in question two potential participants were excluded by this mechanism. It is now becoming accepted that most adults with mild learning disability, given adequate information in the correct form, can give valid consent by themselves for most studies. For those with moderate or severe learning disability there is a need for inclusion rather than exclusion in research. In Scotland the recent Incapable Adults (Scotland) Act 2000 recognises that (in)capacity is a graded and not absolute concept and there are clear mechanisms to both protect and involve people with all degrees of learning disability in research. Currently this is not the situation elsewhere in the UK.

A number of strategies were found useful to facilitate the use of focus groups of people with learning disability. The 'co-facilitator' aided communication (particularly when participants had speech or language problems), helped to create a relaxed atmosphere and noticed and encouraged the less vocal. They gave confidence to participants when dealing with difficult issues and were available to follow these up where necessary. Each group was small (2–4 participants) and met twice – allowing extra time for discussion of complex issues and giving those with communication difficulties an extended period to express their views. To stimulate ideas and memories, the co-facilitator helped participants to discuss issues between groups and one group visited a general hospital. The unstructured nature of the groups was in part justified by the results, which showed important differences between the priorities of adults with learning disability, their families and professional carers. Furthermore, some issues raised had not been anticipated by the researchers and may not have emerged using a predetermined agenda.

In qualitative research, acknowledging the role and influence of the researcher is crucial. The researcher is rarely (if ever) neutral in their influence on the group, and this influence should be explored. In this study, the researcher aimed to get people to recall their experiences in a non-directive way, responding to and probing further into issues brought up by participants. Non-directivity by the researcher was far less easy when working with groups of people with learning disability than with other groups. Participants with learning disability had a marked tendency to give short answers to questions and required increased prompting. Indeed, directive questioning could not always be completely avoided in order to let people describe their experiences. It is thought unlikely that this is significantly different from an individual interview situation. However, there is a need for comparative research between different experiential data gathering methods for people with learning disability. The current researcher's experience was that several participants with learning disability clearly set their own agenda when describing their experiences and opinions, requiring minimal external clarification. The cognitive difficulty of subject areas is also important to consider because this is linked to the tendency for concrete rather than abstract conceptualisation in people with learning disability. Factual issues (such as who spoke to them) rather than opinions about the care they received were more easily related. On reviewing the audiotapes, it became apparent that the researcher also tended to ask participants with learning disability more direct factual questions on the process of general hospital care than experiential questions, such as issues about discrimination. The latter may have been avoided because of a concern not to bring up potentially distressing issues. However, feelings/emotions were frequently discussed. Participants were also made aware that the researcher in this case was a doctor (a trainee in the psychiatry of learning disability), which may have influenced their willingness to discuss issues concerning medical staff.

The audiotapes were transcribed onto a computer word-processing package to which the 'QSR NUD*IST' (Non-Numerical Data Indexing, Searching and Theorising) software package (1997) was applied to facilitate data interpretation. This allows transcripts to be viewed and semi-organised, making manipulation of large amounts of data more manageable and enabling thematic areas to be identified and explored. 'Grounded theory' (Glaser & Strauss, 1967) was then used to underpin the subsequent analysis. The results of the study will be published elsewhere – we have concentrated on the methodology here. Despite the challenges posed by using focus group methodology with people with learning disability, we found it to be a very good way of addressing this research question. Much useful data was gathered on their experiences and views, including from some participants with moderate learning disability and communication problems.

Points to consider when beginning qualitative research with people with learning disability are listed in Box 13.5. Qualitative research with people with learning disability can be interesting and rewarding for both researchers and participants but careful planning is needed to facilitate communication and avoid disappointing, confusing or upsetting participants with learning disability. Qualitative methods provide a framework for exploring complex, novel and previously unresearched topics. The views and experiences of people with learning disability can be investigated, disseminated and used to lead to action and change.

Literature searches for learning disability research

The wider issue of literature searches, web-based search engines and how best to use the available online databases are discussed elsewhere in this volume. These techniques and resources are as important in learning disability research as in any other specialty. However, for many interesting journals the social science and psychology sites may have to be searched as some are not listed by Medline and thus may not be scanned by widely used engines such as Pubmed. Many reference management software packages (two commercial examples of which are Reference Manager and Endnote) now permit direct connection and searching of a wide variety of social, educational and psychological (as well as medical) literature databases from within the packages themselves. An important point is the use of MENTAL RETARDATION as a search term. This is the standard term outside the UK for learning disability. Furthermore, one should be careful in interpreting references which have been identified using LEARNING DISABILITY as a search term, as this refers to specific learning disorders in countries (USA included) using DSM–IV as the principal diagnostic schema.

Conclusion

The opportunities for research within the psychiatry of learning disability are many, and the range of subjects covered probably has no equal within psychiatry as a whole. Psychiatric, behavioural, genetic and neurological

---

Box 13.5 Points to consider when beginning qualitative research with people with learning disability

- Read an introductory textbook on qualitative methods (e.g. Bannister *et al*, 1994; Richardson, 1996). The *BMJ* has published several useful series on qualitative research (e.g. Pope & Mays, 1995)
- Study the literature that has used qualitative methods in research with or relating to people with learning disability
- Appropriate supervision from the early stage of project design, through data gathering to analysis is essential. Help may be sought in particular from colleagues in psychology or social sciences
- Consider how people with learning disability may participate in various aspects of the project
- Be realistic as to the time needed to complete a qualitative research project. Just as the questions posed in qualitative research are often complex, so is the process of exploring them and analysing the results. Computer packages are available that facilitate data analysis but time is needed to learn and use them.

disorders are all associated with learning disability and their origins, natural histories and treatments can be investigated by quantitative and/or qualitative methods. There are also important social and ethical areas that have engendered much debate in which the psychiatric researcher can play a major role. Finally, health service provision is undergoing rapid change from hospital to community to generic services and the role of the psychiatrist in learning disability is sure to be questioned on many fronts in the future. It is only by the establishment of a good research base, in which psychiatrists must play a leading role, that rational and worthwhile improvement in the psychological and medical health of and minimisation of the effects of the cognitive deficits inherent in people with learning disability can be made.

Acknowledgements

Tina Cook, Research Associate, University of Northumbria and Northgate and Prudhoe NHS Trust provided helpful commentary regarding qualitative methodology.

References

Allingham-Hawkins, D. J., Babul-Hirji, R., Chitayat, D., *et al* (1999) Fragile X premutation is a significant risk factor for premature ovarian failure: The International Collaborative POF in Fragile X study – preliminary data. *American Journal of Medical Genetics*, **83**, 322–325.

Aman, M. G. & Singh, N. N. (1985). *Aberrant Behavior Checklist: Residential (ABC–1R)*.New York: Slosson Educational.

Aman, M. G., Burrow, W. H. & Wolford, P. L. (1995). The Aberrant Behavior Checklist–Community: factor validity and effect of subject variables for adults in group homes. *American Journal of Mental Retardation*, **100**, 283–292.

Arvio, M. & Sillanpaa, M. (2003) Prevalence, aetiology and comorbidity of severe and profound intellectual disability in Finland. *Journal of Intellectual Disability Research*, **47**, 108–112.

Atkinson, D., Jackson, M. & Walmsley, J. (1997) *Forgotten Lives: Exploring the History of Learning Disability*. Kidderminster: BILD.

Aziz, M., Stathopulu, E., Callias, M., *et al* (2003) Clinical features of boys with fragile X premutations and intermediate alleles. *American Journal of Medical Genetics*, **121B**, 119–127.

Bannister, P., Burman, E., Parker, I. *et al* (1994) *Qualitative Methods in Psychology: A Research Guide*. Buckingham: Open University Press.

Boer, H., Holland, A., Whittington, J., *et al* (2002) Psychotic illness in people with Prader Willi syndrome due to chromosome 15 maternal uniparental disomy. *Lancet*, **359**, 135–136.

Bowley, C. & Kerr, M. (2000) Epilepsy and intellectual disability. *Journal of Intellectual Disability Research*, **44**, 529–543.

Brown, M. & MacArthur, J. (1999) Discriminating on grounds of need not disabilities. *Nursing Times*, **95**, 48–49.

Cambridge, P. & McCarthy, M. (2001) User focus groups and Best Value in services for people with learning disabilities. *Health and Social Care in the Community*, **9**, 476–489.

Carnaby, S. (1997) 'What do you think?': a qualitative approach to evaluating individual planning services. *Journal of Intellectual Disability Research*, **41**, 225–231.

Cederbaum, S. (2002) Phenylketonuria: an update. *Current Opinions in Pediatrics*, **14**, 702–706.

Chelly, J. & Mandel, J. L. (2001) Monogenic causes of X-linked mental retardation. *Nature Reviews Genetics*, **2**, 669–680.

Cooper, S. A. & Collacott, R. A. (1994). Clinical features and diagnostic criteria of depression in Down's syndrome. *British Journal of Psychiatry*, **165**, 399–403.

Costello, H., Moss, S., Prosser, H., *et al* (1997) Reliability of the ICD–10 version of the Psychiatric Assessment Schedule for Adults with Developmental Disability (PAS–ADD). *Social Psychiatry and Psychiatric Epidemiology*, **32**, 339–343.

Craig, G. M., Scambler, G. & Spitz, L. (2003) Why parents of children with neurodevelopmental disabilities requiring gastrostomy feeding need more support. *Developmental Medicine and Child Neurology*, **45**, 183–188.

Crawford, P., Brown, S. & Kerr, M. (2001) A randomized open-label study of gabapentin and lamotrigine in adults with learning disability and resistant epilepsy. *Seizure*, **10**, 107–115.

Cuskelly, M., Jobling, A. & Buckley, S. (eds) (2002) *Down Syndrome Across the Life Span*. London: Whurr Publishers.

Deb, S. & Braganza, J. (1999). Comparison of rating scales for the diagnosis of dementia in adults with Down's syndrome. *Journal of Intellectual Disability Research*, **43**, 400–407.

Dimitropoulos, A., Feurer, I. D., Roof, E., *et al* (2000) Appetitive behavior, compulsivity, and neurochemistry in Prader–Willi syndrome. *Mental Retardation and Developmental Disabilities Research Reviews*, **6**, 125–130.

Dixon-Woods, M. & Fitzpatrick, R. (2001) Qualitative research in systematic reviews. Has established a place for itself. *BMJ*, **323**, 765–766.

Doody, G. A., Johnstone, E. C., Sanderson, T. L., *et al* (1998) 'Pfropfschizophrenie' revisited. Schizophrenia in people with mild learning disability. *British Journal of Psychiatry*, **173**, 145–153.

Dovey, S. & Webb, O. J. (2000). General practitioners' perception of their role in care for people with intellectual disability. *Journal of Intellectual Disability Research*, **44**, 553–561.

Duggan, L. & Brylewski, J. (2001). Antipsychotic medication for those with both schizophrenia and learning disability. *Cochrane Database of Systematic Reviews*, issue 3. Oxford: Update Software.

Dykes, M. K. & Erin, J. (1999) *A Developmental Assessment for Students with Severe Disabilities* (DASH–2). Austin, TX: Pro-Ed.

Edwards, N. (2003) The Mini PAS–ADD Interview Pack. *Journal of Intellectual Disability Research*, **47**, 493–494.

Emerson, E. (2003) Prevalence of psychiatric disorders in children and adolescents with and without intellectual disability. *Journal of Intellectual Disability Research*, **47**, 51–58.

Endicott, J. & Spitzer, R. L. (1978) A diagnostic interview: the schedule for affective disorders and schizophrenia. *Archives of General Psychiatry*, **35**, 837–844.

Entwistle, V. A., Renfrew, M. J., Yearley, S., *et al* (1998) Lay perspectives: advantages for health research. *BMJ*, **316**, 463–466.

Epstein, C. J. (2002) 2001 William Allan Award Address. From Down syndrome to the "human" in "human genetics". *American Journal of Human Genetics*, **70**, 300–313.

Espie, C. A., Paul, A., Graham, M., *et al* (1998) The Epilepsy Outcome Scale: the development of a measure for use with carers of people with epilepsy plus intellectual disability. *Journal of Intellectual Disability Research*, **42**, 90–96.

Espie, C. A., Watkins, J., Duncan, R., *et al* (2001) Development and validation of the Glasgow Epilepsy Outcome Scale (GEOS): a new instrument for measuring concerns about epilepsy in people with mental retardation. *Epilepsia*, **42**, 1043–1051.

Folstein, M., Folstein, S. & McHugh, P. (1975) Mini-mental state: a practical method of grading the cognitive state of patients for the clinician. *Journal of Psychiatric Research*, **12**, 189–198.

Fombonne, E. (1999). The epidemiology of autism: a review. *Psychological Medicine*, **29**, 769–786.

Fraser, M. & Fraser, A. (2001) Are people with learning disabilities able to contribute to focus groups on health promotion? *Journal of Advanced Nursing*, **33**, 225–233.

Fraser, W. & Kerr, M. (eds) (2003) *Seminars in the Psychiatry of Learning Disability* (2nd edn). London: Gaskell.

Freedman, R. I. & Boyer, N. C. (2000) The power to choose: support for families caring for individuals with developmental disabilities. *Health and Social Work*, **25**, 59–68.

Gibbs, S. (2001) *The Experiences of Adults with Learning Disabilities and Their Carers in General Hospitals* (MPhil Thesis). Edinburgh: University of Edinburgh.

Glaser, B. G. & Strauss, A. L. (1967) *The Discovery of Grounded Theory: Strategies for Qualitative Research*. Chicago, IL: Aldine.

Greenhalgh, T. & Hurwitz, B. (1999) Narrative based medicine: why study narrative? *BMJ*, **318**, 48–50.

Guy, W. (1976) ECDEU *Assessment Manual for Psychopharmacology*. Rockville, MD: National Institute of Mental Health.

Hagberg, B. (2002) Clinical manifestations and stages of Rett syndrome. *Mental Retardation and Developmental Disabilities Research Reviews*, **8**, 61–65.

Hagerman, R. J., Leehey, M., Heinrichs, W., *et al* (2001) Intention tremor, parkinsonism, and generalized brain atrophy in male carriers of fragile X. *Neurology*, **57**, 127–130.

Hall, S., Oliver, C. & Murphy, G. (2001) Self-injurious behaviour in young children with Lesch–Nyhan syndrome. *Developmental Medicine and Child Neurology*, **43**, 745–749.

Harrison, P. & Oakland, T. (2000) *Adaptive Behavior Assessment System* (ABAS) San Antonio, TX: Psychological Corporation.

Hart, S. L. (1998) Learning-disabled people's experience of general hospitals. *British Journal of Nursing*, **7**, 470–477.

Hart, S. L. (1999) Meaningful choices: consent to treatments in general health care settings for people with LD. *Journal of Learning Disabilities for Nursing, Health and Social Care*, **3**, 20–26.

Herxheimer, A., McPherson, A., Miller, R., *et al* (2000) Database of patients' experiences (DIPEx): a multi-media approach to sharing experiences and information. *Lancet*, **355**, 1540–1543.

Jacquemont, S., Hagerman, R. J., Leehey, M., *et al* (2003) Fragile X premutation tremor/ataxia syndrome: molecular, clinical, and neuroimaging correlates. *American Journal of Human Genetics*, **72**, 869–878.

Jones, J. (1995) Why do qualitative research? *BMJ*, **311**, 2.

Jopp, D. A. & Keys, C. B. (2001) Diagnostic overshadowing reviewed and reconsidered. *American Journal of Mental Retardation*, **106**, 416–433.

Kahng, S., Iwata, B. A. & Lewin, A. B. (2002) Behavioral treatment of self-injury, 1964 to 2000. *American Journal of Mental Retardation*, **107**, 212–221.

Kearney, P. M. & Griffin, T. (2001) Between joy and sorrow: being a parent of a child with developmental disability. *Journal of Advanced Nursing*, **34**, 582–592.

Kitzinger, J. (1995) Qualitative research. Introducing focus groups. *BMJ*, **311**, 299–302.

Kitzinger, J. & Barbour, R. S. (1999). Introduction: the challnege and promise of focus groups. In *Developing Focus Group Research* (eds J. Kitzinger & R. S. Barbour) pp. 1–20. London: Sage.

Kjellberg, A. (2002) More or less independent. *Disability and Rehabilitation*, **24**, 828–840.

Kreuger, R. A. (1994) *Focus Groups: A Practical Guide for Applied Research* (2nd edn). London: Sage.

Krinsky-McHale, S. J., Devenny, D. A. & Silverman, W. P. (2002) Changes in explicit memory associated with early dementia in adults with Down's syndrome. *Journal of Intellectual Disability Research*, **46**, 198–208.

Lehmann, J. P. & Roberto, K. A. (1996) Comparison of factors influencing mothers' perceptions about the futures of their adolescent children with and without disabilities. *Mental Retardation*, **34**, 27–38.

Lindop, E. & Read, S. (2000) District nurses' needs: palliative care for people with learning disability. *International Journal of Palliative Care Nursing*, **6**, 117–122.

Llewellyn, G. (1995) Relationships and social support: views of parents with mental retardation/intellectual disability. *Mental Retardation*, **33**, 349–363.

Llewellyn, G., Dunn, P., Fante, L. *et al* (1999) Family factors influencing out-of-home placement decisions. *Journal of Intellectual Disability Research*, **43**, 219–233.

Macaulay, A. C., Commanda, L. E., Freeman, W. L., *et al* (1999) Participatory research maximises community and lay involvement. North American Primary Care Research Group. *BMJ*, **319**, 774–778.

March, J., Steingol, B. & Justice, S. (1997) Follow the yellow brick road! People with learning difficulties as co-researchers. *British Journal of Learning Disabilities*, **25**, 77–80.

March, P. (1991) How do people with a mild/moderate mental handicap conceptualise physical illness and its cause? *British Journal of Mental Subnormality*, **37**, 80–91.

Marshall, D., Moore, G. & MacConkey, R. (2003) Integration and the healthcheck 2000 experience: Breaking through to better health for people with learning disabilities, in association with primary care. In *Learning Disabilities: A Handbook of Integrated Care* (ed. M. Brown) pp. 153–181. Salisbury: APS Publishing.

Matson, J. L. (1995) *The Diagnostic Assessment for the Severely Handicapped II*. Baton Rouge, LA: Scientific Publishers.

May, P. A. & Gossage, J. P. (2001) Estimating the prevalence of fetal alcohol syndrome. A summary. *Alcohol Research and Health*, **25**, 159–167.

McCracken, J. T., McGough, J., Shah, B., *et al* (2002) Risperidone in children with autism and serious behavioral problems. *New England Journal of Medicine*, **347**, 314–321.

Mervis, C. B. & Klein-Tasman, B. P. (2000) Williams syndrome: cognition, personality, and adaptive behavior. *Mental Retardation and Developmental Disabilities Research Reviews*, **6**, 148–158.

Mortimer, A. M. & Bowen, K. (1999) Measuring IQ in schizophrenia research: An update of the Quick Test in estimating IQ decline. *Cognitive Neuropsychiatry*, **4**, 81–88.

Muir, W. J. (2003) Genetics and ethics: the way forward. In *Learning Disabilities: A Handbook for Integrated Care* (ed. M. D. Brown) pp. 93–115. Salisbury: APS Publishing.

Muir, W. J. (2004) Learning disability. In *Companion to Psychiatric Studies* (eds E. C. Johnstone, C. P. L. Freeman, M. S. Sharpe *et al*), pp. 527–578. London: Harcourt Publishing.

Murphy, K. C. & Owen, M. J. (2001) Velo-cardio-facial syndrome: a model for understanding the genetics and pathogenesis of schizophrenia. *British Journal of Psychiatry*, **179**, 397–402.

Mutter, M., Binkert, F. & Schinzel, A. (2002) Down syndrome livebirth rate in the eastern part of Switzerland between 1980 and 1996 stays constant in spite of growing numbers of prenatally diagnosed and subsequently terminated cases. *Prenatal Diagnosis*, **22**, 835–836.

Nicholls, R. D. & Knepper, J. L. (2001) Genome organization, function, and imprinting in Prader–Willi and Angelman syndromes. *Annual Review of Genomics and Human Genetics*, **2**, 153–175.

Nihara, K., Leland, H. & Lambert, N. (1993) *AAMR Adaptive Behavior Scale–Residential and Community* (2nd edn) (ABS–RC;2). Austin, TX: Pro-Ed.

O'Brien, G. (ed.) (2002) *Behavioural Phenotypes in Clinical Practice*. London: MacKeith Press.

Oostra, B. A. & Willemsen, R. (2003) A fragile balance: FMR1 expression levels. *Human Molecular Genetics*, **12**, R249–257

Pope, C. & Mays, N. (1995) Reaching the parts other methods cannot reach: an introduction to qualitative methods in health and health services research. *BMJ*, **311**, 42–45.

Prosser, H., Moss, S., Costello, H., *et al* (1998) Reliability and validity of the Mini PAS–ADD for assessing psychiatric disorders in adults with intellectual disability. *Journal of Intellectual Disability Research*, **42**, 264–272.

Raven, J. C. (1998) *Raven's Standard Progressive Matrices*. London: Harcourt Assessment.

Reiss, S. & Valenti-Hein, D. (1994) Development of a psychopathology rating scale for children with mental retardation. *Journal of Consulting and Clinical Psychology*, **62**, 28–33.

Richardson, J. T. E. (ed.) (1996) *Handbook of Qualitative Research Methods*. Leicester, BPS Books.

Richardson, M. (2000) How we live: participatory research with six people with learning difficulties. *Journal of Advanced Nursing*, **32**, 1383–1395.

Rodgers, J. (1999) Trying to get it right: undertaking research involving people with LD. *Disability and Society*, **14**, 421–433.

Rogers, S. J., Wehner, D. E. & Hagerman, R. (2001) The behavioral phenotype in fragile X: symptoms of autism in very young children with fragile X syndrome, idiopathic autism, and other developmental disorders. *Journal of Developmental and Behavioral Pediatrics*, **22**, 409–417.

Roid, G. (2003) Stanford–Binet Intelligence Scales (5th edn) (SB5). Itasca, IL: Riverside Publishing.

Royal College of Psychiatrists (2001) *DC–LD: Diagnostic Criteria for Psychiatric Disorders for Use with Adults with Learning Disabilties/Mental Retardation* (Occasional Paper OP48). London: Gaskell.

Sanderson, T. L., Best, J. J., Doody, G. A., *et al* (1999) Neuroanatomy of comorbid schizophrenia and learning disability: a controlled study. *Lancet*, **354**, 1867–1871.

Saxton, J., McGonigle, K. L., Swihart, A. A., *et al* (1993) *Severe Impairment Battery*. Bury St Edmunds, Thames Valley Test Company.

Schalock, R. L. & Braddock, D. L. (eds) (1999) *Adaptive Behavior and its Measurement: Implications for the Field of Mental Retardation*. Washington, D.C.: American Association on Mental Retardation.

Senatore, V., Matson, J. L. & Kazdin, A. E. (1985) An inventory to assess psychopathology of mentally retarded adults. *American Journal of Mental Deficiency*, **89**, 459–466.

Shearn, J. & Todd, S. (1997) Parental work: an account of the day-to-day activities of parents of adults with learning disabilities. *Journal of Intellectual Disabilities Research*, **41**, 285–301.

Smith, J. A. (1996) Qualitative methodology: analysing participants' perspectives. *Current Opinion in Psychiatry*, **9**, 417–421.

Sparrow, S., Balla, D. & Cicchetti, D. (1984) *Vineland Adaptive Behavior Scales*. Circle Pines, MN: AGS Publishing.

Stalker, K. (1998) Some ethical and methodological issues in research with people with learning difficulties. *Disability and Society*, **13**, 5–19.

Stalker, K., Duckett, P. & Downs, M. (1999) *Going with the Flow: Choice, Dementia and People with Learning Difficulties*. Brighton: Pavilion Publishing/JRF.

Swain, J., Heyman, B. & Gillman, M. (1998) Research, private concerns: ethical issues in the use of open-ended interviews with people who have learning difficulties. *Disability and Society*, **13**, 21–36.

Tamm, L., Menon, V., Johnston, C. K., *et al* (2002). fMRI study of cognitive interference processing in females with fragile X syndrome. *Journal of Cognitive Neuroscience*, **14**, 160–171.

Tassabehji, M. (2003) Williams–Beuren syndrome: a challenge for genotype-phenotype correlations. *Human Molecular Genetics*, **12** (suppl. 2), R229–237.

Thornton, C. (1996) A focus group inquiry into the perceptions of primary health care teams and the provision of health care for adults with a learning disability living in the community. *Journal of Advanced Nursing*, **23**, 1168–1176.

Walmsley, J. & Johnson, K. (2003) *Inclusive Research with People with Learning Disabilities*. London: Jessica Kingsley.

Wechsler, D. (1999*a*) *Weschler Adult Intelligence Scale* (3rd revision) (WAIS–III UK). London: Psychological Corporation.

Wechsler, D. (1999*b*) *Weschler Abbreviated Scale of Intelligence*. London: Psychological Coroporation.

Wechsler, D. (2004) *Wechsler Pre-School and Primary Scale of Intelligence–Third UK Edition* (WPPSI–III UK). London: Psychological Corporation.

Whittaker, A. (1997) *Looking at Our Services: Service Evaluations by People with Learning Disabilities*. London: King's Fund Centre.

Williams, P. E., Weiss, L. G. & Rolfhus, E. (2003) *Wechsler Intelligence Scale for Children* (4th edn) (WISC–IV). San Antonio, TX: Psychological Corporation, Harcourt Assessment.

Wilson, B. A., Cockburn, J. & Baddeley, A. (2003) *The Rivermead Behavioural Memory Test* (2nd edn) (RBMT–II). Bury St Edmunds: Thames Valley Test Company.

Zarb, G. (1992) On the road to Damascus: first steps towards changing the relations of disability research production. *Disability, Handicap and Society*, **7**, 125–138.

Web links

Norah Fry – http://www.bris.ac.uk/Depts/NorahFry/PlainFacts/index.html
OMIM (Online Mendelian Inheritance in Man – http://www.ncbi.nlm.nih.gov/omim/
ISI, Institute for Scientific Information (2003) Journal Citation Reports (Thomson ISI) – http://www.wok.mimas.ac.uk

CHAPTER 14

Research in psychotherapy

Chris Freeman and Yvonne Edmonstone

Starting out in research can be overwhelming and the idea of beginning that research in the field of psychotherapy can be especially daunting – particularly if only the potential difficulties are considered. This chapter provides an introductory overview and considers both the potential difficulties and advantages. Hopefully, it will convince the reader that there is much to be gained from tackling research in psychotherapy.

Why attempt research in psychotherapy

First, although the debate regarding the existence of significant benefits from specific psychotherapeutic treatments continues (Shepherd, 1984; Bloch & Lambert, 1985), simple clinical curiosity suggests that finding out what is effective and how it is effective is worthwhile. Second, overcoming the particular difficulties inherent in psychotherapy research has led to the development of many techniques that could be carried over into other fields. Acquiring some expertise in these techniques might thus provide wider benefits.

What are the potential difficulties?

Potential difficulties in psychotherapy research are shown in Box 14.1.

Defining psychotherapy treatments

With the wide range of different treatments covered by the term 'psychotherapy', it is essential to be able to define specific treatments precisely if efficacy is to be compared. Moreover, the desired outcome of these treatments is similarly diverse. Consideration of broad categories of treatment, such as behavioural v. psychoanalytic therapy, exemplifies the many differences involved. The behaviour therapist may be looking for changes in behaviour, which can be readily observed, as the desired outcome, but the psychoanalyst may focus on more subtle internal changes. Research in psychotherapy must therefore begin by defining which particular form of psychotherapy is being considered.

It is also necessary to look at how treatment is being delivered. Treatments administered must be consistent between therapists, between sessions and between patients if worthwhile evaluations are to be possible. Only with such consistency can outcome be related to the treatment given rather than to non-specific variables.

These problems can be overcome to a certain extent by the use of treatment manuals, for example *Cognitive Therapy in Depression* (Beck *et al*, 1979). Therapists can then be trained in the techniques as detailed in the manual. Analysis of recorded sessions can be used to assess therapists' adherence to the techniques specified – for instance, using groups of observers to rate video recordings of sessions for therapist competence. When different treatments are being compared, it is obviously important that raters are masked as to the initial treatment intentions.

The level of expertise demonstrated by therapists in relation to the outcome achieved might also need to be considered. When comparing similar patients treated by either lay counsellors or trained therapists, Strupp & Hadley (1979) found no quantitative differences in the outcomes. Strupp (1980) suggested, however, that there may be qualitative differences in the performances of the lay counsellors and trained therapists that are obscured by group comparisons. Detailed analysis of an individual counsellor's 'successful treatment' *v*. 'failed treatment' cases, for example, illustrated some difficulties experienced in dealing with transference issues. These studies still failed to find any significant differences in outcome or to clearly define what the 'qualitative differences' might be.

Such difficulties are many times more complex than the problems encountered in drug treatment studies – consistency in prescribing a particular drug at a particular dose by different practitioners, whatever their experience, is more easily achieved than consistency in administering a particular psychotherapy treatment. It is also considerably easier to ascertain whether the treatment has been administered and complied with by monitoring returned tablets, or blood or urine levels of drug or metabolite.

Specific methods

The use of treatment manuals and the rating of therapeutic competence in recorded sessions can help to ensure that the treatments being provided under the one heading are as near identical as possible. These issues are particularly important when attempts to evaluate actual clinical practice are made. Controlled prospective research trials tend to use experienced clinicians practising in their own fields; just how this compares with what is being given under the same treatment headings at a routine clinical level merits further consideration. There is much potential for the further development of evaluation methods and in using them at a clinical level. There is considerable scope in this area for the trainee involved in research.

Controls in psychotherapy

Establishing control or placebo groups in psychotherapy research may require more sophisticated techniques than establishing the equivalent placebo or non-treatment group for a drug trial. Consider an investigation (Fig. 14.1) where symptom measures taken before and after treatment show some improvement. Simplistically, the improvement could be considered the result of the treatment – however, there are obviously alternative

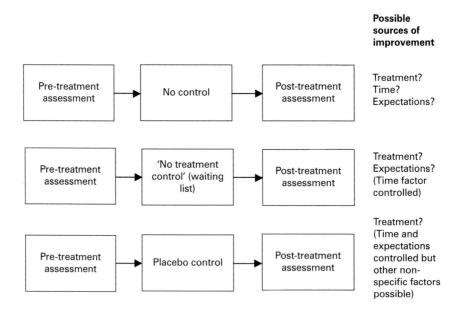

Fig. 14.1 The elimination of possible explanations for the success of a treatment through three experimental designs.

explanations! Perhaps the symptoms were naturally fluctuating or have 'spontaneously remitted' with time, independently of the treatment received? Perhaps the belief that the treatment given would be effective was sufficient to persuade patients to report improvement?

Attempts to eliminate these possible alternative explanations have led to the design of 'no-treatment groups' and 'placebo-treatment groups' as controls. However, unlike pharmacological trials where a drug can be withheld completely or a non-active alternative administered, 'no-treatment' or 'placebo treatment' is more difficult to provide in psychotherapy; however, various strategies have been used.

One possible design to create 'no-treatment controls' is to use those on a waiting list for treatment. All patients then have an initial assessment interview before being placed randomly in either the treatment or waiting-list group. Follow-up assessments then compare any improvements achieved with treatment with any improvements in the waiting-list group.

The difficulties with 'no-treatment' control groups in psychotherapy lie in the fact that the initial pre-trial assessment interviews or explanations given to patients for ethical reasons may in themselves be therapeutic. Extensive assessment interviews might have much in common with the initial stages of treatment. Malan et al (1975) showed that some significant changes can occur in patients after only an initial contact with practitioners. It appears that even placing patients on a waiting list may instil some hope!

To allow changes in the treatment group to be compared with those in the 'no-treatment' control group, the two groups must be similar in their composition, i.e. both the included individuals and their circumstances must be comparable. This is achieved by randomly assigning patients from the same source population initially to each group.

Using a placebo control in drug research studies involves administering a pharmacologically inert substance usually in a triple-blind design, i.e. neither the patient, the prescriber nor the outcome evaluator knows whether the substance given is the active one or not. Attempting to develop equivalent placebo controls in psychotherapy is difficult, because neither the patient nor the therapist can remain ignorant of the treatment. It is also likely that both will have their own opinions and expectations. Similarly, progress assessments run the risk of being contaminated by information gleaned about the treatment from the patients' accounts of their experiences.

Various strategies have been used to create 'no-treatment groups' (Prioleau et al, 1983). For example, the patient may be involved in periods of discussion where the therapist explicitly attempts to direct the patient's conversation towards topics that are assumed to be irrelevant to the psychological problems that had led the patient to be offered psychotherapy. Such a placebo treatment attempts to control for variables such as duration of treatment, meeting regularly with a therapist and having the opportunity to engage in conversation in a particular setting. However, it is still possible that these discussions, even though they do not focus on specific problems, still contain some of the elements of psychotherapy that contribute to its success.

Other researchers have tried to use recreational time spent with the therapist, for example watching videos together or performing simple cognitive tasks, as a control. It is difficult, however, to design controls that remove non-specific factors but still maintain face validity with the patient.

Similar difficulties to those described with 'no-treatment' control groups occur with 'placebo' control groups, in that encouraging expectations of positive outcome or instilling hope probably contributes to effectiveness of treatment – but to withhold it in placebo treatments would again decrease their credibility.

Unfortunately, distinguishing specific treatment factors from non-specific treatment factors is not easily achieved. Attempts to overcome these problems have led to the design of trials comparing one or more active treatments with or without placebo controls (Basham, 1986). The rationale of these designs is that all therapies will have similar non-specific treatment factors, so comparing them directly will remove the need for a placebo control (Fig. 14.2).

A further advantage of these designs is that they more closely mirror clinical practice where the clinician is likely to be faced with the choice of which treatment to give, rather than the choice of whether to give treatment or to withhold it. Things are also made easier from an ethical viewpoint because all patients are being offered some form of treatment. There are many examples of comparative outcome studies in the literature (e.g. Shapiro & Firth, 1987).

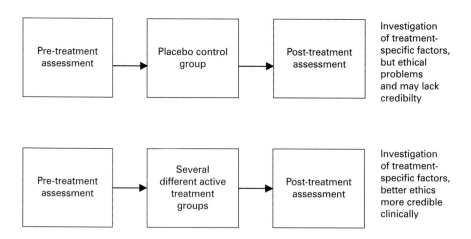

Fig. 14.2 Comparison of active treatments with or without placebo control groups.

Another non-specific factor that it is difficult to make allowances for in study design is investigator bias. Evidence suggests that the attitudes of the investigators do influence outcome. Enthusiasm by what are now called 'product champions' may positively bias the outcome results (Rosenthal & Frank, 1956).

This may explain why some new psychotherapy methods appear to show better results in early studies published by their originators, compared with the less impressive results produced when they are studied by workers without the same allegiance to the method. Masked assessments of outcome and independent replication of studies can help to remove this bias.

When replication studies show less impressive outcome results than the original studies, supporters of specific therapeutic techniques may argue that the difference can be accounted for by lack of therapist training and expertise. However, if the skills used to obtain the results achieved in research are not within the relatively easy reach of the practising clinical psychiatrist, then their usefulness must be questioned.

Power and sample size

Many of the methodological problems faced in psychotherapy research are akin to those found in other branches of psychiatry (see Chapter 8). One particular problem that merits further expansion in this chapter is the statistical power of design, i.e. the probability of rejecting the null hypothesis when it is false or the likelihood of detecting any existing differences. This will depend on the size of the difference being looked for and the number of members in each of the different groups.

In psychotherapy research, even when therapy is compared with no-treatment or waiting-list controls, the magnitude of the placebo response can be quite high, and detecting any differences in outcome requires sufficient numbers in each group. More often, however, comparisons are made between two or more different treatments. Differences in outcome between such groups are likely to be much smaller, and much larger groups will then be needed if these differences are to be detected. For example, a difference of one-third of a standard deviation between mean outcome of one group compared with mean outcome of the other group would require around 150 members in each group for difference to be detected (Donner, 1984). Numbers may need to be further increased to allow for missing data that would ultimately reduce the available sample size.

Very few, if any, of the published studies in psychotherapy research have adequate sample size to detect the differences being looked for. This has led to an upsurge of interest in meta-analysis in an attempt to detect any outcome differences that would otherwise have been missed.

It is important that these 'power issues' are considered from the outset of any proposed research project in psychotherapy, to prevent meaningless 'no difference detectable' results being produced inadvertently.

The larger numbers needed for such comparative outcome studies may be prohibitive to the trainee, but they should not squash any enthusiasm for doing research in psychotherapy. Instead, it is important to remember that there are other methods available, some of which will be looked at in more detail later in this chapter.

Measurements of outcome

Specific rating scales suitable for use in psychotherapy are discussed in Chapter 11, therefore this chapter will consider only the general principles and problems of measurement in psychotherapy research.

Differences looked for in psychotherapy may be small and even with large groups may be missed if the measures chosen are not sufficiently sensitive. They must be sufficiently specific to the problems being treated and relevant to the treatment goals.

Different outcome measures applied to the same clients with the same treatments may yield quite different results. Outcome assessments should, therefore, include several different measures. Some of the dimensions that need to be considered are summarised in Fig. 14.3. – they are discussed in greater detail by Waskow & Parloff (1975).

It is important to choose measures that will most accurately reflect the effects of the treatment that are considered to be most relevant. Different

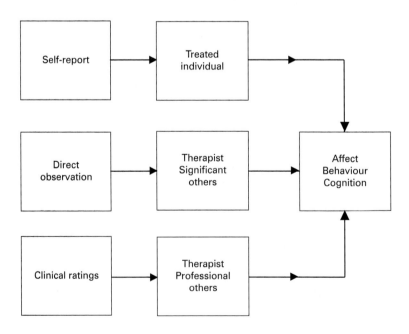

Fig. 14.3 The evaluation of outcome.

values may be given to different aspects of outcome in different treatments (e.g. the outcome looked for by an analytic psychotherapist may be very different from that looked for by a behavioural therapist).

The effectiveness of a treatment method should, ideally, be measured by the extent to which it meets its objectives. However, many of the objectives in psychotherapy have a tendency to be ill defined. Stating that the objective of a particular psychotherapy is 'personal growth', 'transformation', or 'self-actualisation', without ever saying how these might be measured, makes recording accurately whether they have been attained or not very difficult. Outcome measures in psychotherapy may be looking at psychodynamic change, symptom relief, social adaptation or a combination of these.

It has been suggested (Mintz, 1981) that if a patient's initial symptoms do not improve, then treatment has not been successful. Also, if these symptoms do improve, then dynamic and symptomatic assessments converge. However, Malan et al (1968) argued that dynamic assessment must be based on an understanding of the underlying condition and not on the behavioural manifestations alone. Dynamic assessment depends on the judgement of an expert clinician and the formulation of dynamically based measures of improvement that can be independently rated.

Assessing the outcome of behavioural models of psychotherapy may involve the use of more direct outcome measures, such as recording the frequency of symptomatic behaviour either by observer or self-report measures such as patient diaries. The Yale–Brown Obsessive Compulsive Scale (YBOCS; Goodman et al, 1989), which is used to measure change in obsessive–compulsive disorders, is an example of how the time taken up with symptomatic behaviours (obsessive thinking and compulsive rituals) can be measured. It also rates resistance control, distress and secondary avoidance.

The measures chosen to assess outcome in psychotherapy must then be capable of accurately measuring the specific outcome variables, including symptom relief and behavioural changes where applicable. Failure to use appropriate measures to specifically evaluate each treatment being considered in comparative studies may lead to specific differences in outcome being missed and only general similarities being reported.

The timing of outcome studies is also important. It has been argued that long-term follow-up may not be necessary for evaluating psychotherapy (Nicholson & Berman, 1983) because results obtained are generally similar to those in short-term follow-up. However, in principle, outcome research should attempt to address the question of whether or not benefits are maintained. Obtaining long-term data can, however, be a costly and time-consuming exercise. There will always be some treated individuals who are lost to follow-up and some long-term outcomes that are affected by additional treatment received after the study treatment has ended (Malan et al, 1976).

So-called hard measures of outcome are becoming increasingly popular in research. Measures must be clearly definable and measurable; for example, weight gain, change in menstrual function, or salivary amylase levels in treatment outcome studies of bulimia or anorexia nervosa (Fairburn *et al*, 1986). Individual variance must still be considered.

Generalisability of results

Whether or not results achieved in any study can be replicated in clinical practice is a central issue in all psychotherapy research. If results are to be accepted and utilised clinically, the group studied must be representative of the target clinical population and the settings, timings and method used must have clinical equivalents.

Study groups tend to be 'diagnostically neater' than clinical populations where 'boundaries of caseness' may be less distinct. Other difficulties may arise when therapists have different levels of skills and the motives and attitudes to treatment of study participants are different from those of attending clinics. Studies that report statistically significant differences in outcome may be impressive but it is important that they can be applied in the clinic if the real value of the difference is to be appreciated. Always bear in mind that the clinical significance of results may be very different to their statistical significance!

Which methods are used ?

This chapter has looked at five different groups of recurring difficulties inherent in psychotherapy research and at ways of overcoming them. Most of these difficulties have been described in relation to outcome research, but, as mentioned, there are other methods that may be more accessible to the trainee. Some basic principles of outcome research, single-patient studies, process research and meta-analysis will now be considered.

Outcome research

Outcome research sets out to answer the simple but important questions of 'what works ?' and 'which works better ?'. In psychotherapy research the most common designs are pre–post treatment comparison, no-treatment control, placebo control and comparative-treatment outcomes (Box 14.2).

The treatment being studied can be considered as 'whole treatment packages' or divided into separate treatment components. The whole treatment approach has most in common with clinical practice. It does not, however, give any indication of which aspects of treatment have been the most beneficial.

Dividing the treatment into specific components allows all or part of the treatment to be given and the results to be compared. The timing of outcome measures is important. This has allowed for simplification of some treatments for example, in behavioural therapy. Unfortunately, it is

> **Box 14.2** The most common designs in psychotherapy research
>
> - Pre–post treatment comparison
> - No-treatment control
> - Placebo control
> - Comparative-treatment outcomes.

more difficult to use this technique in other types of psychotherapy research because components such as empathy, although easily conceptualised, are difficult to eliminate in practical terms.

Alternatively, treatments can be added on sequentially to each other (e.g. Weissman, 1979). Attempts have also been made to further refine treatments by giving varying 'degrees of treatment' (e.g. intensity) and duration or number of sessions (Shapiro *et al*, 1990).

Efficacy *v.* effectiveness

The term 'effectiveness research' is used to describe outcome investigations that measure the impact of treatment in a routine clinical or naturalist setting. In contrast, efficacy research might be described as 'laboratory-based' experiments. Efficacy research is usually carried out by specially constructed research groups working in an academic environment with selected groups of patients and often specially trained therapists. Most of the evidence we use to guide us clinically is currently efficacy rather than effectiveness based.

Those studies that have compared the two, usually (but not always) show a greater impact for efficacy-based studies. There may be many reasons for this, including clinical samples having more severe problems, less selection and screening in clinical samples, higher drop-out rates and lower levels of motivation for treatment in clinical samples.

One of the important issues for the trainee considering areas of psychotherapy research is that effectiveness studies do not necessarily need to meet the requirements of a randomised controlled trial and need to be carried out locally. The factors that produce the difference, if any, between efficacy and effectiveness may be unique to a particular clinical situation, and quite different ones may operate in other clinical settings.

Single-patient research

Single-patient research provides perhaps a more viable option for the trainee than many larger-scale outcome studies. If carried out correctly it can provide worthwhile scientific data without the need for studies with large cohorts, extensive time or financial commitment of the researcher, or complicated statistics. It should not, however, be seen as simply writing up a case report. There are basic principles to be followed if the results produced are to be worthwhile and informative. The question to be answered must be clearly defined, the measures to be used specifically chosen, and the clinical interventions carefully construed.

Single-patient studies are most obviously applicable to behavioural research and much of the existing literature is in the field of applied behavioural research (Barlow & Hersen, 1973). However, the techniques used have been applied to other disciplines (Peck, 1985).

One of the main advantages of single-patient research is that it can be carried out by the practitioner working in their usual clinical environment. It allows the clinician to attempt to answer questions about their patient, the treatment being administered and the effects of the treatment immediately and in the long term. The main issues in single-patient research are described in Box 14.3.

Methods in single-patient research have been discussed in Chapter 7, so only a few basic principles will discussed here. First, only one patient is being considered. Variability within this individual and its possible correlation with treatment is being investigated.

A stable baseline is normally established before initiating any changes and measuring their effect. Longer baseline assessment times with multiple measures increase the clinician's confidence that there is some stability before any changes observed and that subsequent variations are a result of treatment.

Measures chosen must be scaled to the individual – for example counting frequencies of target behaviours. These measurements will then constitute the main outcome measures in the single-patient study. More general measures such as 'depression' are also of value in generalising the results of the individual to a wider group. Using standardised measurements allows

---

Box 14.3 The main issues in single-patient research

- The problem
    - Precipitating factors?
    - Perpetuating factors?
    - Presentation factors?
- The treatment
    - Is there any improvement?
    - Is it a result of specific or non-specific treatment factors?
    - Is one treatment more effective than another?
- The theory
    - Was the original hypothesis correct?
    - Was the treatment effective for other reasons?

the individual's presentation to be classified. It can then be compared with the presentation of others in homogeneous groups, for example with similar pathology.

Experimental designs for single-patient research generally take one of two forms – either ABA type designs or multiple baseline designs (see Chapter 7).

In summary, single-patient studies offer the chance to scientifically evaluate individual variation and treatment effects. They are particularly applicable to research in behavioural psychotherapy. With careful planning they are well within the capabilities of any trainee interested in research in psychotherapy.

Process research

When looking at the methods of outcome studies, it was noted that information regarding differences in types of psychotherapy might not be detected unless suitably large numbers of patients were studied (Kazdin, 1986). Fortunately, using some of the methods available to study the process of psychotherapy more directly may overcome some of these problems. Detailed analysis of process may answer questions about the underlying process of change which would be obscured in larger outcome studies giving treatment-equivalent results.

There are several methods that allow the components of the therapeutic process in psychotherapy, such as relationship variables, to be carefully studied. Instead of looking at the final outcome of any therapeutic effort, process research concentrates on what is actually happening between an individual patient and therapist during therapy. The main emphasis in process research is on changes in patient behaviour at points during the therapy, not as in outcome research where measures are compared before and after therapy. Process research measures can be both qualitative and quantitative.

Designs using only qualitative measures should not be considered second rate, for in some instances it is more appropriate to collect and consider data qualitatively before any attempt is made to quantify them. In qualitative research it is almost always necessary to use more than one source of data. Any conclusion reached will be more secure if it is backed up by multiple measures, including direct and indirect assessments, objective records and personal accounts, and material from both the participant and observers (Campbell & Fiske, 1959). Investigators must consider which combination of data sources will be the most feasible to use and which will give them maximum confidence in their conclusions.

Special care must be taken by the researcher to consider their personal connection to what is being studied. Psychological interactions need to be understood, but impartiality and commitment to unbiased evaluation must be maintained. Examples of qualitative methods used in process research are qualitative analysis of conversation and account analysis.

Qualitative analysis of conversation can be used to review an individual psychotherapeutic interview (Labou & Fanshel, 1977). Here a description and explanation of the particulars of psychotherapeutic exchange, as well as the more general rules of conversation and the procedures upon which it is built, are sought.

In account analysis, observations of behaviour are supplemented by analyses of individual's accounts of their behaviour (Kraut & Lewis, 1982). This can be extended to look at areas of social interaction. A technique called 'interpersonal process recall' (IPR) has been developed (Kagan, 1984; Barker, 1985) in which a videotape of a specific interaction is replayed to the patient and therapist. The researcher stops the tape frequently to ask the participants for their thoughts and feelings at that point. This technique can yield interesting research data which may show that the perspectives of client and therapist on a single event can be very different (Caskey *et al*, 1984). Potential problems with this method are that it may interfere with therapy and may not accurately reflect the experiences occurring in the actual session. Nevertheless, it does keep the emphasis on direct experiences of the therapeutic process itself and has uses in teaching as well as in research.

Ideally, all process research should consider the perspectives of both therapist and patient, since these can be very different, before, during and after treatment.

The second group of process research methods are quantitative. These allow intensive clinical research which aims to look in depth at the processes of change and interaction in psychotherapy. These methods make use of a rich database derived from repeated and/or multiple empirical measures and statistical analysis of the results.

Quantitative data, like their qualitative equivalents, can be collected by either self-report or observer-rated methods – both have their advantages and problems. Self-report measures emphasise the individual's own account of their psychological state by considering their perceptions, attitudes and feelings. Self-report measures range from unstructured interviews and narrative analysis through to more formalised methods, such as the repertory grid analysis (Kelly, 1985) where the patient is provided with a systematised structure but provides its unique content themself. Self-report measures have the advantages of being flexible and having high personal validity, allowing the participating individuals to express their thoughts and feelings in their own words. They also allow some clinical problems that could not otherwise be easily approached, such as obsessional or paranoid thoughts, to be measured. The main disadvantages are the difficulties in demonstrating any causal relationship between such measures and actual behaviour, and in trying to assess long-term validity.

Observational measures focus from the outside upon the patient's behaviour. They are used mainly to assess behaviour and to monitor behavioural change. Typical observational measures include counts of behaviour frequency, magnitude, intensity or duration and the use of ratings or checklists used by observers. The unit of observation must be meaningful and reliably identifiable. The sampling procedures used must be sufficient to ensure that the types of behaviour being measured do take place during the observations (i.e. the lower the frequency of the behaviour, the more vigilant the observations must be). Problems arise from the fact that the knowledge of being observed might itself influence the behaviour being exhibited. Similarly, observers' reports may be influenced by a knowledge of the results expected. A wide range of application is possible for both self-report and observer-rated measures used individually or in combination (Elliot *et al*, 1985).

Shapiro's Personal Questionnaire is an example of a self-report method that has been used by a number of people to study changes during psychotherapy. It has been specifically designed to facilitate repeated measures over brief periods of time. Using the Personal Questionnaire, Shapiro reported an immediate improvement effect in therapy as rated by the client after behavioural therapy (Shapiro, 1969). However, when a more interpretative approach was used, clear deteriorations were found during psychotherapy using the Personal Questionnaire (Shapiro & Hobson, 1972). It was suggested then that interpretative therapy may be stressful to the patient in the short term but provide long-term benefit.

Further studies using the Personal Questionnaire have attempted to look in detail at specific variables within the therapeutic relationship (e.g. Parry *et al*, 1986). Therapist and patient factors have been extensively studied. Truax & Carkhuff (1967), in their studies on client-centred therapy, suggested that accurate empathy, unconditional positive regard, and genuineness are related to positive outcome – however, they suggested that these were not reliably measured.

The interpersonal context can be focused on further by investigating the 'mutual interactions' or 'inter-expectations' of participants using quantitative methods; again either self-report or observer-rated measures may be used. For instance, the process of 'empathy' can be operantly defined as the extent to which one participant can predict the views or psychological framework of the other. This can again be looked at using repertory grid methods (Ryle & Breen, 1972) or patient and therapist Personal Questionnaire ratings (Shapiro & Post, 1974).

Perhaps the best known example of this type of method is the Interpersonal Perception Method (IPM; Laing *et al*, 1966). This looks at key relationship issues and rates them in terms of agreement, understanding and realisation for each individual. It has been used extensively to investigate marital therapy (Laing *et al*, 1966) and to study changes in the client–therapist relationship during psychotherapy.

Elliot *et al* (1985) have thoroughly investigated the process of change in psychotherapy using quantitative methods. They linked self-report and observational techniques to develop a 'discovery-orientated approach' which is based on the following assumptions:

- psychotherapy process research starts with patient and therapist experiences and perceptions
- it should focus upon significant change events
- these should be studied closely and comprehensively since significant events are infrequent and complex.

Essentially Elliot *et al* attempted to identify significant change events in therapy and to link these to the participant's subjective experiences. They incorporated the IPR techniques of Kagan (1984) and extended these further into comprehensive process analysis. In this analysis a significant event identified by IPR is categorised on multiple quantitative and qualitative measures that assess five aspects of the therapeutic process. These are content, action, style, state-experience and quality. The behaviour of both therapist and patient is analysed and ratings are made by them and by a group of observers. The research group attempts to come to some agreement about plausible mechanisms by which antecedent factors could lead to events before and within a session. These possible mechanisms of change are then looked at in relation to the clinical experience of the group and the individual experiences of the therapist and patient. The use and further development of these techniques may provide an opportunity to clarify important elements in the process of psychotherapy (Rice & Greenberg, 1984). There is much scope for the trainee to become involved in process research.

In today's clinical climate where 'audit' is a keyword, studies looking at what is being provided under the cover of psychotherapy, and how it is being provided, are likely to be given due consideration. Elements that might be given more consideration on a clinical level are therapist variables in terms of expertise and style, frequency of sessions, utilisation of 'between-session patient task-setting' and patient self-monitoring techniques, duration of therapy and appropriate measures of outcome.

Meta-analysis

Meta-analysis is a technique, derived from empirical social science, which is used in an attempt to make sense of existing outcome research in psychotherapy. It is a quantitative rather than qualitative approach.

In the past, traditional reviews of outcome research of mental health treatments, particularly psychotherapy, have differed in their conclusions. Clear guidance for future practice, training and research can only be provided when some agreement is reached. Traditional reviews have been descriptive in style and qualitatively orientated and too many interpretative comments are made. Studies may be excluded from reviews because they are believed to have poor methods; no account is then taken of their findings. The normal format of such reviews is for studies with common characteristics to be grouped together and results of such groups to be described and presented qualitatively. Links between study features and outcomes may be suggested.

Results are often presented in the format of a 'box score' total. Here the number of statistically significant (or positive) findings and statistically non-significant (or null) findings are tallied. Problems occur when results do not attain statistical significance because of inadequate statistical power. An example of such a traditional style review is that of Luborsky *et al* (1975), which cited positive outcome results for psychotherapy. An early example of the use of meta-analysis in psychotherapy research is the review of psychotherapy outcome studies by Smith & Glass (1977).

Meta-analysis attempts to cover, or at least be representative of, all of the existing studies of the topic being reviewed. Sampling procedures are used, in a replicable manner, to obtain a sample of studies from the total number. The quality of the study is considered (also quantitatively) rather than excluding studies evaluated as having poor methods. Each study included is given a score for its methods and these scores are later correlated with the study findings. Other components of each study are dealt with similarly. Generalisations can then be made across studies rather than describing each study individually as in the traditional review. For instance, the literature can be described in terms of such parameters as the types of patients treated, the treatments given and the instruments used to measure outcome.

Quantitative generalisations can also be made about study outcomes. There are several different statistical techniques employed to do this. The most common approach is to measure the effect size, whereby the difference between group means is expressed in standard deviation units. Another method is to test the null hypotheses of no treatment differences across studies by combining the probabilities obtained in each study.

Other methods have been reported. What they all share is the ability to preserve more information about the magnitude of effects obtained in each study than traditional 'box scores'.

Meta-analysis also allows for statistical analysis of components of studies other than outcome. For instance, more complex questions such as outcome predictors can be approached. A summary of the differences between traditional style reviews and meta-analysis is given in Table 14.1 and is discussed further by Shapiro (1983).

Despite its critics (Shepherd, 1984), meta-analysis has become increasingly popular and widely used. It should not, however, be seen as an easy alternative to the 'hands-on approach', but should be used carefully with appropriate consideration to conclusions reached. The researcher should bear in mind the existence of meta-analysis when contemplating how the results of their own work might later be compared with that of others.

Useful resources

There are several books which no psychotherapy researcher should be without. These include the first and second editions of *What Works for Whom? A Critical Review of Psychotherapy Research* (Roth & Fonagy, 1996,

Table 14.1 Differences between traditional style reviews and meta-analysis

Traditional review	Meta-analysis
Qualitative	Quantitative
Selective coverage	More representative coverage
Studies with poor methodology excluded	All levels of methodology evaluated
Studies described individually	Studies described by general features
Narrative statements made about study features, findings and outcome	Quantitative statements using systematised coding used to describe study features, findings and outcome
Results concern only statistically significant outcomes	Magnitude of effects considered
'Box score' tabulation of results – qualitative description of findings and discussion of results	Large and varied data-sets Statistical analysis of results

2005) and *What Works for Whom? A Critical Review of Treatments for Children and Adolescents* (Fonagy *et al*, 2002).

The first edition of *What Works for Whom? A Critical Review of Psychotherapy Research* was based on a large commissioned review of psychological therapies research funded by the UK Department of Health in 1994. The second edition reviews the studies published from then through until the end of 2003. These are very comprehensive reviews covering the efficacy of psychotherapy in nearly all the areas it has been tested. Chapter 2 of the second edition (Research and practice) is a comprehensive review of the methodological considerations that the authors used while conducting their review. Chapter 1 of *What Works for Whom? A Critical Review of Treatments for Children and Adolescents* (Introduction and review of outcome methodology) covers some of the same ground, but has a more extensive comparison of psychotherapy and drug studies and a detailed review of the limitations of meta-analysis.

The reviews in these volumes are not made redundant by the guidelines that are now regularly produced by the National Institute for Clinical Excellence (NICE). The methodology used in the two review processes is somewhat different and NICE excludes many studies that are reviewed by Fonagy & Roth. Evidence-based reviews from NICE are now available for many areas relevant to psychological therapies research, including computerised treatments: depression, post-traumatic stress disorder and obsessive–compulsive disorder.

The Bibles of psychotherapy

Bergin and Garfield's Handbook of Psychotherapy and Behavior Change is now in its fifth edition (Lambert, 2004). This is an invaluable books for the budding psychotherapy researcher. Each edition complements the one before. In each edition there is an update on the major approaches in psychotherapy, but the section on research application in special groups and settings differs from edition to edition. What is most important about these books is that they do not just concentrate on outcome research, they review the research on process in psychotherapy, therapist variables and patient variables.

Relevant studies

This chapter has tried to present both the attractions and the difficulties of research in psychotherapy. To conclude, a brief outline of four relevant studies will be given, looking particularly at the methods used. Consideration of the difficulties inherent in each study and how these were overcome will be made. Examples from four different types of psychotherapy have been chosen: individual behavioural therapy, individual dynamic therapy, group therapy and family therapy.

The fourth study has been included to illustrate how small studies may be more feasible for the trainee – it has also been chosen to illustrate some of the problems that may be encountered in such studies.

National Institute of Mental Health Treatment of Depression Collaborative Research Program (Elkin et al, 1989)

Aims

The American National Institute of Mental Health (NIMH) compared the effectiveness of two brief psychotherapies (interpersonal psychotherapy and cognitive–behavioural therapy (CBT)) with pharmacotherapy (imipramine) plus clinical management and placebo plus clinical management. Its aims were to test the feasibility and value of the collaborative clinical trial model in the area of psychotherapy and to study, within this research model, the effectiveness of two specific forms of psychotherapy for treating non-bipolar, non-psychotic out-patients with depression.

Definition

Treatments were specified in manual form. Training and supervision were given by experts in the respective fields. Treatment integrity was assessed during and at the end of the study. Treatment sessions were videotaped and rated by trainers who were unaware of the groups and clinical experts who were not directly involved in the study.

Controls

The inclusion of a 'psychotherapy placebo' was originally considered. This was rejected for various reasons. It was considered that if the proposed control conditions were far removed from actual treatment, ethical and plausibility questions would be raised, but if the control did meet ethical and plausibility questions, it would constitute a new treatment in its own right! Instead, imipramine with clinical management, considered a proven effective treatment for depression, was used as a reference treatment condition with which to compare the two psychotherapies. Comparison was also made with placebo with clinical management to establish the efficacy of imipramine used in the study conditions and as a partial control condition against which to compare the psychotherapies. The clinical management component approximated a 'minimal supportive therapy' condition and the placebo served as a control both for expectations due to administration of a drug and for contact with a caring supportive therapist.

Power

A power analysis was used to determine the sample size required. The 250 patients were randomly assigned to the four treatment groups. This allowed the differences in pairs of treatments to be detected. However, numbers were not large enough when treatment groups were further divided on the basis of initial symptom severity to detect differences between all treatment interactions.

Outcome measures

Patients were assessed before, during and at termination of treatment, and at 6-, 12- and 18-month follow-up. Assessments were made from several different perspectives: the patient, the therapist, an independent clinical evaluator (unaware of the treatment given) and, whenever possible, a person significant in the patient's life. Measures used from the perspective of the clinical evaluator were the Hamilton Rating Scale for Depression (HRSD; Hamilton, 1960) and the Global Assessment Scale (GAS; Endicott *et al*, 1976), and from the perspective of the patient, the Beck Depression Inventory (BDI; Beck *et al*, 1961) and the Hopkins Symptom Checklist (HSC; Parloff *et al*, 1954).

Generalisability

In this study, each collaborating investigator at three different centres adopted standardised measures for describing and assessing the problem being treated, the characteristics of the treatment interventions, and the nature, rapidity and durability of patient change. This has the advantage of providing a form of immediate replication and makes it possible to test the generalisability of findings across research sites. Generalisations cannot, however, be made beyond the specific patient sample considered, i.e. non-psychotic, non-bipolar, out-patients meeting criteria for a major depressive disorder.

Results

Patients in all four treatment groups showed significant improvements. Imipramine with clinical management was the most effective, placebo with clinical management the least, with the two psychotherapies in between, but generally closer in efficacy to imipramine with clinical management. Patients who were most severely impaired responded much better to imipramine with clinical management, moderately to the two psychotherapies and poorly to placebo with clinical management. Among the patients with less severe illness there was a suggestion that general support may in itself be helpful.

Evaluation of family therapy in anorexia nervosa and bulimia nervosa (Russell et al, 1987)

Aims

This study assessed the efficacy of family therapy in a series of patients with anorexia nervosa and another series with bulimia nervosa. The study consisted of a controlled trial of family therapy compared with a less specific and supportive form of individual supportive therapy.

Definition

All four therapists involved had received equal training in both family and individual psychotherapy. Each treatment was supervised by an expert in each field, with group supervision looking at videotapes of sessions to ensure that the stated forms of therapy were adhered to.

Controls

To allow for possible variations in the experience, skills and enthusiasm of the four therapists involved, each carried out both forms of therapy. The individual therapy was devised as the control therapy. It was not a formal psychoanalytic psychotherapy but was supportive, educational and problem-centred. Patients were randomly allocated to family therapy or control treatment so as to obtain two patient populations that were matched for the type of illness, age at onset and duration of illness (i.e. factors related to severity and prognosis).

Power

A total of 80 patients (57 with anorexia nervosa and 23 with bulimia nervosa), all of whom had been admitted to a specialist unit for weight restoration, were considered. They were divided into four groups based on the factors outlined above before random allocation to treatment. This procedure carried the disadvantage of relatively small numbers of patients within each subgroup. Numbers were reduced further by early drop-outs; however, no alteration in the direction of the main findings was noted when results were reanalysed to include drop-outs.

Outcome measures

The following measures were used to assess the patients when they were first admitted to hospital, before discharge and at the 1-year follow-up visit:

1   the Morgan and Russell Scales for Anorexia Nervosa (Morgan & Russell, 1975) with adaptations for bulimia nervosa; information from patient and informant, if possible, gauging nutritional state (weight),

menstrual function, mental state, psychosexual adjustment and socio-economic status;

2   need for readmission to hospital;

3   the Crown–Crisp Experiential Index (Crown & Crisp, 1979) which includes measures of depression and obsessionality.

Generalisability

The relatively small proportion of patients judged to have recovered from their anorexia nervosa or bulimia nervosa at the end of 1 year of treatment compared with reports from other prognostic studies can be explained by the relatively high proportion of patients with severe illness and the relatively short (1-year) follow-up period. These factors need to be considered when attempting to generalise the results.

Results

Family therapy was more effective than individual therapy in patients whose illness was not chronic and had begun before the age of 19 years. A more tentative finding was the greater value of individual supportive therapy in older patients.

Controlled trial of psychotherapy for bulimia nervosa (Freeman et al, 1988)

Aims

This study evaluated the efficacy of different psychotherapeutic treatments for bulimia nervosa. Cognitive–behavioural therapy, behaviour therapy, group therapy and controls were compared.

Definition

The two therapists involved in the study gave both types of individual treatment to reduce the likelihood of any differences resulting from therapists. The groups were run by both therapists. Structured formats were developed for each type of treatment. This permitted flexibility to cope with patients who progressed at different rates. All treatments consisted of 15 weekly sessions of about 1 h. Treatment sessions were recorded and discussed regularly. Occasionally, review of videotapes was used to ensure adherence to the programme and groups were viewed through a one-way screen.

Controls

Women on a waiting list were assigned as controls. They were assessed more briefly than participants in an attempt to minimise the potential non-specific therapeutic effects of assessment. They kept an eating diary and completed the BITE (Henderson & Freeman, 1987) questionnaire. A further appointment was made for 15 weeks later, the patients having been assured that by that time the waiting list would have been cleared and they could then start treatment. Patients were allocated to the different treatment groups by restricted randomisation. In order that patients did not have to wait unduly before starting treatment, the ratio of randomisation was altered as a new group was about to begin.

Power

Power calculations were used to determine the sample size necessary. Of the patients, 20 were assigned to waiting-list control, 30 to behaviour therapy, 30 to group therapy and 32 to cognitive–behavioural therapy. Drop-out rates were similar between treatments.

Outcome measures

Measures were taken at assessment, halfway through treatment and at the end of treatment. Patients' weekly eating diaries were also assessed. Weekly rates of bingeing, self-induced vomiting and laxative abuse were compared. The eating disorders questionnaires used were the BITE, the eating attitudes test (EAT; Garner & Garfinkel, 1979) and the eating disorders inventory (EDI; Garner et al, 1983). In addition, associated psychopathology was gauged using the Motgomery–Asberg depression rating scale (MADRS; Montgomery & Asberg, 1979) and self-report scales for self-esteem, depression and anxiety.

Generalisability

The study highlighted the relative looseness of DSM–III criteria for bulimia nervosa and the need to use other available diagnostic interviews. Most patients were first and direct referrals, reflecting the fact that the centre involved was the only clearly defined resource for these patients in the area. Other units may receive different types of referrals. The treatments provided were felt to be feasible in a clinical National Health Service setting.

Results

At the end of the trial, the controls had significantly higher scores that the treated groups on all measures of bulimic behaviour. In terms of behavioural change, all three treatments were effective. Most of the advantages that were found were for straightforward behavioural therapy. There appeared to be no advantage in adding cognitive elements. Group therapy was the least satisfactory but was still successful. It appears that bulimia nervosa is amenable to treatment by structured once-weekly psychotherapy in either individual or group form.

Multiple treatment approach to the group treatment of insomnia: a follow-up study (Davies, 1989)

Aims

This study evaluated the effectiveness of psychological methods in the group treatment of insomnia. The group treatments used were cognitive–behavioural strategies, sleep education and gradual drug withdrawal.

Definition

Each of the three treatment groups was given similar group therapy comprising the same treatment elements by the same psychologist for 11–13 sessions.

Controls

The main criticism of this study is that it used no control groups, which prevents a firm conclusion about the long-term effectiveness of group therapy for insomnia being drawn.

Power

Only 15 participants were included in the study. A larger sample would provide more data on such variables as the effect of age and gender on the treatment of insomnia.

Outcome measures

Outcome measures were administered before and after treatment and at follow-up 1 year after treatment had ended. Four questionnaires were used; the Leicester Sleep Questionnaire (Davies, 1989), which looked specifically at sleep difficulties, and the Aston Symptom Check List, (Aston, 1984), General Health Questionnaire (Goldberg, 1972) and Coping Response Questionnaire (Billings & Moos, 1981), which attempted to assess general health, the use of coping strategies and the level of anxiety and benzodiazepine-associated symptoms. Results were based on participants' own estimates and self-monitoring records. More objective measures would have been interesting.

Generalisability

Participants were 15 consecutive referrals to the psychologist from general practitioners in one health centre where the psychologist was based. They were thus typical of that practice, but numbers were small and no attempt was made to evaluate the effects of variables such as age and gender on treatment response.

Results

Generally the results indicate that group therapy was successful in improving quality and quantity of sleep and that this improvement was maintained after an interval of 1 year. However, the results need replicating with larger numbers and suitable controls.

Summary

The above four studies highlight some of the difficulties inherent in psychotherapy research but also show some ways in which these have been overcome and progress has been made. Such research is essential if significant steps are to be taken towards understanding and improving the effectiveness of psychotherapy.

References

Aston, H. (1984) Benzodiazepine withdrawal: an unfinished story. *BMJ*, **288**, 1135–1140.

Barker, C. (1985) Interpersonal process recall in clinical training and research. In *New Developments in Clinical Psychology* (ed. F. N. Watts). Chichester: Wiley.

Barlow, D. & Hensen, M. (1973) Single-case experimental designs: uses in applied clinical research. *Archives of General Psychiatry*, **29**, 319–325.

Basham, R. B. (1986) Scientific and practical advantages of comparative design in psychotherapy research. *Journal of Consulting and Clinical Psychology*, **54**, 88–94.

Beck, A. T., Ward, C. H., Mendelson, M., *et al* (1961) An inventory for measuring depression. *Archives of General Psychiatry*, **4**, 561–571.

Beck, A. T, Rush, A. J., Shaw, B. F., *et al* (1979) *Cognitive Therapy of Depression*. New York: Guilford Press.

Billings, A. G., & Moos, R. H. (1981) The role of coping responses and social resources in attenuating the stress of life events. *Journal of Behavioural Medicine*, **4**, 139–157.

Bloch, S. & Lambert, M. J. (1985) What price psychotherapy? A rejoinder. *British Journal of Psychiatry*, **146**, 96–98.

Campbell, D. T. & Fiske, D. W. (1959) Convergent and discriminant validation by the multitrait-multimethod matrix. *Psychological Bulletin*, **56**, 81–105.

Caskey, N., Barker, C. & Elliot, R. (1984) Dual perspectives: clients' and therapists' perceptions of therapist responses. *British Journal of Clinical Psychology*, **23**, 281–290.

Crown, S. & Crisp, A. H. (1979) *Crown Crisp Experiential Index*. London: Hodder & Stoughton.

Davies, R. (1989) A multiple treatment approach to the group treatment of insomnia: a follow-up study. *Behavioural Psychotherapy*, **17**, 323–331.

Donner, A. (1984) Approaches to sample size estimation in the design of clinical trials – a review. *Statistics in Medicine*, **3**, 199–214.

Elkin, I., Shea, M. T., Watkins, J. T., *et al* (1989) National Institute of Mental Health Treatment of Depression Collaborative Research Program – General effectiveness of treatments. *Archives of General Psychiatry*, **46**, 971–983.

Elliot, R., James, E., Reimschuessel, C. *et al* (1985) Significant events and the analysis of therapeutic impact. *Psychotherapy*, **22**, 620–630.

Endicott, J., Spitzer, R., Fliess, J., *et al* (1976) The Global Assessment Scale. A procedure for measuring overall severity of psychiatric disturbance. *Archives of General Psychiatry*, **35**, 837–844.

Fairburn, C. G., Kirk, J., O'Conner, M., *et al* (1986) A comparison of 2 psychological treatments for bulimia nervosa. *Behaviour Research and Therapy*, **24**, 629–644.

Fonagy, P., Target, M., Cottrell, D., *et al* (2002) *What Works for Whom? A Critical Review of Treatments for Children and Adolescents*. London: Guilford Press.

Freeman, C. P., Barry, F., Dunkeld-Turnbull, J., *et al* (1988) Controlled trial of psychotherapy for bulimia nervosa. *BMJ*, **296**, 521–525.

Garner, D. M. & Garnfinkel, P. E. (1979) The eating attitudes test: an index of the symptoms of anorexia nervosa. *Psychological Medicine*, **9**, 273–279.

Garner, D. M., Olmstead, M. P. & Polluy, J. (1983) Development and validation of a multi-dimensional eating disorder inventory for anorexia nervosa and bulimia. *International Journal of Eating Disorders*, **2**, 15–34.

Goldberg, D. P. (1972) *The Detection of Psychiatric Illness by Questionnaire*. London: Oxford University Press.

Goodman, W. K., Price, L. H., Rasmussen, S. A., *et al* (1989) The Yale–Brown Obsessive Compulsive Scale (YBOCS). Part I – Development, use and reliability. Part II – Validity. *Archives of General Psychiatry*, **46**, 1006–1016.

Hamilton, M. (1960) A rating scale for depression. *Journal of Neurology, Neurosurgery and Psychiatry*, **23**, 56–62.

Henderson, M. & Freeman, C. P. (1987) A self-rating scale for bulimia. The BITE. *British Journal of Psychiatry*, **150**, 18–24.

Kagan, N. (1984) Interpersonal process recall: basic methods and recent research. In *Teaching Psychological Skills* (ed. D. Larsen) Monteney: Brooks/Cole.

Kazdin, A. E. (1986) Comparative outcome studies of psychotherapy: methodological issues and strategies. *Journal of Consulting and Clinical Psychology*, **54**, 95–105.

Kelly, G. A. (1985) *The Psychology of Personal Constructs*, Vols 1 and 2. New York: Norton.

Kraut, R.. E. & Lewis, S. H. (1982) Person perception and self-awareness: knowledge of one's influence on one's own judgements. *Journal of Personality and Social Psychology*, **42**, 448–460.

Labou, W. & Fanshel, D. (1977) *Therapeutic Discourse*. New York: Academic Press.

Laing, R. D., Phillipson, H. & Lee, A. R. (1966) *Interpersonal Perception*. London: Tavistock.

Lambert, M. J. (ed.) (2004) *Bergin and Garfield's Handbook of Psychotherapy and Behavior Change* (5th edn). New York: Wiley.

Luborsky, L., Singer, B. & Luborsky, L. (1975) Comparative studies of psychotherapies: is it true that "Everyone has one and all shall have prizes"? *Archives of General Psychiatry*, **32**, 995–1008.

Malan, D. H., Bacal, H. A., Heath, E. S., *et al* (1968) A study of psychodynamic changes in untreated neurotic patients. I. Improvements that are questionable on dynamic criteria. *British Journal of Psychiatry*, **114**, 525–551.

Malan, D. H., Sheldon Heath, E., Bacal, H. A., *et al* (1975) Psychodynamic changes in untreated patients. II. Apparently genuine improvements. *Archives of General Psychiatry*, **32**, 110–126.

Malan, D. H., Balfour, F. H. G., Hood, V. G., *et al* (1976) Group psychotherapy: a long-term follow-up study. *Archives of General Psychiatry*, **33**, 1303–1315.

Mintz, J. (1981) Measuring outcome in psychodynamic psychotherapy. *Archives of General Psychiatry*, **38**, 503.

Montgomery, S. A. & Asberg, M. (1979) A new depression scale designed to be sensitive to change. *British Journal of Psychiatry*, **134**, 382–389.

Morgan, H. G. & Russel, G. P. M. (1975) Value of family background and clinical features as predictors of long-term outcome in anorexia nervosa. Four year follow-up of 41 patients. *Psychological Medicine*, **5**, 355–371.

Nicholson, R. A. & Berman, J. S. (1983) Is follow-up necessary in evaluating psychotherapy? *Psychological Bulletin*, **93**, 261–278.

Parloff, M. B., Kelman, H. C. & Frank, J. D. (1954) Comfort, effectiveness, and self-awareness as criterion for improvement in psychotherapy. *American Journal of Psychiatry*, **111**, 343–351.

Parry, G., Shapiro, D. A., & Firth, J. (1986) The case of the anxious executive: a study from the research clinic. *British Journal of Medical Psychology*, **59**, 221–233.

Peck, D. F. (1985) Small N experimental designs in clinical practice. In *New Developments in Clinical Psychology* (ed. F. N. Watts). Chichester: Wiley.

Prioleau, I., Murdock, M. & Brody, N. (1983) An analysis of psychotherapy versus placebo studies. *Behavioural and Brain Sciences*, **6**, 275.

Rice, L. N. & Greenberg, L. S. (eds) (1984) *Patterns of Change; Intensive Analysis of Psychotherapy Process*. London: Guilford Press.

Rosenthal, R. & Frank, J. D. (1956) Psychotherapy and the placebo effect. *Psychological Bulletin*, **53**, 294–302.

Roth, A. & Fonagy, P. (1996) *What Works for Whom? A Critical Review of Psychotherapy Research*. London: Guilford Press.

Roth, A. & Fonagy, P. (2005) *What Works for Whom? A Critical Review of Psychotherapy Research* (2nd edn). London: Guilford Press.

Russell, F. M., Szmukler, G. I., Dare, C., *et al* (1987) An evaluation of family therapy in anorexia nervosa and bulimia nervosa. *Archives of General Psychiatry*, **44**, 1047–1056.

Ryle, A. R. & Breen, D. (1972) The use of the double dyad grid in the clinical setting. *British Journal of Medical Psychology*, **45**, 383–389.

Shapiro, D. A. & Hobson, R. F. (1972) Change in psychotherapy: a single case study. *Psychological Medicine*, **2**, 312–317.

Shapiro, D. A. & Firth, J. (1987) Prescriptive v. exploratory psychotherapy. Outcomes of the Sheffield Psychotherapy Project. *British Journal of Psychiatry*, **151**, 790–799.

Shapiro, D. A., Barkman, M., Hardy, G. E., *et al* (1990) The Second Sheffield Psychotherapy Project: rationale, design and preliminary outcome data. *British Journal of Medical Psychology*, **63**, 97–108.

Shapiro, M. B. (1969) Short term improvements in the symptoms of affective disorder. *British Journal of Social and Clinical Psychology*, **8**, 187–188.

Shapiro, M. B. & Post, F. (1974) Comparison of self-ratings of psychiatric patients with ratings made by a psychiatrist. *British Journal of Psychiatry*, **125**, 36–41.

Shepherd, M. (1984) What price psychotherapy? *BMJ*, **288**, 809–810.

Smith, M. L. & Glass, G. V. (1977) Meta-analysis of psychotherapy outcome studies. *American Psychologist*, **32**, 752–760.

Strupp, H. H. (1980) Success and failure in time limited psychotherapy – with special reference to the performance of a lay counsellor. *Archives of General Psychiatry*, **37**, 831–841.

Strupp, H. H. & Hadley, S. W. (1979) Specific vs. non-specific factors in psychotherapy. A controlled study of outcome. *Archives of General Psychiatry*, **36**, 1125–1136.

Truax, C. B. & Charkuff, R. R. (1967) *Towards Effective Counselling and Psychotherapy*. Chicago, IL: Aldine.

Waskow, I. E. & Parloff, M. B. (1975) *Psychotherapy Change Measures* (DHEW, no. 74–120). Washington, DC: US Government Printing Office.

Weissman, M. M. (1979) The psychological treatment of depression: evidence for the efficacy of psychotherapy alone, in comparison with and in combination with pharmacotherapy. *Archives of General Psychiatry*, **36**, 1261–1269.

CHAPTER 15

Historical research

German Berrios

Societal and biological changes cause shifts in the definition and clinical presentation of mental illness. Successful management of mental illness therefore depends upon the periodic updating of clinical categories, therapeutic devices and concepts. Empirical research provides the information for review of clinical categories and therapies; concepts are updated by means of philosophical and historical research. Up to the Second World War, this task was mostly undertaken within the discipline but since then professional philosophers and historians have become involved. It is not only that their *métiers* have become highly technical but that young trainees are increasingly discouraged from doing philosophy or history by the view that psychiatry should be a form of applied neurobiology. Hence, the current generation of trainees should be forgiven for thinking that psychiatry is 'evidence-based neurobiology' and that the concept of 'evidence' is now crystal clear. As this chapter will show, things are more complicated.

The current rhetoric of science conceives the scientist as an untainted seeker of truth. The truth, in turn, is found out by interrogating 'Mother Nature'. Within this purview, the psychiatrist has to decide (at this serious level of inquiry there are no longer algorithms, statistical packages, or Cochrane guidelines to dictate how to think!) *who* or *what* within psychiatry is going to play the role of Mother Nature! Few psychiatric researchers get to this stage and those who do quietly shake in their intellectual boots. Should 'nature' be the patient's DNA, cerebral blood flow, the entire brain, or perhaps (heaven forbid) the 'person as a whole'? The choice of candidate has important implications in terms of what categories and frames to use and training to pursue. When it comes to the choice of object of inquiry, 'evidence-based' medicine is of little help because the definition of evidence depends on (rather than dictates) the object of inquiry.

Thus, decisions as to which conceptual 'scaffolding' is the most creative for psychiatry, and what counts as 'fact', 'rule' and 'evidence', must be taken. Who does the deciding and what are their warrants? Since the 19th century this has been done by a small, changing clique with access to perks, rewards, and the resorts of power. There has never been a mechanism whereby the clinical troops (to which most of us belong) are actually consulted. This vaticanisation of psychiatry started in Continental Europe but has been taken up enthusiastically everywhere else.

The history of psychiatry was born in the same elitist milieu. Basking by the fires of a weekend tryst, the princes of psychiatry might on some occasion have felt that the past of their subject ought to be sung. Knowing what was good for them, shivering minstrels would have spun glorious yarns about their princes and their successes but would have been careful about questioning their right to be decision-makers in the first place.

Mercifully, things have since changed and the psychiatric historian of today waits upon no prince. They want to know about the conceptual and *moral* warrants of princely powers, about the sources of their money and the pressure groups they really represent. This approach started in the 1960s when Foucault (1972) first introduced the idea that the historian should be the scourge of psychiatry. Their exaggerations and pseudo-historical productions, however, for a time alienated the psychiatric brotherhood. Things have improved and the clinician–historians are now asked to attend the high table of science and allowed to tell their *roman d'épouvante*.

It is through the work of historians (not geneticists or neuroimagers) that the psychiatric brotherhood has learned that the conceptual scaffolding of psychiatry may on occasions be tinkered with for purposes other than the good of patients. Although by no means perfect, the new historical approach is imbued with the idea that history *must* also contribute to the development of clinical psychiatry. How to write this redemptive and revisionist type of history is the central teaching of this chapter.

Defining the history of psychiatry

The history of clinical psychiatry may be defined as the study of the way in which biological signals, their behavioural expressions and descriptions, and their psychosocial envelopes interact within specific historical contexts. To estimate the extent to which earlier meanings (terms, concepts and behaviours) are preserved when clinical categories are transferred from one discourse to the next, historian and clinician need to know how descriptive and nosographic rules are formulated. For example, can it be assumed that 'mania', 'melancholia' and 'hypochondria' mean the same in 2006 as they did in 1800? How can differences be made explicit? One of the objectives of historical nosography is to decode the rules controlling psychiatric discourse, and make explicit the drafts upon which it is based.

Historical research differs from clinical research in that in the former the question asked and the research technique employed may determine what counts as 'object' of inquiry and as evidence. Depending on how the object is defined, the historian of, say, 'schizophrenia' will find that earlier centuries offer nothing or a great deal. Current clinical researchers, on the other hand, find their object of inquiry determined by 'operational' definitions (e.g. DSM–IV). Those very definitions are anachronism to the historian.

This does not mean, of course, that the DSM–IV definition of schizophrenia cannot itself be made an object of historical inquiry. It can (and should), but the resulting tale will have little to do with the history of *dementia praecox* (as defined by Kraepelin (1910, 1915) or Morel(1860)) or with that of *intellectual insanity* (as defined by Esquirol (1838)). It will, however, have much to do with the social factors that led a group of psychiatrists in the North East of the USA to arrive at this definition of the disease.

A question arises: does the historian need to posit an *invariant element* successfully to 'trace back' the history of a mental disorder? Would the finding of an enduring neurobiological or psychodynamic marker render the psychosocial context less important? It would seem that this is a vain hope as the history of how an apparently invariant condition such as Alzheimer's disease was constructed shows. Trans-historical invariants are vulnerable to challenge, particularly from the social constructionist perspective. After all, it has been argued with plausibility that so-called natural facts do not and cannot exist independently from the language of description; that is, facts are not 'given' but 'created'.

Metaphors and techniques

Two metaphors seem to control the understanding of historical nosology. One pictures the clinician as cataloguing species (diseases) in a garden (i.e. assuming ontological invariance); the other envisages the clinician as a sculptor carving shapes out of formless matter (i.e. creating 'clinical forms'). The garden approach encourages the search for a 'discoverer' who with his powerful eye overcomes all misleading descriptions. The creationist approach requires that the vision guiding the sculptor be 'contextualised'. The latter activity may range from severe 'social-constructionism' to milder forms of social accounting which leave some room for notions such as scientific progress.

The clinical historian must also specify whether the intention is to deal with the history of *terms* (say, delirium or mania), or *concepts* (say, attentional theories of schizophrenia) or *behaviours*. Although not always easy in practice, this distinction is useful, particularly to the beginner. For example, historical semantics and etymology (say, of the word *melancholia*) are unlikely to provide any information on the history of the actual biological signals involved (say, early wakening, psychomotor retardation or constipation) or on the concepts involved. Likewise, what could be called behavioural palæontology (i.e. the study of the actual behaviours throughout time) will say little on the history of the terms or concepts involved.

The concept of calibration

Together with clinical and statistical research, the history of clinical psychiatry is essential to the calibration of psychiatric nosology. Calibration here means readjustment of descriptions to: (a) changes affecting the biological foundation of symptoms (caused, for example, by genetic mutation); (b) shifts in psychological theory leading to new conceptualisations of behaviour; and (c) variations in the social import of disease. Professional historians have a contribution to make not only to psychiatric culture but to clinical knowledge. Building on the belief that mental disorders are complex and distorted reflections of dysfunctional brain sites and states, they should seek to determine which past 'psychiatric' phenomena were noise and which were actual expressions of biological signals modulated by individual grammars and cultural codes.

Throughout history, psychiatric nosology has shown periods of stability and change. Change is associated with much soul-searching, but stability is taken for granted. The historian should also ask why some 'diseases' remain in a steady state for a considerable time. Are biological invariants more responsible for disease stability than cultural devices such as symbols, myths, or 'mentalities'? Self-styled calibrators of the nomenclature of psychiatry often show ignorance of the conceptual history of mental disorders. In general, professional historians have been more preoccupied with the social history of psychiatry, and this has encouraged the growth amongst clinicians of a 'do-it-yourself', low-standard historical industry. Another objective of this chapter is to correct this trend.

That psychiatric understanding and creativity are enhanced by knowledge of their history was clear to 19th century alienists. Some such as Calmeil, Morel, Trélat, Semelaigne, Kirshoff, Winslow, Ireland, Mercier, Bucknill and Tuke wrote special works on psychiatric history. Most of the others, such as Pinel, Heinroth, Esquirol, Guislain, Prichard, Connolly, Griesinger, Lucas, Falret and Dagonet included historical chapters in their classical textbooks.

However, few alienists from this period did as well as Feuchtersleben (1847):

'All professional men labour under a great disadvantage in not being allowed to be ignorant of what is useless ... every one fancies that he is bound to transmit what is believed to have been known'.

He proposed that only the empirical sciences should be allowed to dismiss the past as a mere 'history of errors'. As to the other sciences (which included medical psychology), Feuchtersleben wrote:

'the history of a science [is] properly the science itself'.

The new science of psychiatry 'belonged to both spheres' or types of science:

'That part of it which was philosophical contained an abstract of that state of philosophy in every age, while that which is empirical has by no means attained such precision and clearness as to render a knowledge of previous opinions superfluous'.

In their use of historical information, writers of 20th-century psychiatric textbooks have fared less well. Historical chapters in modern textbooks rarely include (unlike clinical chapters) *references to recent research*; they simply rehearse the oft-told tale of a mythical continuity of ideas starting with Hippocrates and leading to Aretæus, Galen, Platter, Linné, Cullen, Chiarugi, Pinel, Griesinger, Kraepelin, Freud, Jung and Schneider. Although, perhaps, of help in dealing with examination questions, this presentation creates the impression among psychiatric trainees that the history of clinical psychiatry is no longer a research field for everything is known, and that it is bereft of concepts and theories.

On 'conceptual history'

Of all historiographic approaches available, what is called 'conceptual history' is the most apposite to deal with scaffoldings and the other serious matter treated in this chapter. It can be applied to the study of the main interacting frames of psychiatry: descriptive psychopathology, aetiological theory, pathogenesis and taxonomy. Descriptive psychopathology refers to the language of description; aetiology to the causes of disease; pathogenesis to the manner in which disrupted brain mechanisms generate mental symptoms; and taxonomy to the rules governing the classification of disease. Ideological forces within and without psychiatry have partaken in the generation and maintenance of these frames. For example, descriptive psychopathology (i.e. 'semiology') owes much to 18th-century linguistics and theory of signs; aetiological theory and pathogenesis to developments in general medicine, microscopy and 19th century psychological theory; and taxonomy is partly based on 17th- and 18th-century metaphors of order. It goes without saying that these interacting frames only gain full meaning when replaced onto the canvas of the 19th century *practice* of alienism. The latter provides explanatory elements ranging from the evolutionary and biological to the socio-political – as rightly required by social historians. Conceptual historians start from the premise that the 'meaning' of mental disorder is as dependent upon knowledge of its biological origins (i.e. the source of the distorted biological signal) as it is upon knowledge of the psychosocial envelopes. In other words, most 'psychiatric' phenomena are the final expression of a biological signal modulated by personal and cultural grammars.

It follows that the stability of descriptive psychopathology and of the disease categories that populate psychiatry is a function of the rate at which biology and language change (i.e. descriptions and diagnoses are kept stable as much by symbols, myths and other constructs as they are by actual biological invariants). Indeed, psychiatrists have not yet developed accurate ways of deciding on the relative contribution of each. For example, although 'manipulative behaviour' may be fully the result of a human interaction – and hence be 'social' in origin, 'grand mal seizures', 'delirium' and 'hallucination' can be considered as fundamentally 'biological' phenomena.

Pre-19th-century literature is rich in descriptions of insanity but little is known about the *conceptual frames* that propped them up. More is known about the 19th century, but the great changes that transformed the nature of psychiatry remain only partially understood. These include: (a) the transformation of 'insanities' into psychoses; (b) the narrowing (and eventual disappearance) of the 'neuroses' as a general category; and (c) the fragmentation of the old monolithic descriptions of insanity into what is now called mental 'symptoms'.

What is descriptive psychopathology?

Descriptive psychopathology is here defined as a 'language' comprising a syntax, lexicon and rules of application. Because descriptive psychopathology imposes order on a universe of complex behavioural forms, it is also a 'cognitive system'. For each term (purportedly dealing with a self-contained piece of behaviour or 'symptom'), descriptive psychopathology is expected to contain 'caseness' rules (i.e. ways of determining whether a given 'symptom' is present or absent). Symptoms (conceived of as referents or signifiers) are defined by means of decision-making routines which are profitably analysed in terms of signal-detection theory. At a basic level, symptoms are assumed to result from a 'fracturing' of insane behaviour. Consequently, observers may differ in the way in which this task is done. Indeed, before estimations of interrater reliability (e.g. the kappa values) were available, 19th-century alienists used consensual (qualitative) rules to determine *when* a symptom was present. For example, they might appeal to the higher tribunal of 'common sense', to the 'obvious' nature of some disordered behaviours and occasionally to intuition and the 'clinical eye'. When such aids failed, as not infrequently happened in court, particularly in relation to the predication of intentionality, impasses might occur as to how symptom recognition could be achieved.

Absence of a recognisable descriptive psychopathology is a striking feature of psychiatric discourse before the 19th century. However rich in literary detail, earlier references to insanity (or germane terms such as dementia) were made in terms of 'holistic' categories. One explanation may be that detailed descriptions were unnecessary or inconvenient because 'insanity' fulfilled in those days a different social or legal function. For example, any assumption that there might be a continuity between mad and normal behaviour – often made by descriptive psychopathology – would have threatened the 'all-or-none' concept of 'total insanity' which was so important before the 19th century. Furthermore, since Greek times, psychiatric categories were founded on descriptions of polar 'overt' behaviours and of social competence, and left little room for nuances and transitions.

The creation of descriptive psychopathology took about 100 years. It started during the second decade of the 19th century and was completed just before the First World War. It has changed little since. This means that the success of current clinical and research endeavours does depend, and not to a small extent, on the quality of a conceptual machinery tooled during the 19th century. The 20th century has, no doubt, refined the psychiatric discourse by the introduction of techniques of statistical calibration and decision-making. However, the historical question remains: how did 19th-century alienists manage to extract, based on longitudinal observation of what often were institutionalised patient cohorts, stable descriptions and classifications? Five factors will be explored in this regard: (a) the descriptive and medico-legal obligations of medical officers which were gradually introduced into 19th century asylums; (b) the availability of psychological theories; (c) the changing importance of the notion of *sign* and *symptom* in medicine; (d) the introduction of *subjective* symptomatology; and (e) the adoption of a *temporal* dimension in the description of abnormal behaviour.

Explaining and testing

During the early years of the 19th century, there was a simultaneous drive to build asylums for the insane in various European countries. Once built, these institutions created social and scientific consequences of their own. First, they encouraged the accumulation of those with mental illness within confined physical spaces. Overcrowding and lack of medical care occasioned decimation through intermittent infections and pressed the *need* for a regular medical presence. In Great Britain, this was made good by the 1828 Asylums Act. The incorporation of medical practitioners into asylums generated, in turn, new changes. They brought with them the habit (and the medico-legal obligation) of monitoring and documenting clinical change. As long as this need related to the physical state of patients there was no problem for, during the early 19th century, there already existed recognised methods of history-taking. It was otherwise in regard to mental state. Perusal of clinical logbooks from the pre-1840s shows a *poverty* of description consonant with the absence of 'symptom lists'. Early asylum doctors were thus forced to improvise and borrow, and their activity can be said to be an important factor in the creation of a 'semiology' of mental illness. After 1850, however, a change is noticed in the quality of descriptions.

In this regard, it is important to point out that although on occasions accounts of madness can be found before the 19th century that include elegant descriptions of mental states, they cannot be said to amount to a *common* language of description (i.e. shared by all physicians), nor were they intended to be. What emerged from the 19th-century descriptive enterprise is totally different, namely a common language based on an *analytical and pictorial epistemology* dealing with symptoms independently and assuming that the *same* symptom could be seen in different forms of madness. The creation of such language of description (descriptive psychopathology) led to a shift in the perception of madness. It could be claimed, of course, that it was the other way around, namely, that changes in the perception of madness (e.g. its medicalisation) led to treating these phenomena as if they were brain lesions expressed in signs and symptoms. This might have been so at a general level, but the point made here is that once the old monolithic notion of insanity was broken up, semantic interpretation concentrated on individual symptoms and on the way they clustered together. Consequently, the general semantics of *insanity* became unimportant. Changes in the 'semiology' of medicine are no doubt important to this process. But the *sine qua non* for this change was the availability of psychological theories in terms of which behavioural profiles could be constructed.

Summary and the future

Psychiatry needs concepts and concepts are studied by the history and philosophy of psychiatry. As changes take place in the presentation and construction of mental illness, psychiatrists must decide on how to define their object of inquiry and resist the agenda imposed by the neo-liberal establishment. Psychiatry is not only about DNA or brains but about people and hence about symbols, meanings and semantics. This means that the psychiatrist must be a conceptual polyglot (i.e. feel at home both in neurobiology and the human sciences and if he cannot or does not want to do that, he must at least be respectful of those who do).

The advantage of knowing about the history of the discipline is that it renders the psychiatrist irreverent and sceptical of the ready-made solutions offered by the pharmaceutical, genetic, neuropsychological or neuroimaging industry. Mental diseases and symptoms remain complex constructs and change secularly. The insanity and hallucinations of today are very different from those of the 18th century. The rub here is that there is evidence that the former is not 'truer' than or 'superior' to the latter. If the psychiatrist has not understood this basic truth they have understood little of the discipline and should perhaps reconsider their calling.

This is even worse in the case of the trainee whose future is in the hands of mandarins and whose only chance to escape the slavery of the present and gain a broad and balanced perspective is to read deeply into the history of psychiatry. It is important to add that such reading might even open the floodgate of his/her creativity.

Anyone can do empirical research. Nowadays, it consists in little more than the application of strict algorithms (as journal editors do not tire to tell us) to patient or tissue samples. Any deviation, whether of classification system, research technique, statistical evaluation, fashionable topic, etc., is punished by non-publication. Mandarins decide what is good and bad research and by their criteria it is easy to condemn a large area of psychiatric thinking as useless, obsolete, old-fashioned, invalid, unreliable, etc. The latter includes phenomenological descriptions, identification of new symptoms, historical work, psychotherapy, psychosomatic concepts and even research that does not cost any money. On account of this, the fact bears repetition that performing historical research is the only chance that the psychiatrist has to escape the view that 'newest is bestest' and to create the concepts and management approaches that their patients demand.

References

Esquirol, E. (1838) *Des Maladies Mentales Considérées sous les Rapports Médical, Hygienique et Médico-Legal*. Paris: Baillière.

Feuchtersleben, E. (1847) *The Principles of Medical Psychology* (translated by H. E. Lloyd & B. G. Babington from the first German edition, 1845). London: Sydenham Society.

Foucault, M. (1972) *Histoire de la Folie a l'Age Classique*. Paris: Gallimard.

Kraepelin, E. (1910–1915) *Psychiatrie. Ein Lehrbuch für Studierende und Ärzte, Klinische Psychiatrie*. Leipzig: Barth.

Morel, B. A. (1860) *Traité de Maladies Mentales*. Paris: Masson.

For instances of work based on a variety of historiographical techniques see the past 16 years of the journal History of Psychiatry (http://hpy.sagepub.com). For a history of mental diseases see: Berrios G. E. & Porter R. (eds) (1995) A History of Clinical Psychiatry, London: Athlone Press; for a history of psychopathology see: Berrios G. E. (1996) A History of Mental Symptoms. Cambridge: Cambridge University Press.

Index

Compiled by Caroline Sheard